Wolfgang Bengel
Mastering Dental Photography

To Beatrix, Christian, and Susanne

Mastering Dental Photography

Wolfgang Bengel, Dr med dent

Bensheim, Germany

Quintessenz Verlags-GmbH

Berlin, Chicago, London, Copenhagen, Paris, Milan, Barcelona, Istanbul, São Paulo, Tokyo, New Delhi, Moscow, Prague, Warsaw

Die Deutsche Bibliothek – CIP Einheitsaufnahme

Bengel, Wolfgang:
Mastering dental photography/Wolfgang Bengel. –
Berlin; Chicago; London; Copenhagen; Paris; Milan; Barcelona; Istanbul; São Paulo;
Tokyo; New Delhi; Moscow; Prague; Warsaw: Quintessenz-Verl., 2002
ISBN 3-87652-383-4

quintessence books

Printing: Druckerei Schlüter Vertriebsgesellschaft mbH, Schönebeck (Elbe)

ISBN 3-87652-383-4
Printed in Germany

Contents

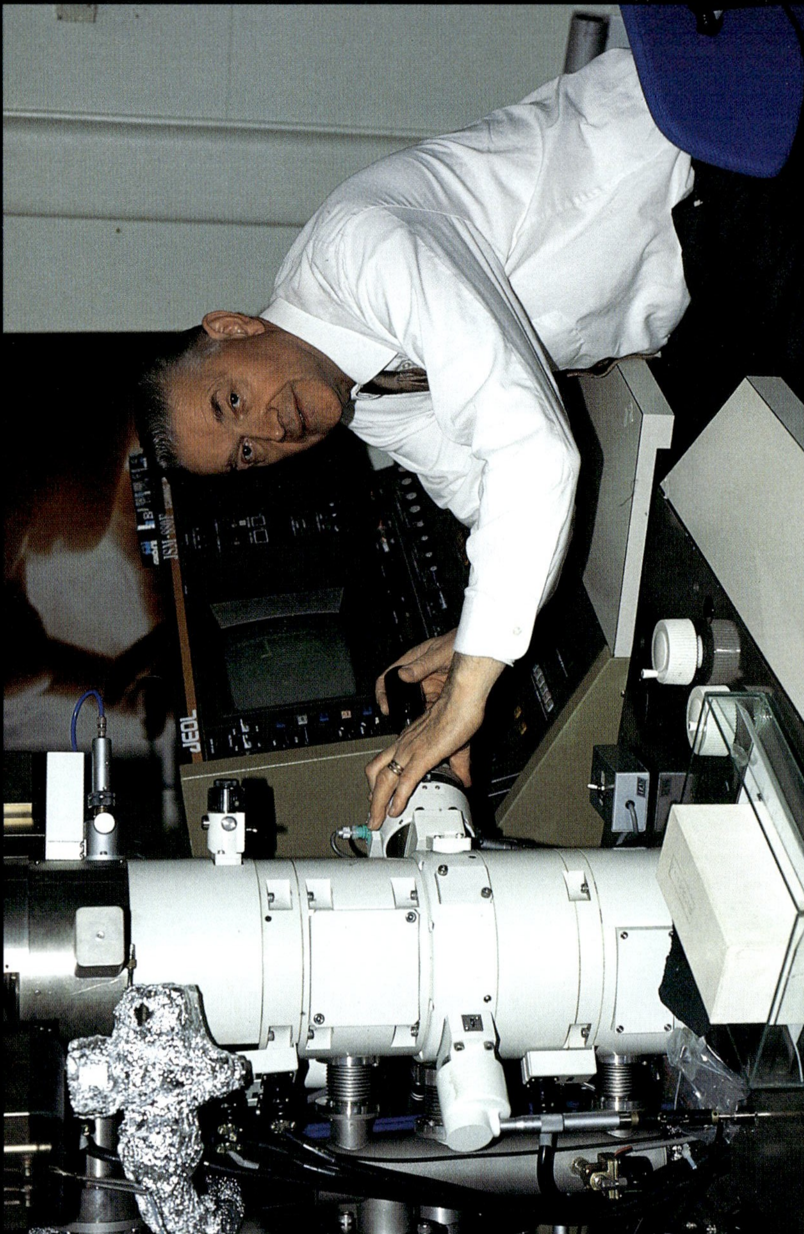

Foreword

Photography has played a significant role in medicine from the very beginning. One of the first photographs, taken over 150 years ago, was a microscopic picture of a human bone.
Today, photography is no longer merely a substitute for drawings, but has become a valuable diagnostic tool. It allows us to see things which are completely invisible to the human eye.
Photography and other visual media have not only undergone rapid technical development in the past 150 years, but even in their infancy had begun to influence our lives. Today, pictures play a dominant role in our visually-oriented age. Some photographs were so powerful that they changed history and altered or at least influenced man's actions in important issues.
Photography has always played an important part in dentistry in improving documentation in the practice and communications between the dentist and other colleagues in the medical field. Sight is the most important sense for the dentist, and thus dentists tend to present things visually, also in order to improve communications with their patients.

Nevertheless, there are a number of pitfalls and stumbling blocks in dental photography. Dentists can save themselves a lot of time and money by reading this book before starting to apply photography in their practices.
Wolfgang Bengel first published a book on dental photography 16 years ago. This new book is far more practically oriented. It is the result of 15 years of experience as a lecturer and seminar leader. Hundreds of pictures show not only his results, but also the way in which they were achieved. Moreover, they also demonstrate that even this facet of dentistry can be done with pleasure.

Lennart Nilsson
Stockholm, Autumn 2001

◄ Lennart Nilsson, a legendary scientific photographer in his own time, seated at a scanning electron microscope in his laboratory at the Karolinska Institute, Stockholm.

Preface and Acknowledgements

My first book on dental photography was published in 1984. Much has changed since then, not only on the technical front, but also in the use of pictures and their place in the media.

After the book was published, I had many opportunities to become much more closely acquainted with photography in a broad range of applications, through hands-on photography courses and discussions after lectures. Thus I began to consider writing a new book that was primarily practical; it was to be far less theoretical and much more geared to the dental practice.

As the basic principles of photography have not substantially altered, these would be discussed to the degree necessary for an understanding of the subject as a whole. New technical developments, such as digital photography and intraoral video systems, would be added. In contrast to the earlier work, the image rather than the text is at the forefront. This work is not a revision of the first book but a completely new one.

Writing such a book relies on the help of others. I would like to thank Mr ZTM Kohlbach for providing dental casts to illustrate technical photography. These were particularly helpful because they were also the basis for the successful chairside communication program known as Dental Explorer. I would like to thank my colleagues in my practice for their patience during this project. Also, I would like to thank my family for their understanding and support and my father for reviewing the manuscript. I am grateful to the photographic industry for its support in providing information and pictures of products. In particular I would like to thank Mr Dehner from Olympus, Mr Schwedhelm from Yashica, Mr Hübschen from Kaiser, Mr Hiesinger from Novoflex, and Mr Bayard and his colleagues from Kodak, each of whom helped me with the subject of digital photography.

I would like to thank Mr Haase of Quintessenz-Verlag for the opportunity once again of publishing a book, and Mr Janßen for his care in adapting the graphics. As with the first book, Ms Steinmeyer was responsible for production of this work; I would like to thank her especially for her attention to detail and her patience.

Bensheim, Autumn 2001

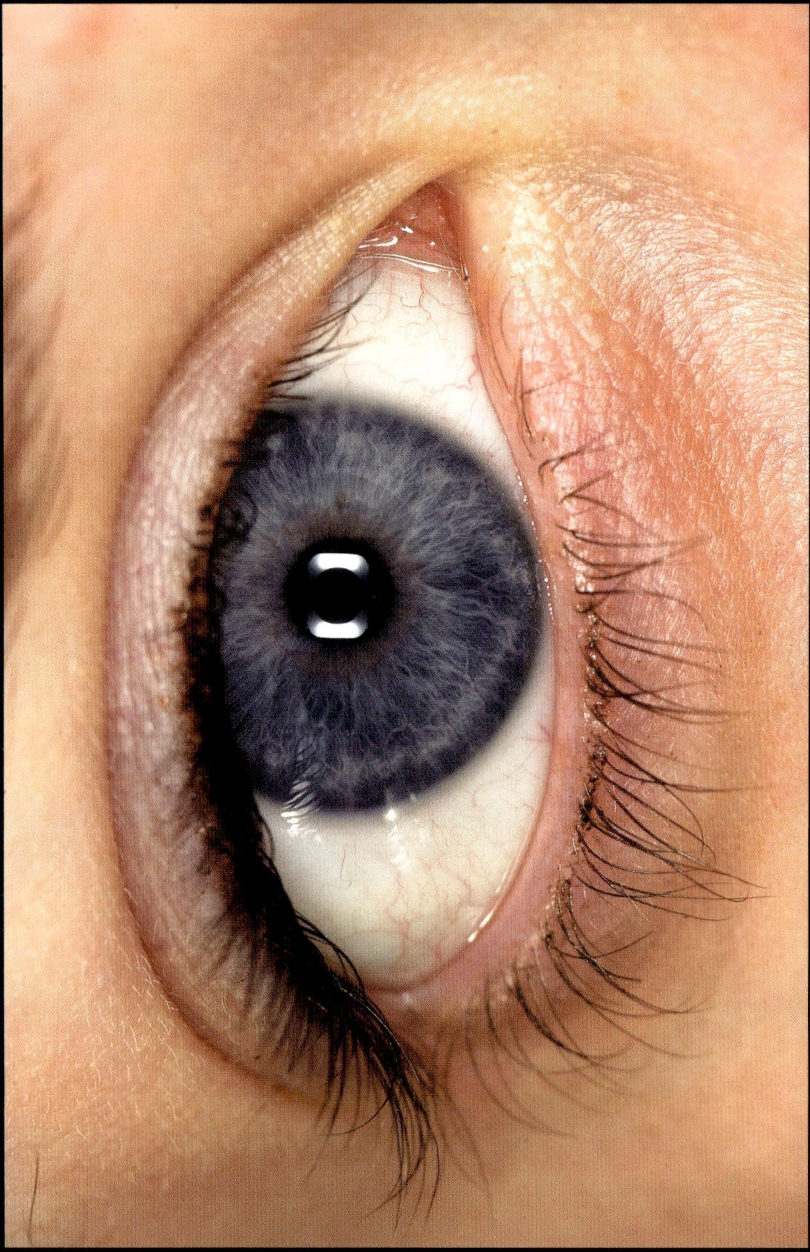

Introduction: Man – Image – Medicine

Man is a visual animal. When our ancestors slowly began to walk erect and our eyes moved from the sides to the front of our skulls, we began to see in three dimensions – not necessarily a disadvantage for a species which swung rapidly from branch to branch through the treetops. At the very latest, when we began to walk on two legs and left the forests to conquer the steppes and the rest of the world, vision became our absolute primary sense. This is still the case today.

◄ The eye is the most important sensory organ of man, the visually oriented animal. This biological neurocomputer is far more complex than the often-used analogy of „eye –camera". Though the front parts of the eye – the cornea, iris and lens – are primarily used to project the image, the retina behind them – the connection to the brain – converts these images so that these colors, forms and movements are converted into data for the brain. These strike the million or so ganglia in the retina and are transmitted to the appropriate areas of the brain via the optic nerve. About 30 areas of the brain are involved in processing visual information.
Some phenomena of light and visual perception are illustrated and explained at the beginning of each chapter of this book. These "gratuitous" images are related only to each other and not to the chapters they head (Photo taken with Nikon Coolpix 990, macro setting).

Today, now well advanced in the visual age, the image is beginning to replace the word. Images need only to be recognized, but words must be understood. An image always lends authenticity, whereas even the strongest proof cannot assault the bulwark of mere assumptions.
Images can inform and also engender emotions. Images, many of which have since become icons, played a large role in ending the Vietnam War. The image of the Earth taken from space has bolstered the perception of our world as a unified and vulnerable system than has many a politician's speech. Lennart Nilsson's images of life in the womb showed us that human beings have to be regarded as such from the very beginning and had a great impact on the debate about abortions more than pronouncements by the church.
Images create their own credibility, even if they lie like mad. Images can manipulate and deceive. "What do you want to believe, facts or your eyes?" asked a media advisor of former US President Ronald Reagan when he was asked about the obvious discrepancy between politics and staging. Even 400 years after Copernicus we do not appear to be revolving, but the sun still sets. Images linger longer than words, a finding of media research, on which the media are based. "A punch in the eye is worth more than three on the ear," is an adage from boxing which also applies to teaching.
Images are perhaps the only remaining way of understanding aspects of our highly complex world,

though indeed only by drastically reducing factual relationships even to the point of narrative fiction. Unfathomable complexity is reduced to simple concepts and perspicuity.
In the meantime, the images we have created, especially televised ones, have long since begun to influence us. As the principal cultural medium, television determines the models, the receptivity and processing of information. Viewed sceptically by the older generation, younger generations grow up which are becoming used to, and probably already are, to such soporific and distracting perceptions of rapidly changing images replacing one another. While books created a culture of language, even as a mass medium, television images are a mosaic of visual impressions devoid of context, disparate fragments of images held together only by a fictitious correlation. Speeches and intellectual exchanges have been replaced by podium discussions and talk shows in which relaxed debate has been superseded by rapid-fire bons mots.
Imagery, the dominant medium, has also influenced the principles of our media culture even where it is not pre-eminent, such as in this book.
What is true of people in general is especially true in medicine. Images have always been used in this field. When medicine was considered magic, images were too. Images were always created using the prevailing technology. Leonardo da Vinci's anatomical studies are still the pinnacle of artistic expression. The very first photographs also included those for the study of medicine. Medical images today not only portray what we see, but what is invisible to the naked eye.

Why Dental Photography?

Dentistry is one of the branches of medicine which has always used photography. There are many reasons for this.

Documentation

The main aim of dental photography is for documentation to supplement treatment. This includes photographs which show the processes and stages of treatment (Fig. 0.1).
As a general rule, images should be made before every irreversible and invasive procedure. This results not only in a stock of interesting dental records, but also provides forensic ones as well. In many instances disagreements between dentist and patient can also be avoided in this way.
Images should always be made after trauma. This is not only for the dentist's legal protection, but also for the patient's. Dental photography is also useful for checking during treatment and recidive examination of pathological changes in the mucous membranes. Unusual and fleeting results of an examination can be documented to underpin an initial diagnosis. Since stomatology will be increasingly important in the coming years, these aspects will gain greater significance than before. It should be as natural for anyone interested in stomatology to have a camera at hand at all times as an X-ray machine has been for decades.

Communication

"A picture is worth 1,000 words" is a true and often quoted maxim. Conditions in hard and soft tissue can be quickly and easily photographed, facilitating communications between dentists, doctors and laboratories. Images give dental technicians important information about structure and color of teeth, allowing them to individually match crowns to adjacent teeth. Even when the choice of color cannot be communicated to the laboratory directly in this way, photography can go a long way toward optimizing dental technicians' work. A pre-operation image sent along with a tissue

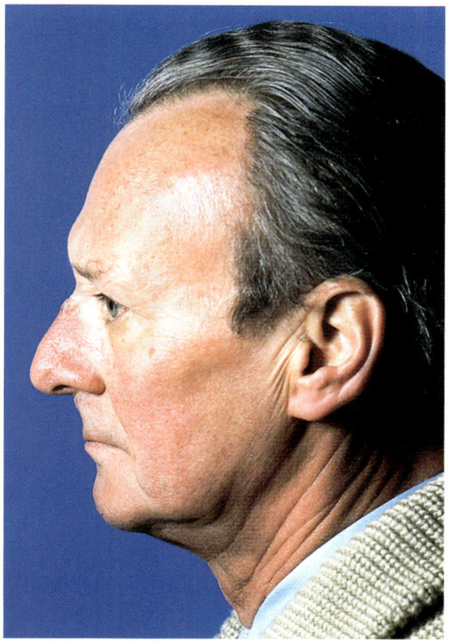

Fig. 0.1 Documentation is the most important application for dental photography. Photography should be done before any irreversible treatment. The illustration was made before prothesis work.

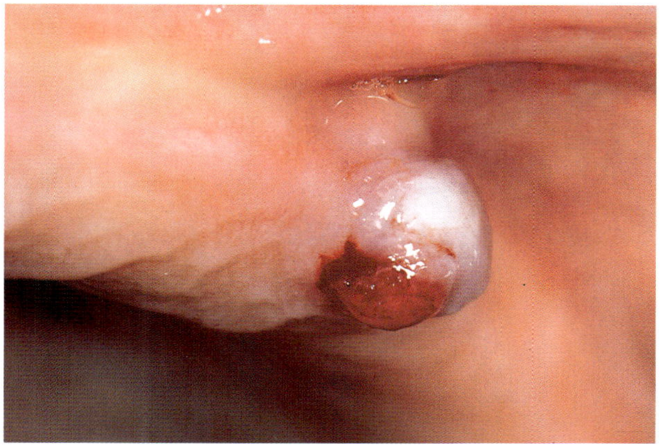

Fig 0.2 Photography aids in communication between dentist and patient. Preliminary excisions and surgical removal of changes in the mucous membrane should always be documented beforehand.

sample to a pathologist can provide important information and support his diagnosis (Fig. 0.2).
Images also play an important role in patient consultations. The image not only allows the dentist to communicate information to the patient, but gives the patient a far better opportunity to express and articulate his or her wishes and desires.

Self-check

Quality control will become more important to dentists in the coming years. Photography will also gain importance. Even without institutionalised quality control, photography will continue to aid the dentist as a self-check measure. Anyone who has photographed the stages of his or her treatment and then enlarged and projected the results is able to confirm this (Fig. 0.3). Images are also a key element in case presentations as part of training or as part of quality control.

Illustrations

It is almost inconceivable that lectures and publications on dentistry would be presented without images. These images are taken either for other reasons or specifically for the purpose (Fig. 0.4).

Marketing a practice

The concept of marketing a practice is often misused. Many recommendations by self-appointed "marketing experts" appear all too crass and are quickly seen through by patients. Marketing in the

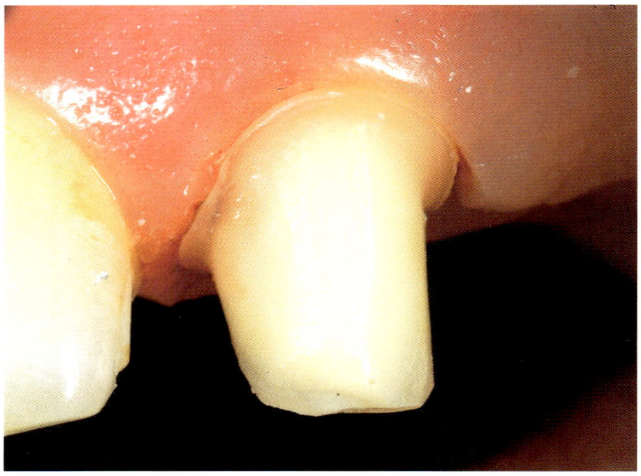

Fig. 0.3 An important consequence of dental photography is the ability for self-checking.

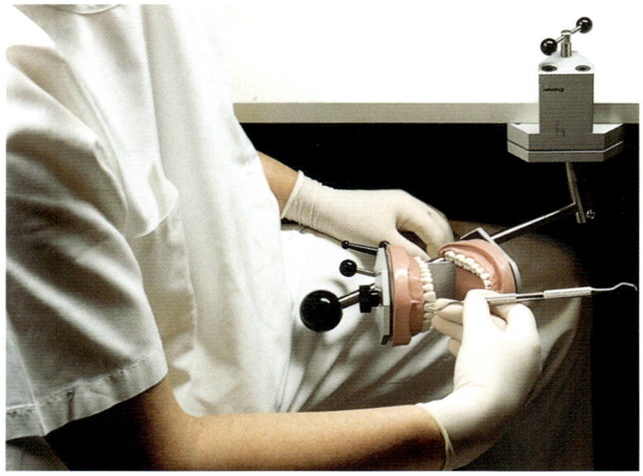

Fig. 0.4 Dental photography is very useful for illustrating the dentist's own lectures and publications.

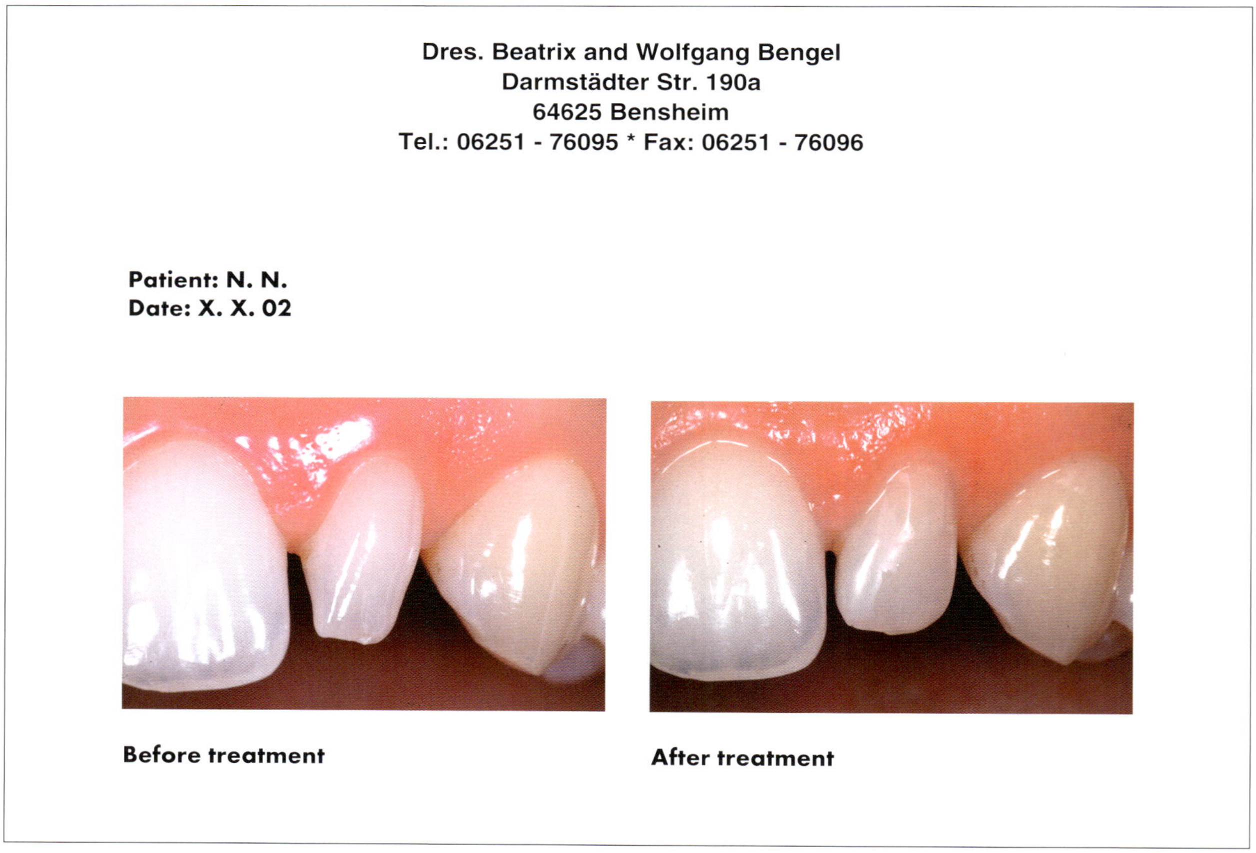

Dres. Beatrix and Wolfgang Bengel
Darmstädter Str. 190a
64625 Bensheim
Tel.: 06251 - 76095 * Fax: 06251 - 76096

Patient: N. N.
Date: X. X. 02

Before treatment

After treatment

Fig. 0.5 The juxtaposition of images taken at the onset and end of treatment not only emphasizes the importance of such work to the patient, but it is also an understated but highly effective marketing means.

positive sense can allow a patient to directly compare the beginning and results of treatment. Two images, printed side-by-side, are generally sufficient for this and can be given to the patient. Very little text is needed. Patients frequently also show these images to friends and acquaintances: there is probably no better low-key but effective marketing tool than this (Fig. 0.5).
Finally, images also contribute to enjoyment and furtherance of the profession of dentistry, which becomes increasingly important in an advancing career (Fig. 0.6).

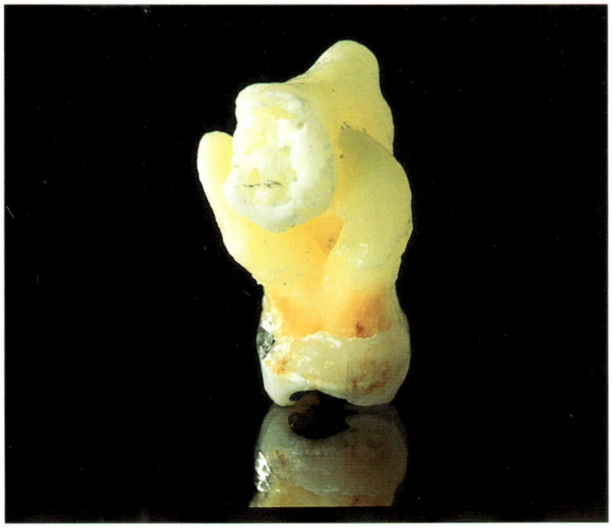

Fig. 0.6 Photographing interesting results or curiosities bolsters interest in dentistry.

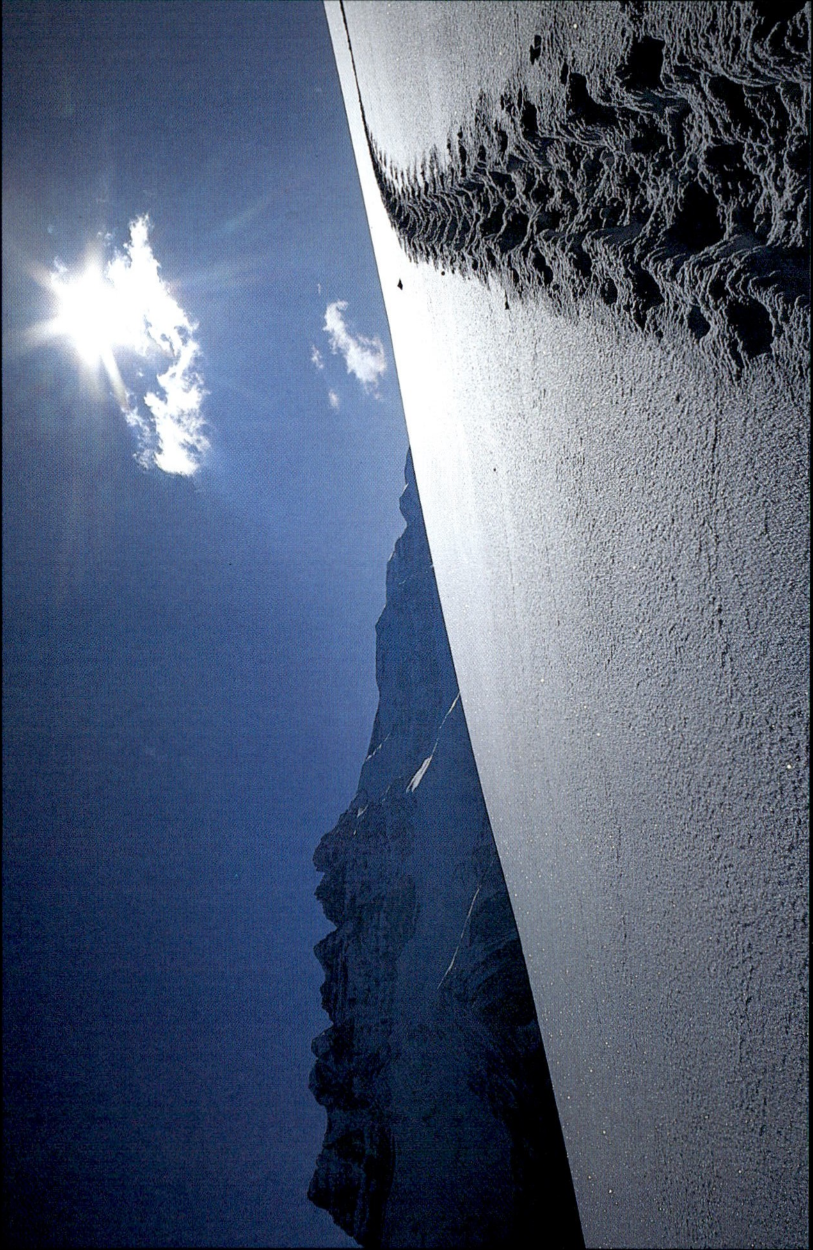

1 Fundamentals of Photography

1.1 Requirements of Dental Photography

The applications mentioned in the introduction result in requirements for images, both in their technical aspects and image composition.

1.1.1 Technical requirements

Technical requirements should present no fundamental problems with the current quality of photographic equipment and films. These include image sharpness, sufficient depth of field, suitable reproduction ratios, correct exposure and illumination - even in the mouth - and correct color rendition. These requirements are discussed in detail below.

◄ The portion of sunlight our eyes can see is perceived as white light. In reality, it is composed of all the colors of the rainbow: violet, blue, green, yellow, orange and red. During the course of human evolution our eyes have obviously adapted ideally to sunlight. The sun's highest radiation is at wavelengths at yellow-green (around 0.55 μm). The human eye's sensitivity also peaks at yellow-green.

1.1.2 Image composition

The requirements for the composition of the image are more difficult to meet and most mistakes are made in this regard. These requirements are not so much creative ones, such as in composition, which applies the golden mean, but three specific areas:

- ✓ Appropriate magnification ratio
- ✓ Reduction of image contents
- ✓ Ability to reproduce photographic conditions

One of the most common mistakes made, not necessarily only in dental photography, is having the camera positioned too far away from the subject. The rule of thumb, "Get close to the subject," is also true in this case. A reproduction ratio of 1:2 or greater should be the rule.

Slides, which mostly are shown too briefly when used to illustrate lectures, should have a very simple composition in order to allow the viewer to take in their entire contents. Book illustrations are less critical, since the reader can peruse them at his or her leisure. Since it is never clear when a photo is taken what its ultimate use may be it is best to take it in such a manner that its contents can be perceived quickly. This means reducing the contents, either through an appropriate scale or through selective focusing. Furthermore, it is always possible that a photograph taken almost by chance could become part of a series of illustrations. Thus it is essential that the most important photographic parameters such as reproduction ratio, viewing angle

and center of the photograph can be reproduced. The goal is not necessarily to be able to precisely recreate these images, but to recreate the conditions under which photographs have been taken which allow the viewer to quickly analyze images in a series without having to reorientate himself or herself with each subsequent image because they have been taken from a different perspective.
Object photography also has these requirements. The background is particularly important in this case and should be as uniform as possible in order to avoid a confusing presentation. Image series with different colored backgrounds are not only visually disturbing but are also easily recognized as having been pieced together.

1.2 Photographic Equipment

The requirements cited above for a good dental photograph result in those for the camera system itself. In particular these are:

- ✓ Adequate reproduction ratio
- ✓ Sufficient working distance
- ✓ Enough depth of field
- ✓ Even illumination (also within the mouth)
- ✓ Correct exposure, independent of reflections from subject
- ✓ Correct color rendition
- ✓ Easy to use
- ✓ Cost-effective

In the following the main camera system components are discussed with a view toward procuring the best possible equipment to meet the requirements.

1.2.1 Camera body

There is complete agreement that the single lens reflex camera is most suited to medical photography (Fig. 1.1). Certain instant cameras such as the Polaroid Macro 5 SLR can be used for a limited number of applications.
Medium format cameras are not applicable due to cost, especially because of their expensive lenses, etc. They are also more difficult to use than an 35 mm SLR. These also produce images which are more than adequate for our purposes. Moreover, projection systems at international conferences are also tailored to 35mm format.
Rangefinder cameras are not suitable for close-up photography as they suffer from viewfinder par-

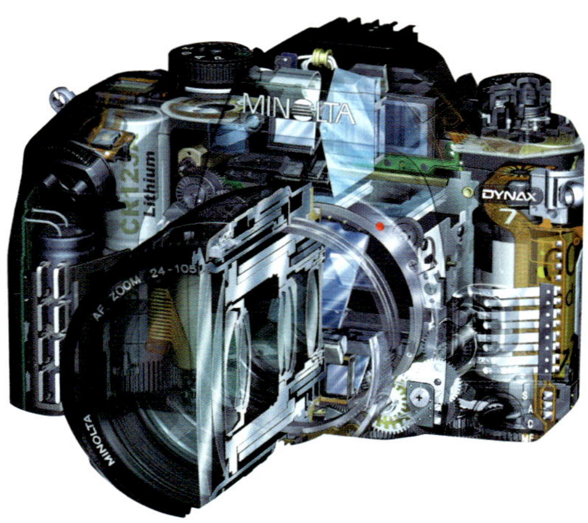

Fig. 1.2 Cross section of a modern single lens reflex camera (Illustration: Minolta).

allax (Fig. 1.2). This means that the image in the viewfinder and the actual one are not identical. Lenses for rangefinder cameras are also not suitable for close-up photography.
It is not necessary to choose the most expensive model in a product range, since the requirements for the camera itself, are, from a technical standpoint, relatively straightforward. Every major camera manufacturer is able to offer such a camera. It makes more sense to spend the money saved on lenses and flash equipment.
The 35mm camera should offer the following:

Winder/motor
Automatic film advance makes work considerably easier since the camera does not have to be removed from the eye after every exposure to wind the film on manually. This saves time, since the largest amount of time is taken up with determining the correct focus and image area. A considerable amount of time is saved when taking a number of exposures one after the other, which should be the rule.

Manual exposure/aperture-priority automatic exposure control
Correct exposure of film is always the result of two factors: aperture and exposure time. A large aperture is coupled with a faster shutter speed and vice versa (Fig. 1.3). SLRs generally allow the exposure to be selected manually or automatically, in which case various auto-exposure modes can be chosen. The method of choice in this instance should be aperture-priority automatic exposure control, in which the aperture is selected and the appropriate shutter speed determined and set automatically by the camera. To use the aperture-priority mode, set the camera to the symbol "A" for aperture priority (Fig. 1.4). Setting the shutter automatically has the advantage of being able to select the aperture and thus influence the critically important depth of field (see below). Depth of field is determined above all by aperture and reproduction ratio. The ability to set the exposure manually ("M" symbol) is important in copy work, but less so in clinical photography.

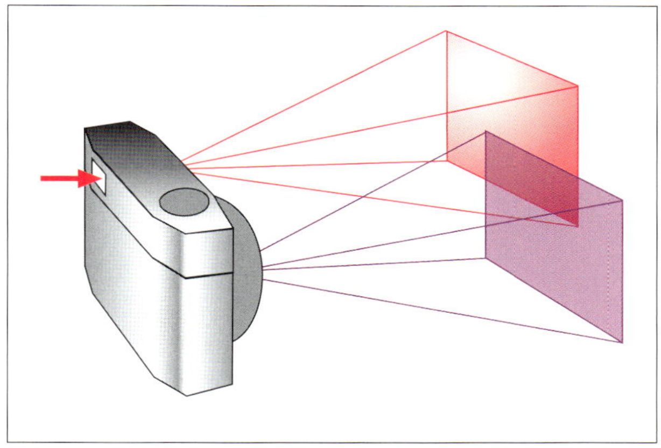

Fig. 1.2 With a rangefinder camera, the image in the viewfinder and that on the film do not correspond at close range (viewfinder parallax).

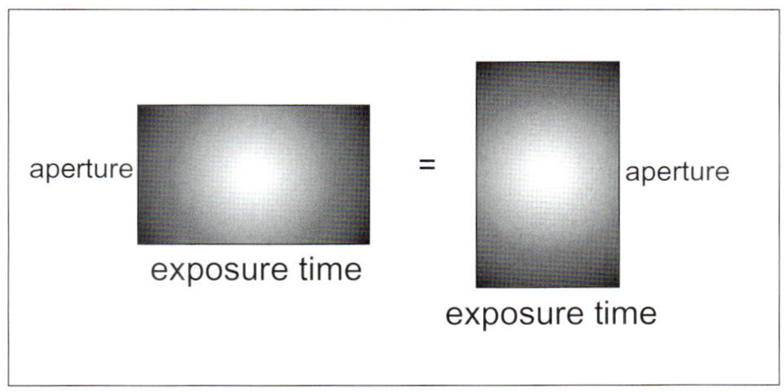

Fig. 1.3 Exposure is always the product of aperture and exposure time. Short exposure time and large aperture achieve the same result as long exposure time and a large aperture.

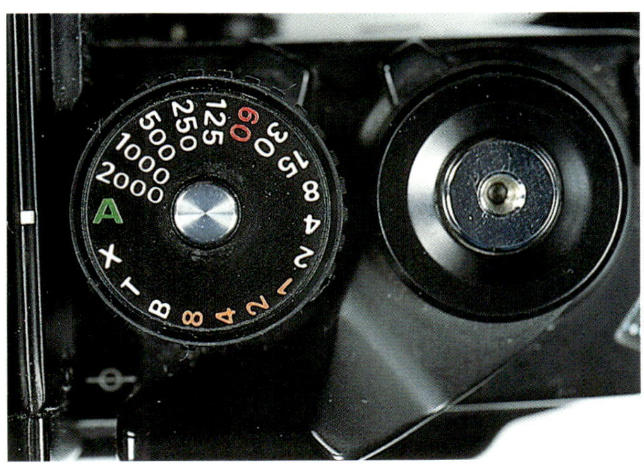

Fig. 1.4 The automatic exposure setting of choice for our purposes is aperture priority ("A" symbol) since it allows control of depth of field.

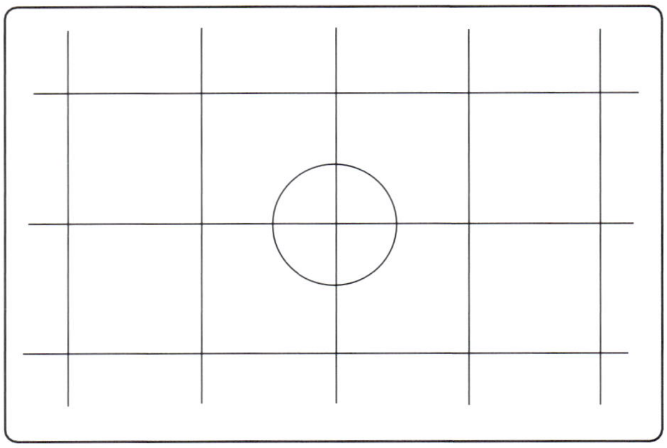

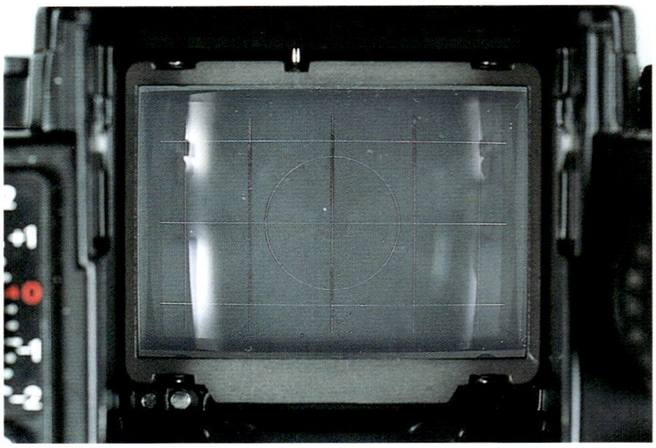

Fig. 1.5 An interchangeable focusing screen is important for dental photography. Focusing screens with a grid, illustrated in (a) and shown from above in a camera (b).

Focusing screens

The focusing screen is part of the focusing system. The mirror projects the image onto the screen; this image is corrected via the pentaprism so that it is the right way up and corrected for left-to-right reversal, allowing us to view the image through the viewfinder.

Standard focusing screens in most cameras are fine matte screens with a split-screen range finder surrounded by a microprism ring. Both of these are intended to aid focusing, but in close-up photography they are somewhat of a hindrance since they tend to darken. Moreover, the function of a split-screen range finder system depends on being able to focus on straight lines, which practically do not occur in clinical photography.

Thus it is advisable to replace the standard focusing screen with a fine matte focusing screen with an engraved grid (Fig. 1.5 a,b). This grid is very helpful in positioning the camera horizontally. The center of the image can be determined exactly with the aid of the crosshairs. The amount of work saved by using such a system is such that the decision to buy a particular camera system should be based on whether an interchangeable focusing screen is available or not for the particular camera body. Many camera systems, such as the Yashica Dental Eye III, have such a focusing screen fitted as standard.

Data back

Later filing of images with patients' records or chronological filing can be greatly facilitated by adding numbers or dates to the images. Almost all camera systems have data backs available and some as a standard feature. Generally data are placed in the lower right hand corner of the image. The more sophisticated method is the insertion of this data on the unexposed space between two frames, as is possible with some more expensive camera models. This means that the effect of the image is not compromised but that the data is still available.

Depth of field preview button

Depth of field is always critical in close-up photography (see below). This can be checked visually in the viewfinder only if the camera has a depth of field preview button. In focusing, the lens aperture is normally fully open to achieve the brightest image in the viewfinder. Pressing the depth of field preview button stops the lens diaphragm down to the aperture which is set (working aperture). Although the image becomes darker, it is possible to visually check the depth of field, an important factor in object photography.

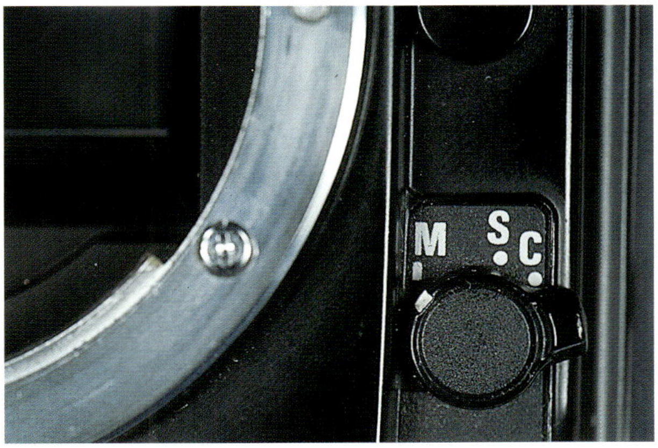

Fig. 1.6 For clinical photography the autofocus function of modern SLR-cameras should be switched off.

Autofocus

Modern cameras and their lenses allow autofocusing. This feature is important in sports and action photography and also for copy work.

However, in clinical photography this autofocus function should be turned off and focusing should be done manually (Fig. 1.6). Since most in this field is done hand-held, it is difficult to avoid a small amount of camera shake. This would mean that the lens motor would continually have to refocus the lens. An even more important reason for switching off the autofocus mode is the fact that the autofocus focusing point is in the center of the viewfinder in most cameras. However, the closest point of the subject is often in the center, such as in the case when photographing a set of teeth. If this point is focused on, the greatest part of the depth of field, that is, that in front of the distance for which the camera is focused, is not used (see below). Thus it would not be possible to have the entire set of teeth in focus. For this reason any new cameras purchased should have autofocus, but this feature should be switched off in clinical photography.

Useful accessories

Most camera systems offer a range of accessories, though only a limited number of these appear of use for our purposes.

These useful accessories, for instance, include dioptric adjustment lenses if this feature is not built-in. Another useful accessory is eye cups which keep out extraneous light and substantially improve the image in the viewfinder.

1.2.2 Lenses

Dental photography is mostly close-up photography, calling for macro lenses. Zoom lenses with a macro setting are not suitable for this purpose, since these can be set only to a reproduction ratio of about 1:4.

To focus on an object which is closer to the camera than "infinity" the ring on the lens is turned to increase the distance between the center of the lens and the film plane. Most normal lenses are designed to produce a maximum magnification ratio of approximately 1:10 to 1:7. The lens can not be moved further away from the film plane. If the photographer wishes to focus on a subject which is closer, the distance between the lens and the camera must be bridged so as to allow no light leakage (Fig. 1.7). This can be achieved in various ways, for instance by using extension rings, bellows unit, macro tubes, etc. This is easiest with macro lenses which generally have the means by which the lens can be extended further than normal. More modern designs permit greater magnification through the use of floating elements; an-

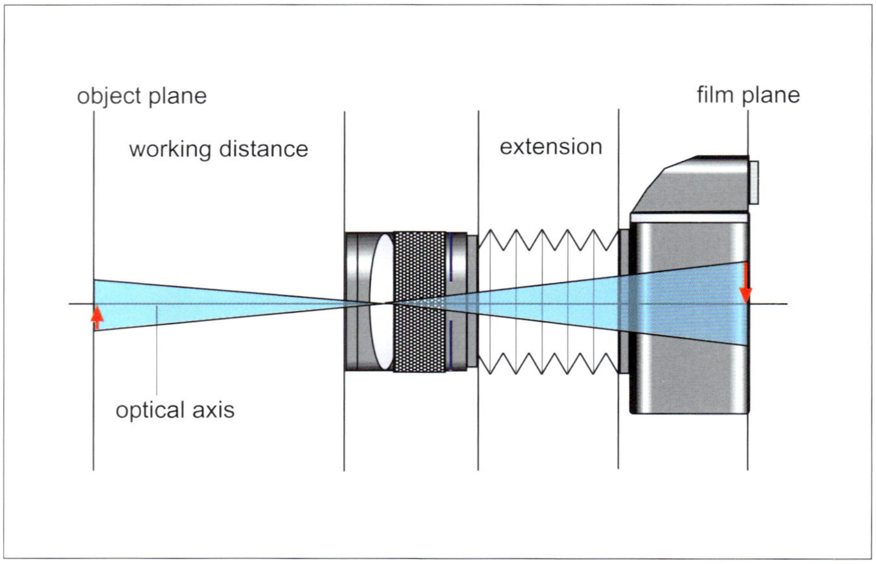

Fig. 1.7 Close up photography is achieved by increasing the distance from the lens to the film plane. This longer length must be light-tight, for example, by using bellows.

other advantage of these macro lenses is their ability to compensate for image problems endemic to close-up photography. These lenses are designed and corrected for close-up photography (Fig. 1.8). If the macro lenses also have an integrated ring flash or sector flash these are termed medical lenses (e. g. Nikon-Medical, Yashica Dental Eye III).

Normal lengths of macro lenses are 50mm, 100mm and 200mm; the 100mm lens is best suited to our purpose.

The lens determines a number of optical and image parameters and thus it is more important to use a more expensive lens than a more costly camera. Lenses influence the following parameters:

- ✓ Image quality (image sharpness, color rendition, contrast)
- ✓ Magnification
- ✓ Working distance
- ✓ Depth of field (via aperture setting and magnification)

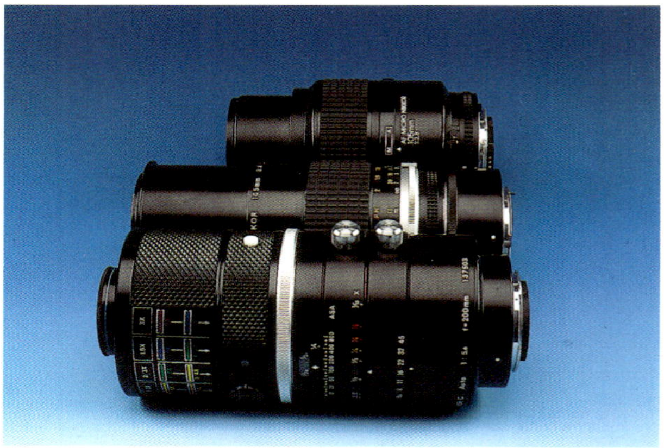

Fig. 1.8 Nikon macro lenses. In front the old 200mm medical lens, in the middle a 105mm macro lens which achieves a magnification of 1:2 and behind the new 105mm AF macro lens which achieves a magnification of 1:1. Despite the greater magnification it is physically shorter than other lenses, since it has floating lens elements. However, this also has a shorter subject-to-camera distance.

Image quality

Optical requirements such as image sharpness, color rendition and contrast should present no problems given the quality of today's lenses. It is also not necessary to use original manufacturers' lenses. Lenses of independent makers differ only in specifications but not in image quality from those of the original manufacturers.

Reproduction ratio

Reproduction ratio is defined as the size of the subject relative to the image on the film. A reproduction ratio of 1:2 means that the subject on the slide or negative is half its actual size. A reproduction ratio of 2:1 means that the subject is two times its real size (Fig. 1.9).

In dental photography the following reproduction ratios are important (approximate):

1:10	Portrait photography (Fig. 1.10)
1:2	Image of a set of teeth (Fig. 1.11)
1:1	Front teeth with partial canines or premolars and molars filling the format (Fig. 1.12)
2:1	Two upper front teeth (Fig. 1.13)

Given the same aperture, the depth of field decreases with greater magnification; with the same focal length the reproduction ratio also decreases.

The reproduction ratio is engraved on many lenses and can therefore be easily preset.

Most macro lenses have a magnification of 1:2 or, better, 1:1. Greater magnification requires special accessories. Compact bellows units, macro tubes, teleconverters and close-up lenses are generally used in clinical photography.

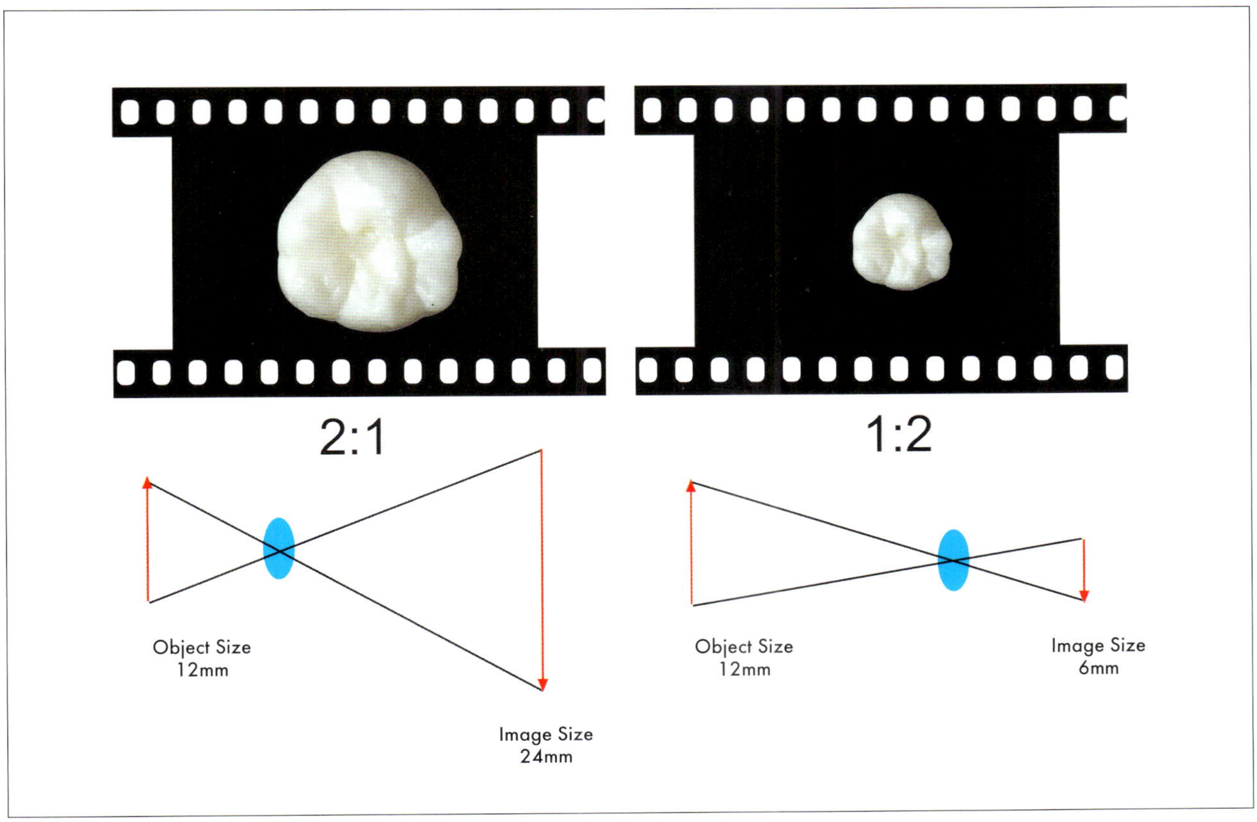

Fig. 1.9 At a magnification of 1:2 the object size is twice the size of the image. At a magnification of 2:1 the image is twice the size of the object.

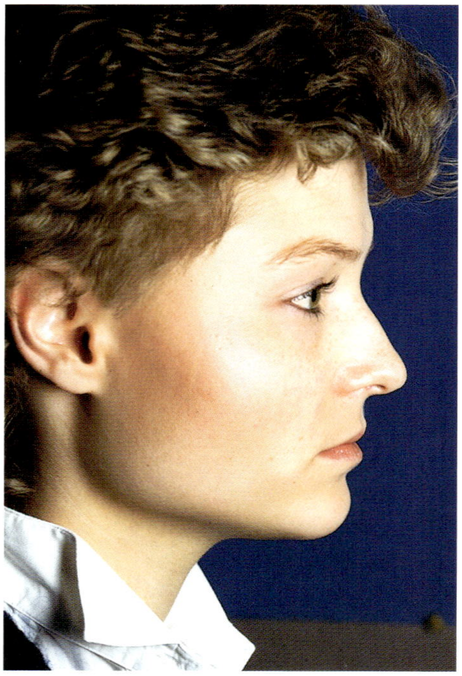

Fig. 1.10 Magnification of about 1:10.

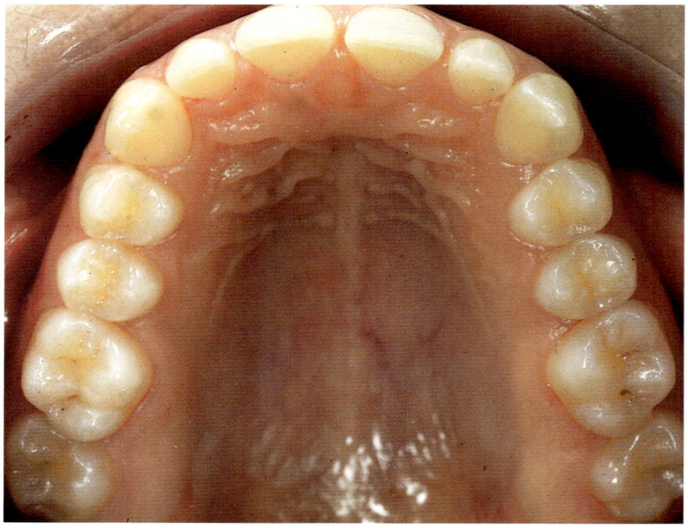

Fig. 1.11 Magnification of 1:2.

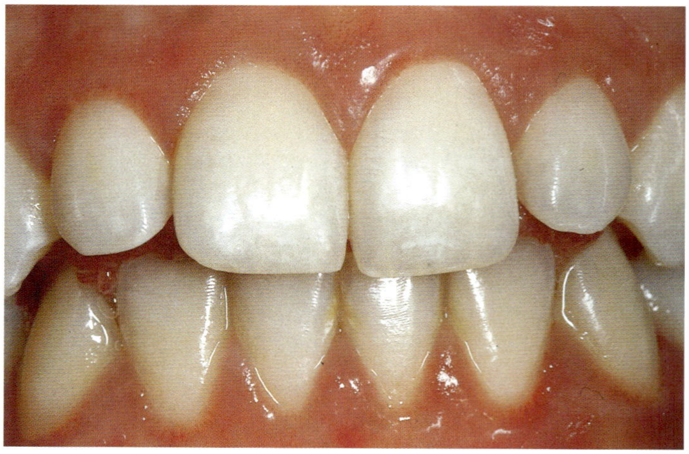

Fig. 1.12 Magnification of 1:1.

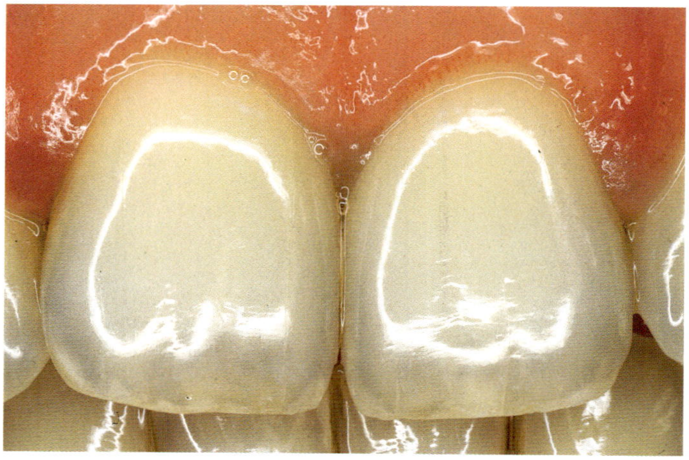

Fig. 1.13 Magnification of 2:1.

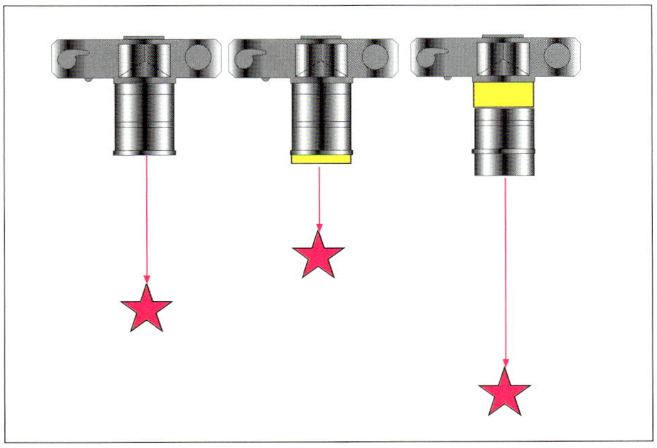

Fig. 1.14 A close-up lens reduces the overall length of the optical system. This leads to a shorter working distance. In contrast, a teleconverter (on the right) increases the overall length and thus the working distance.

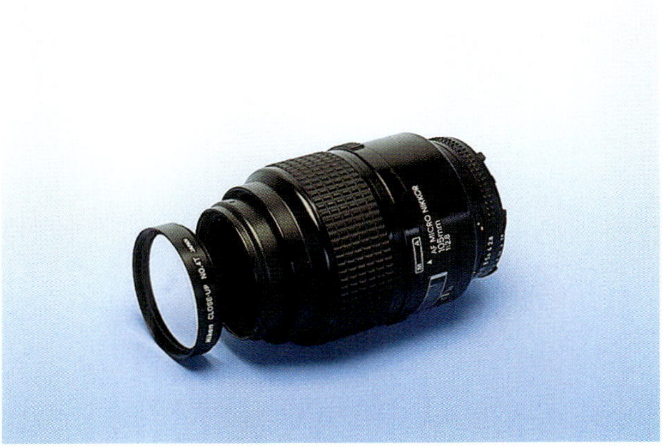

Fig. 1.15 Nikon 105mm AF-Micro Nikkor lens with 4T close-up lens.

Close-up lenses

Close-up lenses act like "spectacles" in front of the camera lens. This means that they reduce the focal length of the lens, thus reducing the subject to camera distance. This enables larger images. Close-up lenses are used for instance on cameras with medical lenses to achieve the maximum reproduction ratio of 2:1.

Close-up lenses have the advantage of being light, easy to use and for the most part relatively inexpensive. Optically, there is no resulting loss of light. Close-up lenses sometimes result in loss of image quality. Thus it is recommended to use close-up lenses with built-in correction for image quality such as achromat lenses corrected for chromatic aberrations, or such close-up lenses which are designed for the particular optical system, e.g. Yashica Dental Eye, Medical Nikkor. There is also another disadvantage caused by their functional principle. As the focal length of the lens plus close-up lens combination is reduced compared to the straight lens the subject to camera distance is also reduced (see below) (Fig. 1.14). If the lens is set to infinity the focal length of the overall system is equal to that of the close-up lens. Thus it generally makes sense to use close-up lenses only when the basic focal length of the macro lens being used is no less than 100mm. Otherwise this would present difficulties with lighting and perspective.

An example of a recommended system is the Nikon 4T close-up lens with the 105mm Micro AF lens (Fig. 1.15), which allows a maximum reproduction ratio of 1.4:1. In the case of a photograph of the front teeth, the two middle incisors and half of the two adjacent incisors are shown. The working distance in this combination is about 70mm, which already presents some difficulties for photographing the side teeth.

Teleconverters

Teleconverters are simple to operate and are therefore frequently used in dental photography. They are a sort of intermediate lens. Fitted between the camera and lens, they increase the lens' focal length (Fig. 1.16). The most frequently used converters are 2x, which double the focal length. Since this does not affect the minimum focusing distance the result is images in greater magnification. Combining a macro lens with a maximum reproduction ratio of 1:1 plus a 2x teleconverter produces an overall result of 2:1. The ability to set the lens to infinity is retained.

A general disadvantage is that the rays of light, which travel from the lens toward the film, are

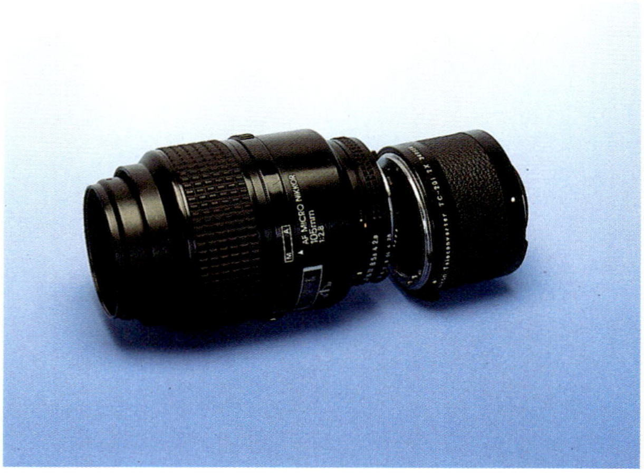

Fig. 1.16 Nikon 105mm AF-Micro Nikkor with TC 201 teleconverter.

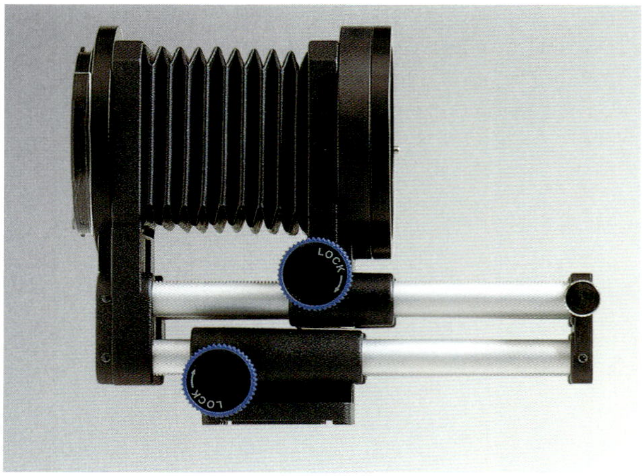

Fig. 1.17 The Novoflex automatic bellows unit is a "portable" solution for dental photography (Photo: Novoflex).

spread by the converter. This reduces the intensity of light on the film surface. A 2x converter loses two f-stops and a 1.4x converter one stop. Teleconverters are thus to be recommended only when the flashgun being used is sufficiently powerful; otherwise the aperture has to be opened up.
Teleconverters reach their limitations with lenses of around 100mm. Lenses with focal lengths above that when used with converters result in too great a focal length and camera-to-subject distance. (see below).
In dental photography there is generally no need to sacrifice optical quality through the use of teleconverters since most photography is done with lenses which are stopped down to f/16 or f/22, thus eliminating most image errors. However, if a lens of a lower quality is used the faults are intensified by the converter.
A recommended combination is using the TC-14A with the 105mm Micro Nikkor, which allows a reproduction ratio from 1.4:1 to infinity.

Auto macro tubes

Among other close-up equipment produced by Olympus is the auto macro tube, which is a cross between a bellows unit and converter. It consists of telescopic tubes which permit infinite adjustable changes in magnification. The auto macro tube is used in close-up photography with short mount lenses of 135mm and 80mm. This system is easy to use and produces good results. Its disadvantage is that it can be used only with Olympus equipment.

Bellows units

Bellows units allow infinite adjustment of the image distance and thus the magnification. Normal bellows are too clumsy for use in clinical photography. The Novoflex Automatic Bellows are an exception; these are compact and offer direct auto aperture coupling (Fig. 1.17).
The main advantage of increasing the image distance to achieve greater magnification is that good optical quality is achieved, regardless of whether this increase is achieved through the use of a bellows unit or auto macro tubes. The disadvantage is the loss of light, since the intensity of illumination is inversely proportional to the square of its distance from the light source (Fig. 1.18).
For example, at a reproduction ratio of 1:1 the object width and the image width are equal to double the focal length of the lens. The loss of light is thus two stops.

Fig. 1.18 The intensity of illumination is inversely proportional to the square of its distance from the light source.

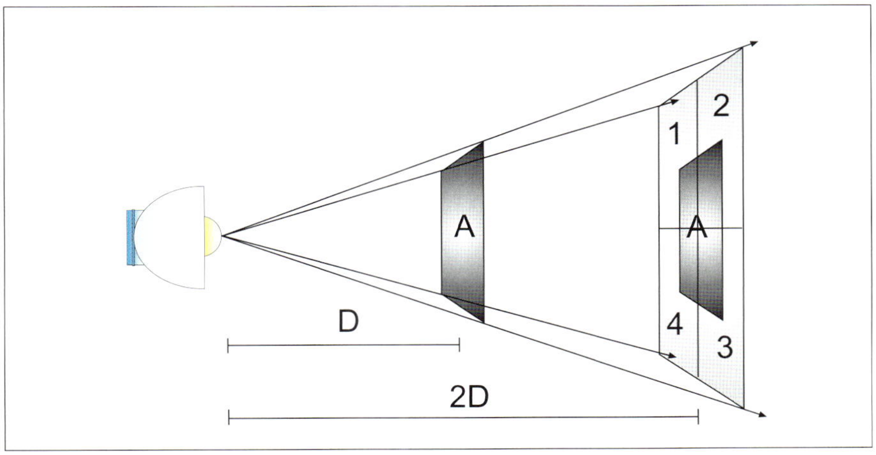

Extension tubes

In dental photography extension tubes should be used only as a last resort. They increase the distance between the lens and the film and thus increase magnification. These are generally sold in sets of three and can be used individually or in combination.

The shorter the focal length of the lens the stronger their effect is; for our purposes this is not an advantage, since we use longer focal length lenses (Fig. 1.19).

Because the light must travel further to reach the film there can be a loss of up to two stops. The subject-to-camera distance is also reduced, although not as much as in using close-up lenses. It is also no longer possible to focus on infinity.

The use of extension tubes is not very practical, since it is no longer possible to infinitely vary the magnification.

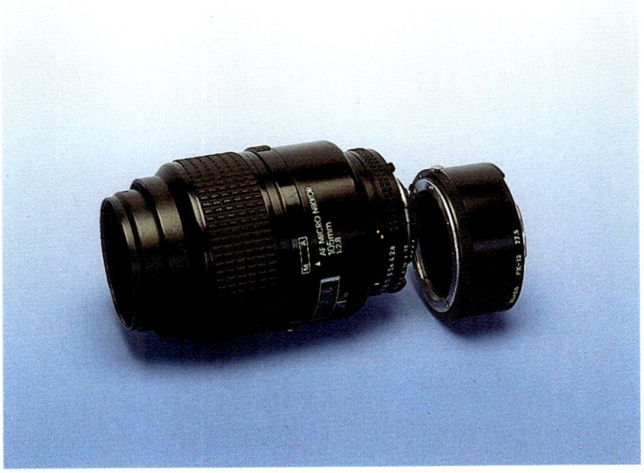

Fig. 1.19 Extension tubes are a compromise solution in dental photography since they do not permit infinite adjustment of the working distance.

Working distance

Working distance is defined as the distance between the subject and the front of the lens (Fig. 1.20). This value is determined by the focal length of the lens and the required magnification. For a particular reproduction ratio, the longer the focal length of the lens the greater the subject-to-camera distance. At a reproduction ratio of 1:1 the subject-to-camera distance is about double the focal length of the lens in conventional lens design. Lenses with floating elements have a significantly shorter subject-to-camera distance.

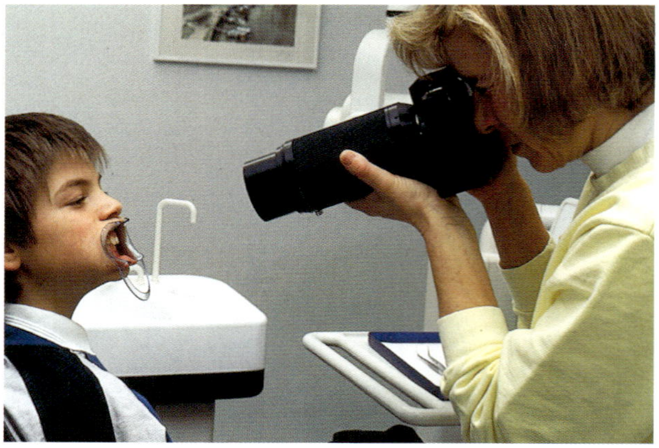

Fig. 1.20 The working distance is defined as the distance between the front edge of the lens to the most forward part of the subject, here the front teeth of the patient. The distance depends on the magnification ratio and the focal length of the lens.

Working distance too great

A subject-to-camera distance which is too great has various disadvantages. The distance between flashgun and subject, for instance, is too great. This means that a high-power flashgun must be used, which is problematical in the case of macro flashguns. Another disadvantage of a large subject-to-camera distance is that small camera movements have a greater effect on the field of view than with shorter ones. It is difficult or even almost impossible to fill the frame exactly.

Working distance too short

If the subject-to-camera distance is too short this can lead to hygienic problems when taking pictures; this is to be strictly avoided, particularly in photography during operations. In dental photography this is merely uncomfortable for the patient if the camera is too close. In intraoral pho-

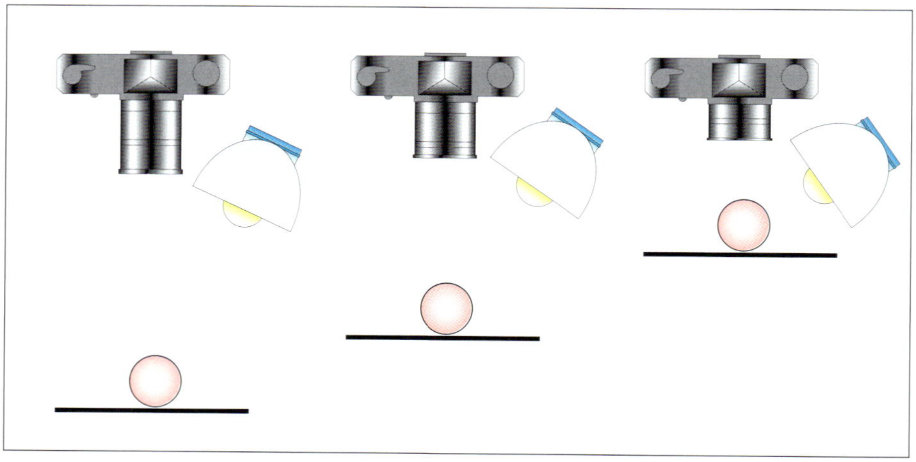

Fig. 1.21 Reducing the working distance means the light comes more from the side. This is problematical for objects in body cavities.

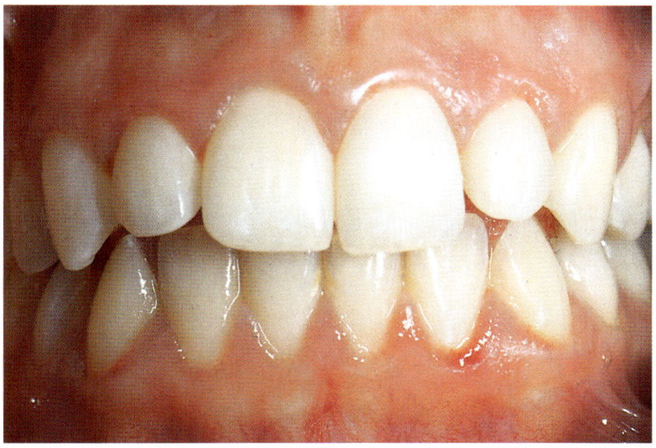

Fig. 1.22 Here the working distance was too short for the side lighting, with the resulting shadows in the right molar area.

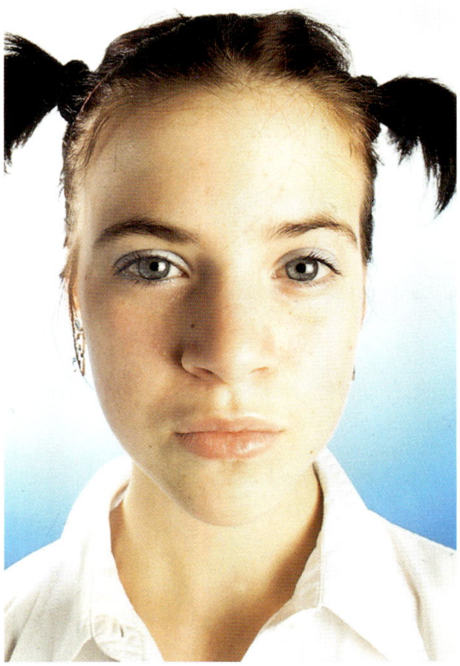

Fig. 1.23 The short working distance resulting from using too short a lens leads to obvious distortion in the portrait.

tography in particular, in which the objects are hidden in the mouth, too short a working distance can create problems in lighting if a ring flash is not used (Fig. 1.21). In this case only the front teeth are properly illuminated. The side teeth generally have shadows from the cheeks or the lips or are illuminated only by the light which falls on them after being reflected by the mucous membranes of the cheeks (Fig. 1.22).

A good rule of thumb for achieving uniform illumination in the mouth is that the working distance should be at least 1.5 times that of the diameter of the ring flash or the distance of the two flash reflectors. Another disadvantage if the working distance is too short is image distortion, which results from an incorrect viewing distance. An eye viewing the subject from the same distance would see the same distorted perspective. The result is that parts of the subject closest to the lens are disproportionally large. In the case of a set of teeth the incisors would appear larger than they would from a greater distance. A portrait would be completely useless because the patient's nose would appear too large (Fig. 1.23).

For these reasons in dental photography a macro lens with a focal length of about 100mm has proven most useful.

Macro lenses of 50mm are to be recommended only in combination with a 2x teleconverter. For the reasons cited above, pictures taken with an intraoral video camera are not suitable as basis for a treatment simulation (dental imaging), since most intraoral video cameras have wide angle lenses.

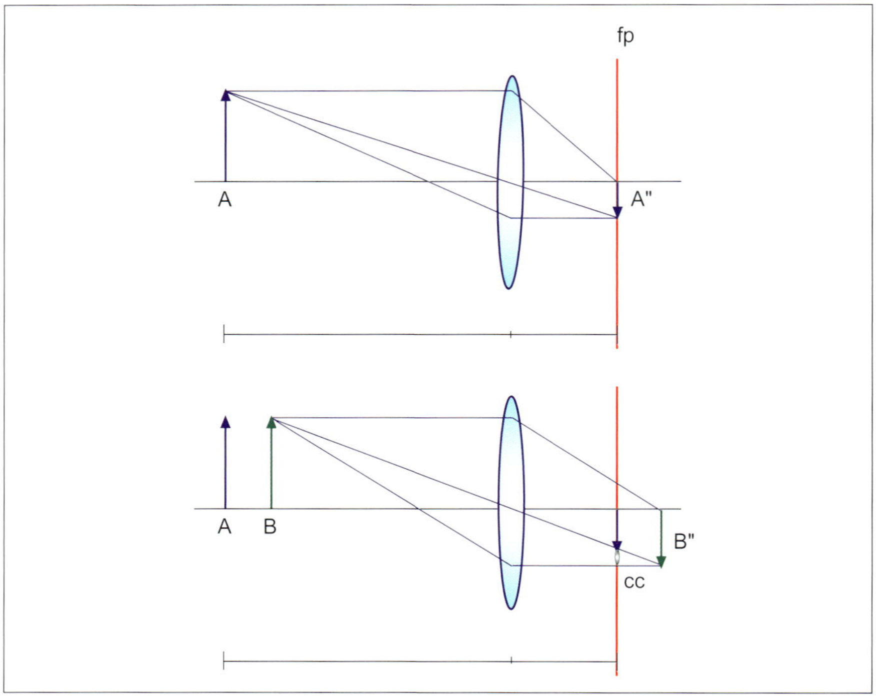

Fig. 1.24 A correctly focused object (A) leads to a sharp image on the film plane (A″). An object which is closer (B) would be sharp behind the film plane (B″). The image point of the top of the object is not exactly focused as a point, but as a so-called circle of confusion. If this exceeds a certain size we perceive the image as being unsharp.
fp = film plane
cc = circle of confusion

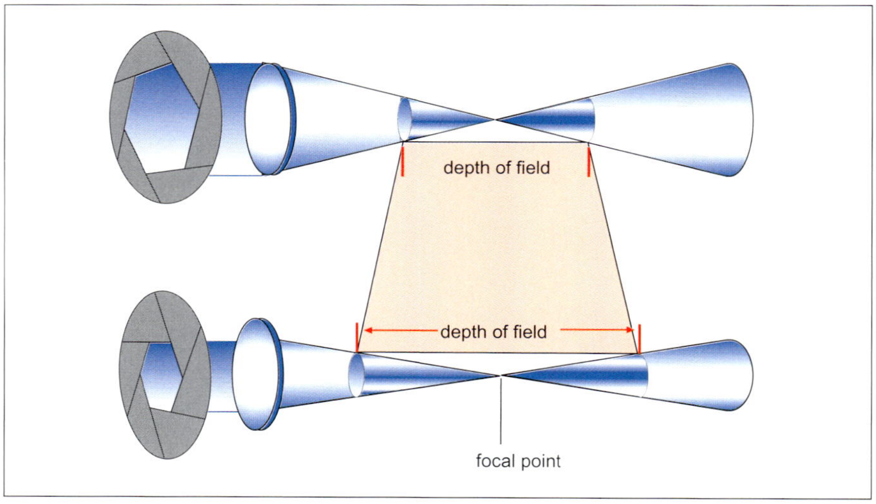

Fig. 1.25 Stopping down the aperture reduces the beam. The diameter of the circles of confusion becomes smaller and the depth of field increases.

MR	Aperture 5.6	8	11	16	22	32	45
1:10	41	59	81	117	161	234	1260
1:5	11.2	16	22	32	44	64	90
1:2	2.2	3.2	4.4	6.4	8.8	13	18
1:1	0.75	1.07	1.47	2.13	2.9	4.27	6.0
2:1	0.28	0.40	0.55	0.80	1.10	1.60	2.3
3:1	0.17	0.24	0.33	0.47	0.65	0.94	1.33

Table 1.1 Depth of field in relation to magnification ratio and aperture. Measurements in millimeters.
MR = Magnification Ratio

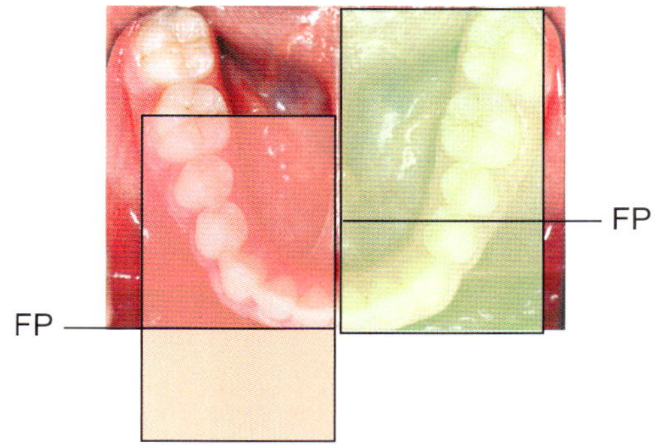

Fig. 1.26 The overall depth of field extends about one third in front of and about two thirds behind the focusing plane (FP). If the closest point in a set of teeth is focused on, the depth of field in front of the focusing plane is lost.

Depth of field

When focusing on a tree standing in a meadow, it is obvious that a certain distance in front of and a greater distance behind the tree is still in focus. This area, which is still perceived as sufficiently sharp, is termed depth of field (Fig. 1.24). Depth of field depends on the aperture and magnification. The smaller the aperture (and the higher the aperture number), the greater the depth of field. Depth of field reduces sharply with greater magnification, so that depth of field in the magnification ratios involved in dental photography is only millimeters (Fig. 1.25).

In dental photography this means that photos can be taken generally only using small apertures. "Standard" apertures should be f/16 or f/22. These require high power flashguns, which is not always the case with ring or macro flashguns.

If necessary, a higher speed film (ISO 200) can be used; this yields one more stop than using ISO 100 film.

It is especially important that depth of field is not sacrificed. It should therefore be kept in mind that the entire depth of field is both in front of and behind the focusing plane. In normal photography approximately one third of the overall depth of field is in front of this and two thirds behind. In close-up photography with a reproduction ratio of 1:1 this ratio changes, with 50% of the total depth of field in front of and 50% behind the distance focused on. This means that if the closest part of the subject is focused on, about 30–50% of the overall depth of field is in front of the subject and thus not used (Fig. 1.26). In photographing a set of teeth from the front, the photographer should not focus on the center of the image (contact point of the central incisers, but on the canines. Only in this way can the entire depth of field be used; otherwise it is not possible to keep a set of teeth in sharp focus from front to back.

In object photography the problem of shallow depth of field can in many instances be overcome by placing the object parallel to the film plane. This is possible only to a certain extent in intraoral photography.

1.2.3 Flashguns

Clinical dental photography is undertaken almost exclusively with the aid of flash, unlike in object or portrait photography.
The undoubted advantages of flash photography are:

- Short duration of flash, eliminating camera shake
- Great intensity of light, allowing smaller apertures
- Color temperature has the characteristics of daylight, allowing use of slide film balanced for daylight
- Flashguns are compact, permitting hand-held photography
- Little heat, no stress to patient

The main difficulty in using flashguns is assessing of the amount of light and estimating the light-shadow-distribution of the image, the latter being determined by arrangement and form of the flashguns.

Assessing of the correct amount of light/flash exposure

When using flashguns the camera must be set to the correct flash synchronization speed (usually 1/60th second, 1/125th second or 1/250th second). When the shutter release is pressed the reflex mirror is locked up, then the front and rear shutter curtain move along the slide film to be exposed. The gap between the shutter curtains is determined by the exposure time which is set, in this case the flash synchronization speed. At short exposure times the gap is small and at slower shutter speeds it is larger. If exposure times are set which are shorter than the flash synchronization speed only a strip of the film is exposed. If the exposure times are too long, the influence of the ambient light can have an adverse effect.
At the correctly set synchronization speed the amount of light falling on the film is determined purely by the amount of flash light. There are a number of ways of setting this amount.

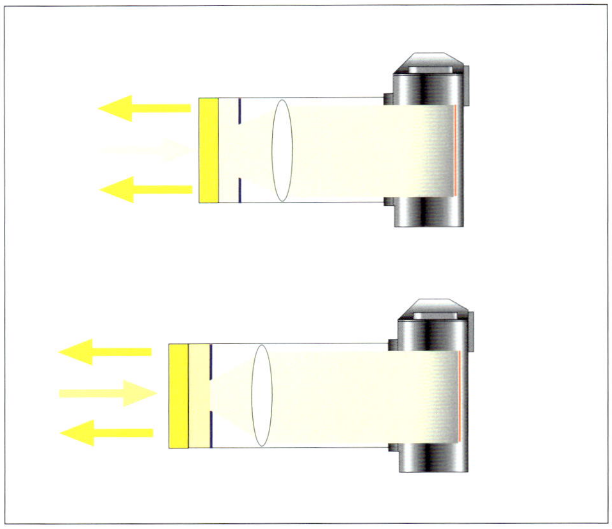

Fig. 12.7 In a medical lens, setting of the magnification and aperture are coupled. A larger magnification is combined with a smaller aperture. Since with a greater magnification the distance between flash and object is shorter, and therefore more light is reflected by the object, this leads to the same amount of light falling on the film despite the smaller aperture.

- ✓ Manually setting the aperture
- ✓ Automatic lighting with medical lenses
- ✓ Computer flash
- ✓ Through the lens (TTL) flash control

Manually setting the aperture

At a specific reproduction ratio and a given lens aperture the amount of light reflected from an object with normal reflectivity (normal subject) back to the camera is always the same, as the object-camera-distance and the amount of light produced by the flash are always the same, too. For a particular camera system the correct aperture can be determined and summarized in a table for various reproduction ratios and thus for various subject-to-

camera distances. These apertures then have to be set manually before every exposure. With a little bit of experience it is possible in this straightforward manner to achieve good results which can be reproduced.
This method of setting the flash output must be used with older camera systems and manual flashguns.

Flash units of medical lenses

Medical flash units also determine exposure in a similar manner, but automatically. The reproduction ratio is first set and the exact plane of focus is determined by moving the camera back and forth. Setting the reproduction ratio on the lens automatically sets the corresponding aperture, which can not be manually adjusted. Automatic setting of the aperture is possible, since the reproduction ratio which is set determines the corresponding subject-to-camera distance. When using medical lenses the output from the flashgun is always at full power. The amount of light falling on the film is determined only by the automatically set aperture (Fig. 1.27). Setting the amount of flash in this manner is foolproof and also is not adversely affected by the varying reflectivity of the subject.

Computer flash

Many flash units have a light sensor which is on the flash and which measures the amount of light falling towards the camera. If the computer flash determines that sufficient light is being reflected, the flash is turned off. Thus the amount of light is determined primarily not by the aperture, but by the duration of the flash. The principal advantage of this type of flash is that within certain limits various apertures can be set. Thus the size of the depth of field can be influenced. Another advantage is that the capacitor is not completely drained each time. This shortens the time between flashes, since the capacitor remains partially charged. Such flashguns can have certain inaccuracies in close-up work if the amount of light entering the lens and thus striking the film and that hitting the flash sensor is not the same. This would result in incorrect exposures. Also, light-absorbing accessories such as bellows units and polarizing filters are not taken into account.

TTL flash

TTL flash (through the lens controlled) was originally patented by Minolta, then taken over by Olympus in 1976, and now offered by every camera manufacturer.

Fig. 1.28 With TTL flash metering the light reflected from the subject passes through the lens to the film; part of this light is reflected by the film surface and strikes a sensor in the base of the camera. The sensor measures the amount of light, transfers the data to the camera's computer, which cuts off the TTL flash when sufficient light has struck the film plane.

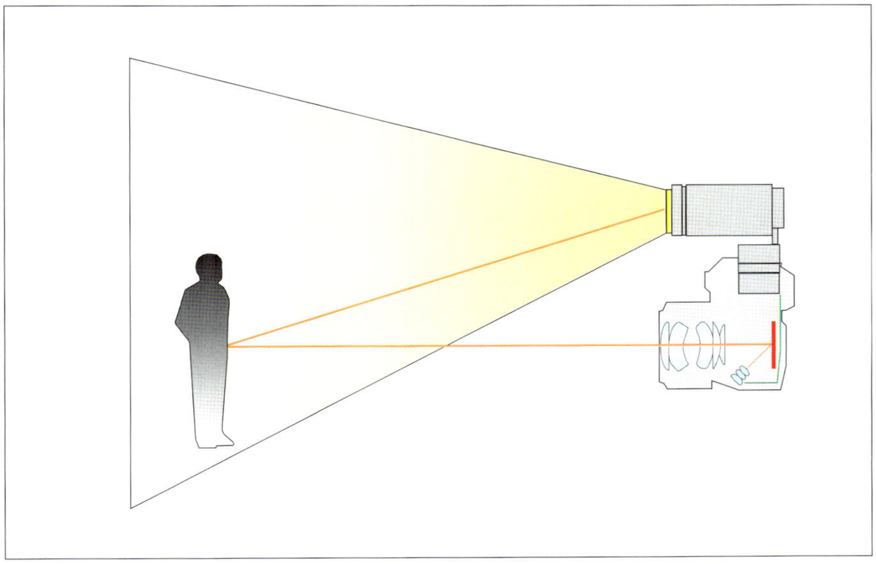

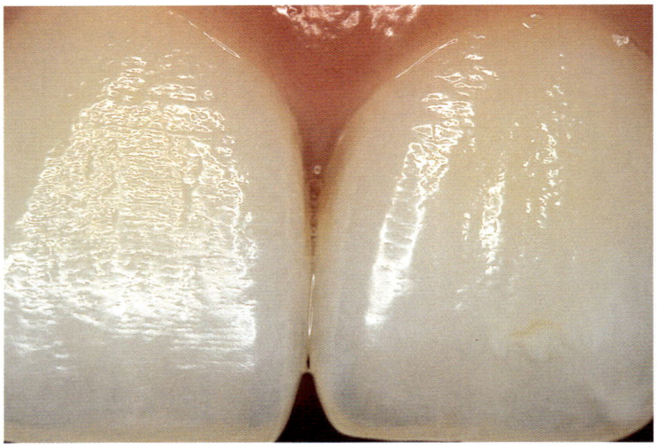

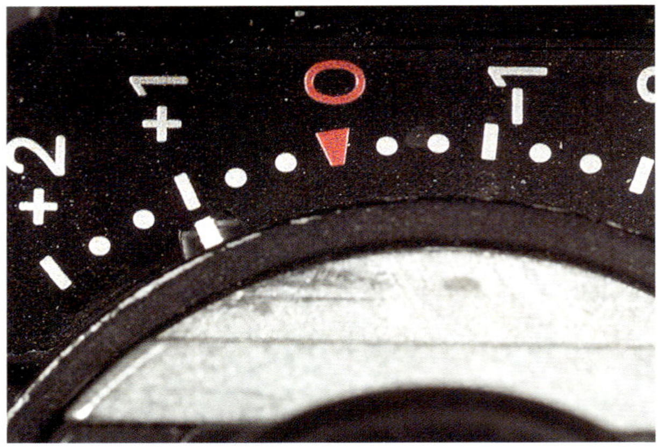

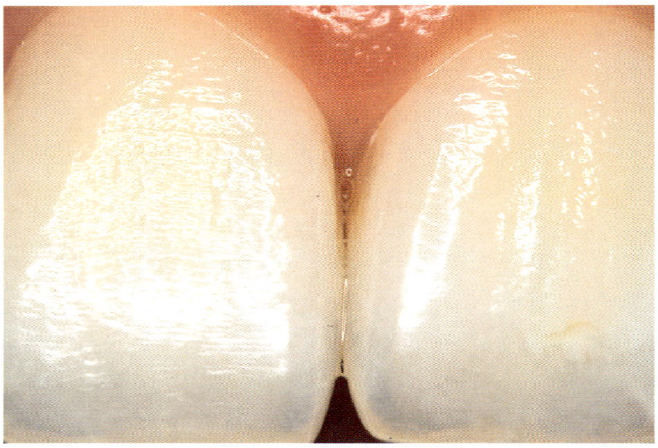

Fig. 1.29 A bright surface which almost fills the frame leads to an underexposed result (a). An exposure compensation (plus-correction) must be manually set (b) to achieve correct exposure (c).

TTL means that for flash metering, only that amount of light is measured which strikes the film through the lens and is reflected from the film surface onto a sensor, generally placed on the camera base. Thus the flash sensor of the computer flash system mentioned above has in practice been installed in the camera itself (Fig. 1.28).

The advantages of this are obvious. Even in close-up work there is no light parallax. Only that light which was effective for film exposure is measured. Thus it is possible to control the aperture (and thus the depth of field) and use light-absorbing accessories such as polarizing filters or bellows units without the danger of incorrect exposure. This type of flash photography has taken the guesswork out of close-up photography. It is also possible to control several flash units through a TTL unit. Naturally TTL flash also has disadvantages.

Since the camera does not "know" what it is taking, a mid-range exposure is selected corresponding to a medium gray level. If the subject has very bright highlights the exposure in the rest of the image is reduced so that the overall exposure is equal to that of a subject with medium reflectivity. Thus, for example, reflections from metal operating instruments can cause such underexposure that the image is unusable. If the image is almost completely filled with white teeth the image can likewise be too dark.

This must be taken into consideration and can be corrected by using the so-called plus correction on the exposure setting of the camera (Fig. 1.29 a–c). The amount of correction depends on the surface and the brightness of the white objects.

In intraoral photography, in which there are always white surfaces from teeth, it generally pays to set the aperture to +1/3 of a stop. When teeth fill the entire content of the frame (e.g. a photo of

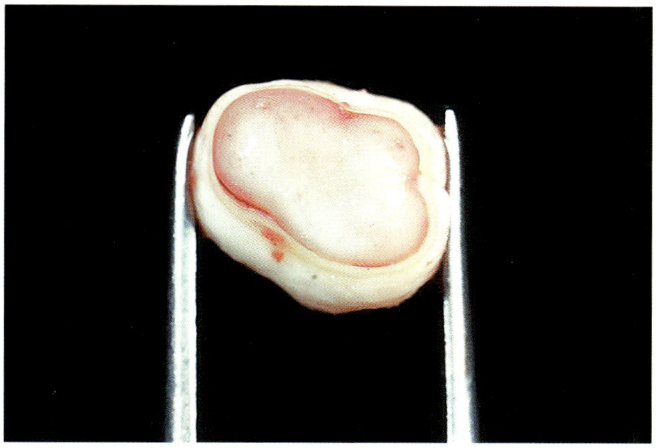

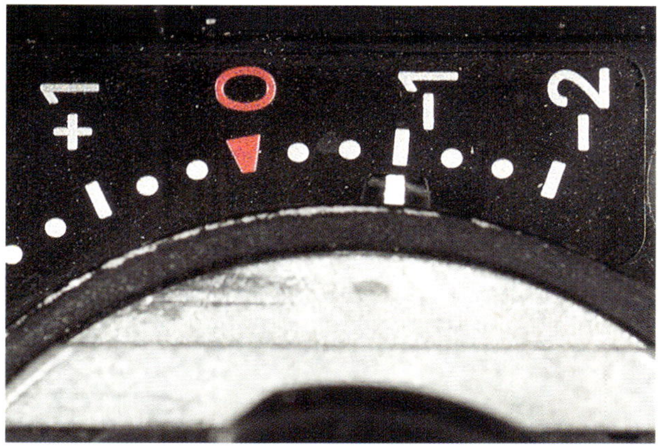

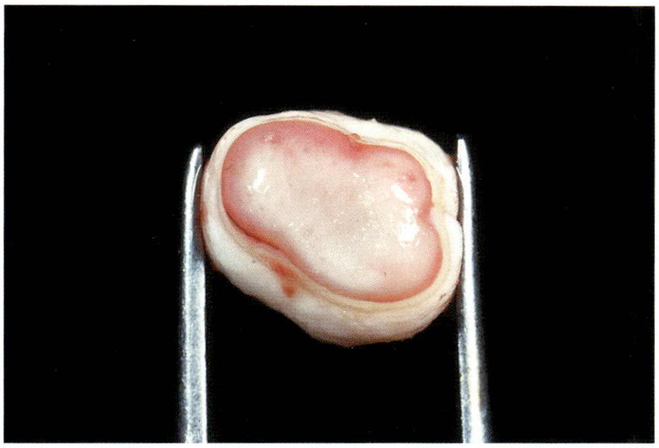

Fig. 1.30 A small object such as this tooth germ against a black background is overexposed (a). Manually setting a minus correction (b) leads to a correct exposure (c).

the middle two upper incisors in a reproduction ratio of 2:1) an exposure correction of one aperture is required.

Conversely the same sort of approach must be taken with subjects which are darker than average. The amount of light must be reduced to prevent the object being overexposed (Fig. 1.30 a–c).

Lighting – Effects of light

In addition to light measurement problems, lighting the subject and assessment of light and shadow distribution present further principal problems of flash photography. These can be assessed through the viewfinder when constant lighting is used, but is not possible with flash due to its short duration. The lighting effect is dependent on the form of the flash reflectors and their arrangement. There are a number of types available for flash photography.

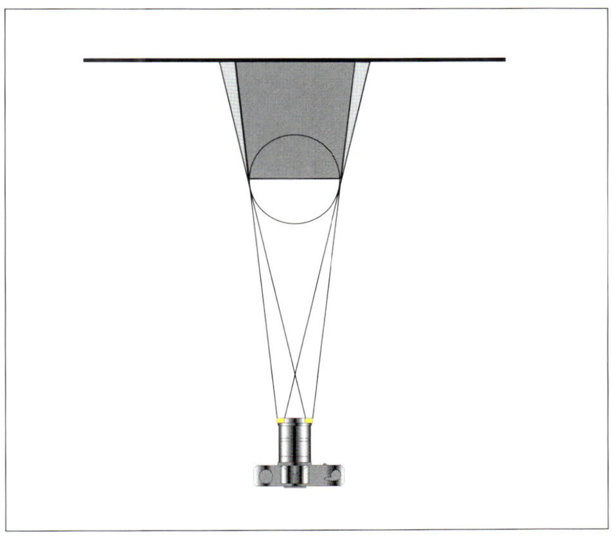

Fig. 1.31 The light from a ring flash surrounds the optical axis. This results in a ring-shaped shadow zone surrounding the subject and a flat, shadowless image of the subject.

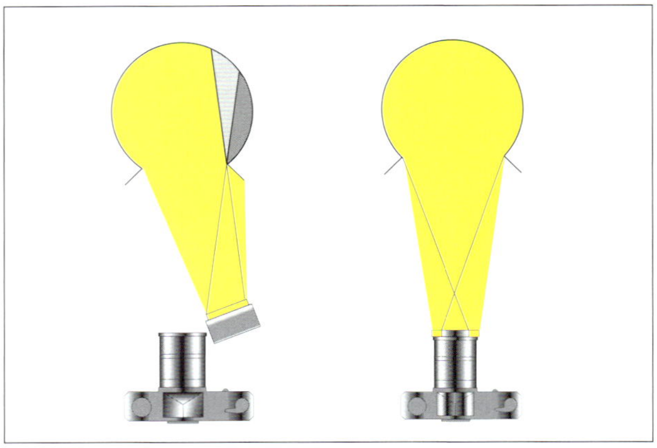

Fig. 1.32 Ring flashes are ideal for illumination of body cavities. If it is not closely enough placed to the lens, illumination by a point flash may result in shadows.

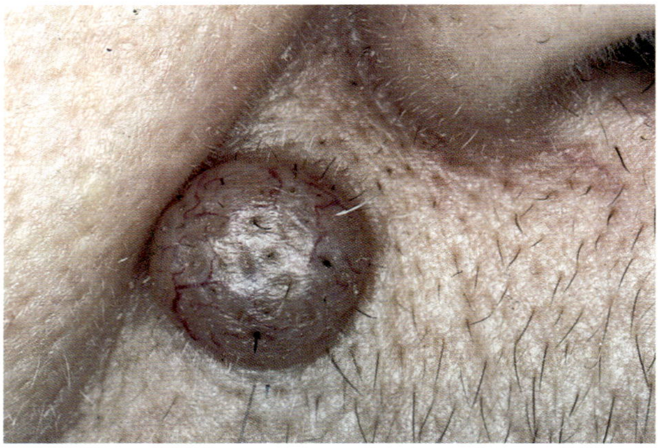

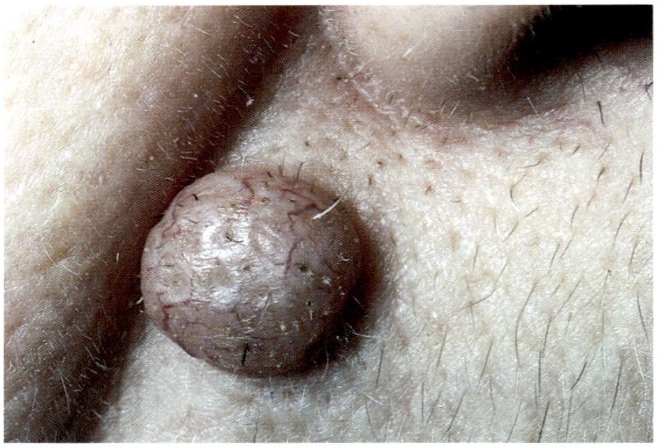

Fig. 1.33 Using a ring flash results in correct color rendition, but a flat representation of the naevus. Side-lighting results in better depth and plasticity (b).

Ring flash, sector flash

Ring flashes are widely used in taking images in body cavities, and thus also in the mouth; these are found in systems such as medical lenses. These types also include sector flashes, in which two to four individual flash tubes are arranged around the lens (Fig. 1.31). In the case of a genuine ring flash one flash tube surrounds the lens. Sector flashes with four flash reflectors and ring flashes are not that different in terms of light output. In both of these types the light practically surrounds the optical axis. The main advantage of this arrangement is that even relatively inaccessible objects deep in the oral cavity can be perfectly lit, even when partially obscured by the lips or cheeks (Fig. 1.32). Thus inexperienced photographers are able to produce correctly exposed and illuminated images in inaccessible areas. Another advantage of this type of front illumination is natural color rendition.

However, ring flashes have the disadvantage of producing an image almost without any shadows. Images tend to look flat and frequently not very brilliant. The shadows, which are necessary to create a three-dimensional effect, are lacking (Fig. 1.33 a,b).
This does not substantially affect images taken in the mouth since the light is always partially obscured here anyway and the characteristics of the ring flash are not evident. For this reason images taken with ring flash can generally only be distinguished through direct comparison with images taken with side lighting.
The quality of the image can be improved by putting a finger over parts of the ring flash or an individual flash tube, or, if possible, turning them off. This lends more direction to the light and the image gains plasticity and depth (Fig. 1.34 a–c). The Nikon SB-29 Speedlight has two flash tubes, which ensures good illumination. The Yashica Den-

Fig. 1.34 Snapshot from a photographic workshop. Covering over one of the three flash reflectors (a) achieves a small improvement in plasticity. Photo b shows the scars on the mucous membrane illuminated by three flash tubes. In Photo c the lower left one was covered. This achieves greater plasticity than by covering the tube at the 12:00 position (Photos b and c: B. Sommer).

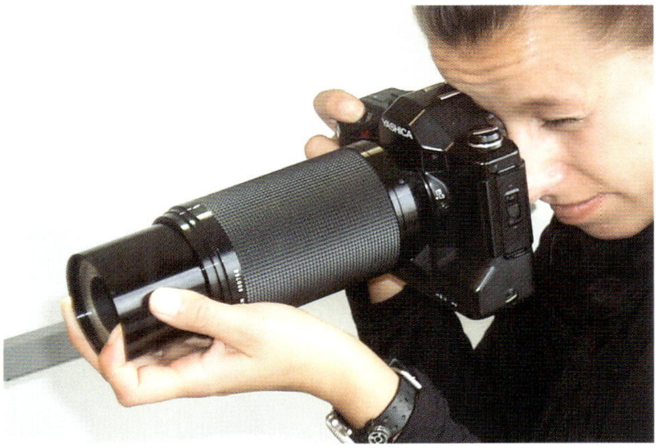

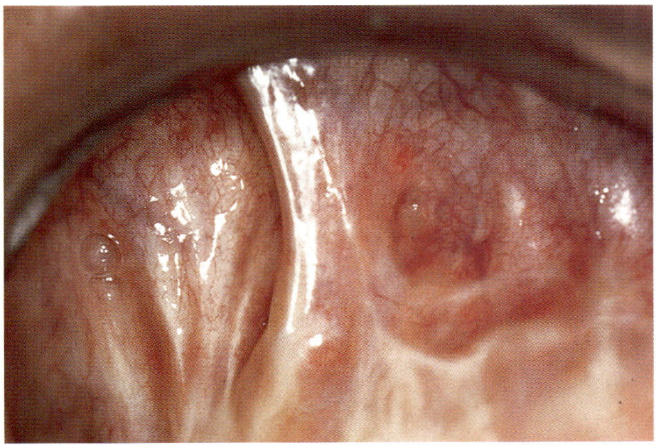

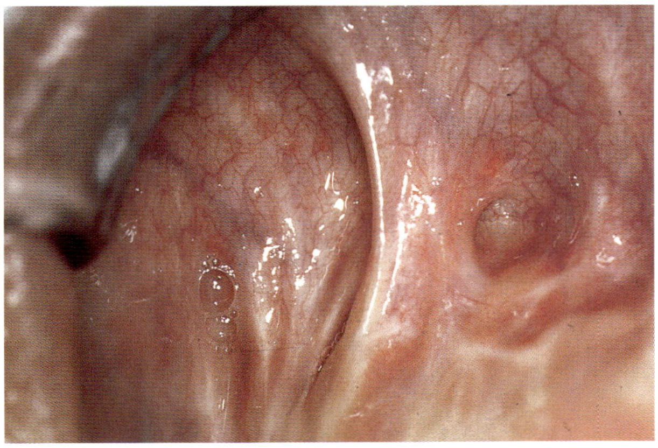

tal Eye has three flash tubes; the upper one can be switched off, thereby improving the plasticity of the illumination.

In general, ring flashes are relatively low powered. When used with teleconverters or other extension accessories it may therefore be necessary to use faster film.

Point flash

A point light source from the side produces a directional light with strong shadows which aids in the three dimensional appearance of the final image. Depending on the part of the mouth which is to be photographed the position of the side lighting has to be altered before each exposure. This requires some experience. Overall front views require the flash to be located at the 12:00 o'clock position; for side lighting the positions are at 3:00 and 9:00 o'clock. With very short subject-to-camera distances the flash must be located very close

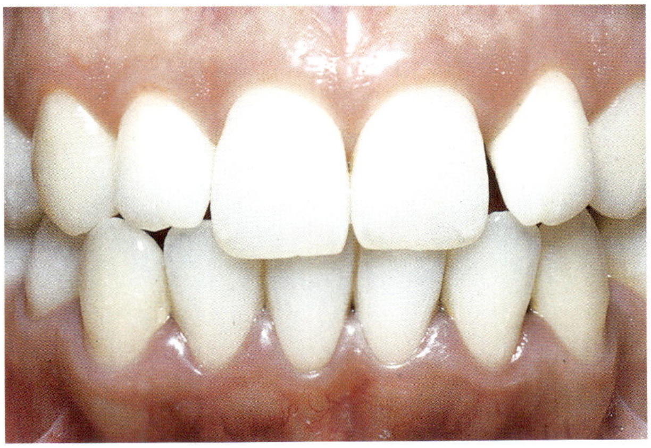

Fig. 1.35 Flashguns positioned to the side can cause irritating shadows if they are not mounted close to the optical axis of the lens and so that they can be rotated. In a front view, however, the flash should be at the 12:00 position.

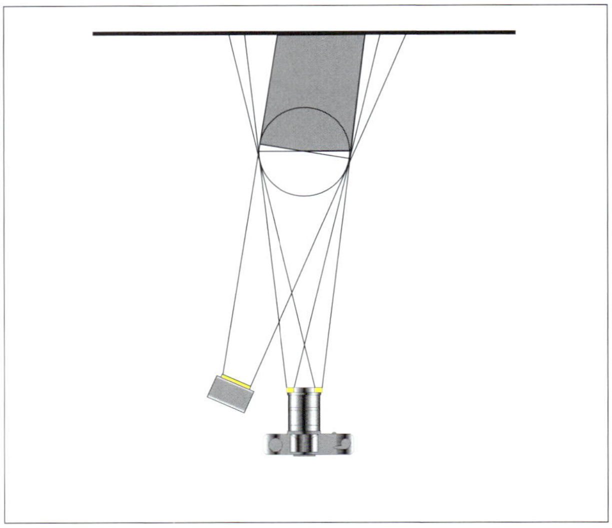

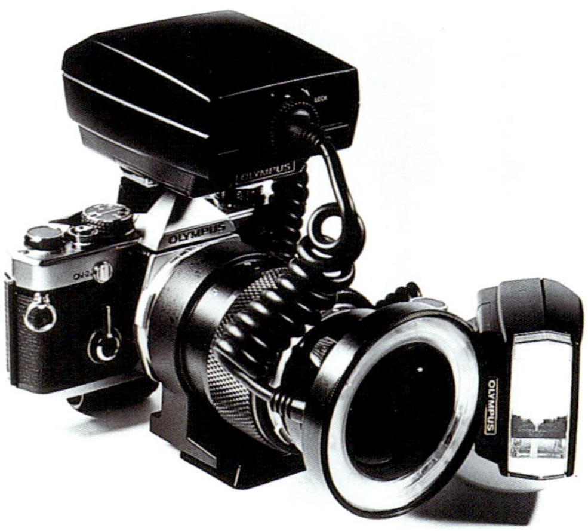

Fig. 1.36 The combination of ring and side flash is not commonly used. (a) shows the light-shadow distribution in diagrammatic form, (b) shows a point-ring-flash combination with Olympus components.

to the optical axis to avoid casting disturbing shadows (Fig. 1.35). For this purpose a rotatable side flash unit which is mounted close to the lens would be suitable.

Combinations

To compensate for the disadvantages of ring and side flash, or to combine their advantages, several flash units can be combined.
The use of ring and side flash together is not that prevalent (Fig. 1.36 a,b). Dine in the USA offers a flash unit with both point and ring flash.
More often used are dual flash systems with two flash units to be mounted to the left and right of the lens (Fig. 1.37 a,b). The resulting light is intense

Fig. 1.37 Using a bilateral flash(a) provides high light-output and even illumination. An example of such a flash bracket system is the Duoflash from Novoflex which is available for current SLR cameras with TTL flash (Photo: Novoflex).

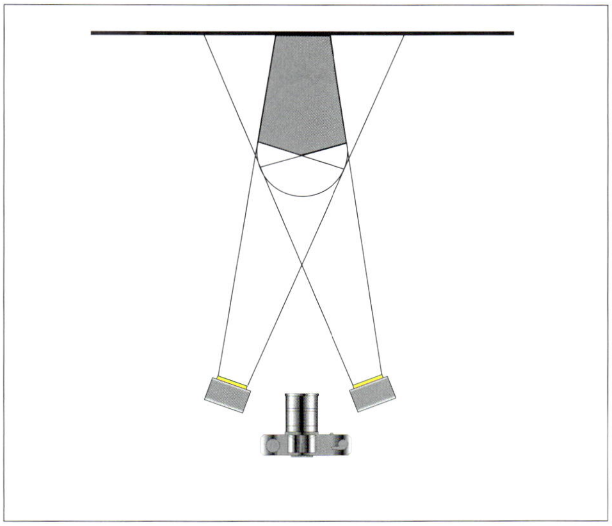

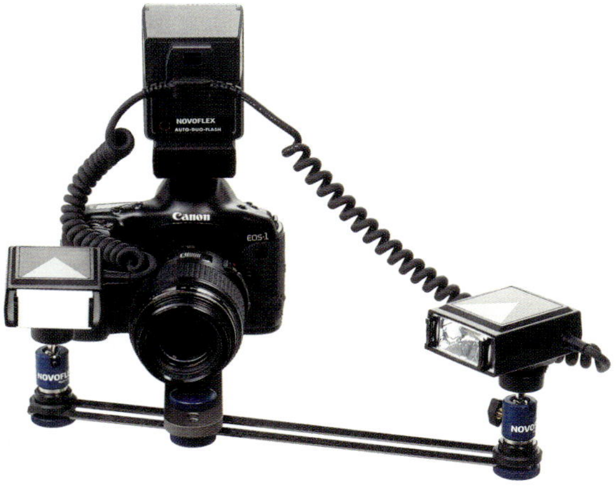

enough to allow the lens to be stopped down quite far, having a positive effect on depth of field. This set-up achieves even illumination even deep in the mouth cavity while at the same time yielding greater plasticity of the image. However, in order to achieve the best possible results the direction of the flash heads has to be checked and adjusted before each exposure, depending on the subject-to-camera distance. The output from one of the two flash tubes can be reduced by using a diffuser. The use of dual flashes also requires some experience on the part of the operator if uniformly good results are to be achieved.

Summary: the deeper the object is in the oral cavity and the greater the magnification ratio, the more suitable a ring flash is. Side flash should be used for images taken outside the mouth. Ring flash should be avoided for object or portrait photographs. The use of a bilateral flash system is op-

timum, but requires a certain amount of experience on the part of the user. Moreover, they are heavier and clumsier to use than ring flashes.
A disadvantage of many macro flash units is their low output. This is indicated by their guide number. A low guide number, such as 8, can mean that faster film speeds such as ISO 200 must be used in order to achieve small enough apertures.

1.2.4 Film

The selection of film plays a significant role in the overall result.

Color transparency film
The film of choice for medical documentation is color transparency film. Slides have the advantage of being the most versatile. Once developed, the results can be seen directly without the aid of any other means. High quality prints can be made from slides and slides are well suited for publications. Nothing surpasses color slides for projection. They can also be easily digitised through scanning and stored on photo CDs.
Slide films differ in their light sensitivity and color characteristics. Standard slide films today are those rated at ISO 100 or ISO 200. There are a great number of these commercially available. Slide film with lower speed (ISO 50 or 64) is sharper, though this can be perceived only through the best possible projection means or large format prints.
Some slide films have problematic color characteristics. Films designed for amateurs have high color saturation; these films are not so suitable for intraoral photography, since the gingiva color is reproduced too strongly, making the gingiva appear livid or somewhat inflamed. In this case a film which has less strong and cooler colors should be used. If the photographer is concerned with achieving consistent results, then professional films should be used. The basis of every film is the layer of gelatin in which the light-sensitive silver halides are embedded. This gelatin undergoes maturation, during which a stage is reached in which color rendition and other technical specifications are optimized. In the case of the emulsions of professional films, the maturation of the gelatin is interrupted by placing the film in the refrigerator, where it is kept until use. Using this type of film makes sense only if the photographer stores the film in the refrigerator to preserve its characteristics. At storage temperatures of about 4 to 6 degrees C° its ageing is considerably slowed. At temperatures of about freezing (–18 degrees C°) this ageing process practically ceases.
Similarly, these films should be developed only in special laboratories. Overnight developing "around the corner" is not necessary a guarantee of the uniformly high quality that can be expected of professional films.

Proven films are Ektachrome 100 HC, Agfachrome RSX II 100, Ektachrome EPR 64, Kodachrome 64, Ektachrome 100 Plus Professional, Ektachrome 100 S Professional, Fujichrome Provia 100 F Professional and Fujichrome Velvia (for object photography, but not for intraoral photography).

Black and white films
Black and white films have lost much of their relevance for medical documentation in recent years and their use is now more the exception rather than the rule.

Color negative films
It makes sense to use color negative films only if it is planned from the outset to produce prints. One instance of this would be routine documentation of profiles and portraits by orthodontists. Otherwise color slides are to be preferred.

Special films
Special films are available for special purposes. Their use is generally the exception rather than the rule in normal dental practice.
Slide duplicating films are especially low contrast films with which slides can be duplicated (which see).
Some films have generally lost their application with the advent of computer graphics to produce slides for slide presentations. These include Agfa Ortho 25, a black and white lith film, as well as

Kodak Vericolor SO-279 Slide Film which allows multicolored text to be placed on slides without computer graphics.
Black and white slide film (Agfa Scala) is sometimes used by lecturers to show form as separate from color. This also tends to be an attention-getter, since black and white film is quite unusual today.
The Polachrome series of instant slide films have lost much ground due to the use of computer graphics.

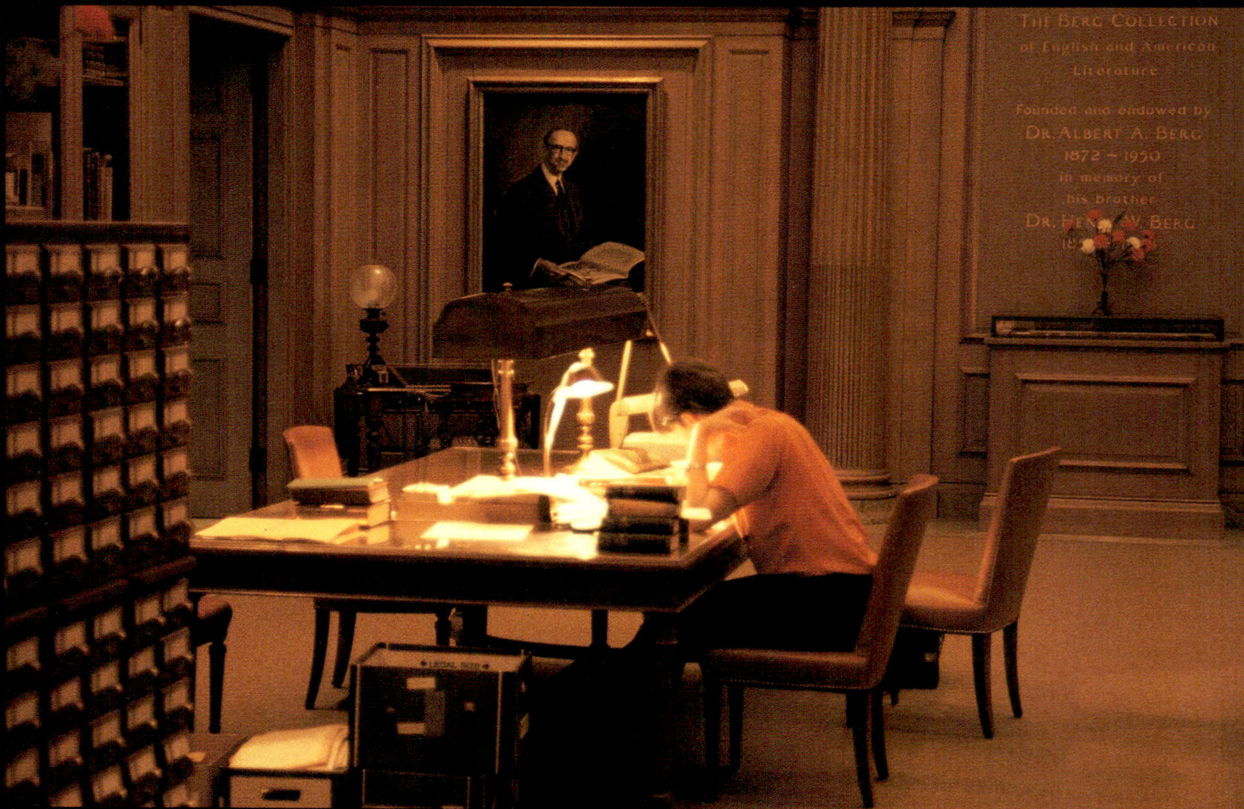
THE BERG COLLECTION
of English and American
Literature
Founded and endowed by
DR. ALBERT A. BERG
1872 ~ 1950
in memory of
his brother

2 Camera Systems Appropriate for Dental Photography

The following listing is not intended to be complete, but only details current systems available without evaluating them. Here, only conventional systems are considered. Digital camera systems are discussed in Chapter 12.

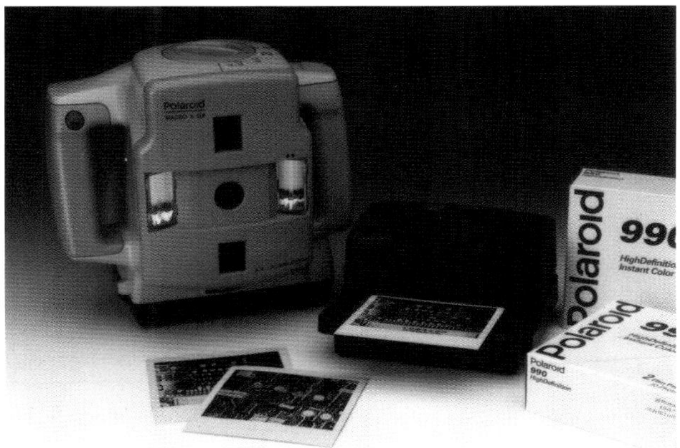

Fig. 2.1 Polaroid Macro 5 SLR instant camera.

2.1 Instant Cameras

2.1.1 Polaroid Macro 5 SLR

Fully automatic single lens reflex camera for close-up photography, with five fixed magnification settings, from 0.2x to 3x (five built-in lenses). Two integrated flash units, which can be switched off (Fig. 2.1). Computerized, automatic exposure setting. Data function. Snap-on accessory lenses for 5x enlargement. Uses Polaroid Type 990 film.

Focusing is done via two light points which are caused to converge by changing the working distance. When photographing the upper jaw the camera can sometimes focus on the palate instead of the occlusal plane.

The Macro 3 SLR, with less functionality, is available as a "cut down" version of the Macro 5 SLR. It permits magnification ratios of 1:1, 2:1 and 3:1, but not profile and enface photographs.

◄ Artificial light, here the ambient and the desk light in a New York library, is not white, although we see it as such (color adaptation by the brain). Slide film balanced for daylight however shows the reddish-yellow color of the light more faithfully than our eyes do.

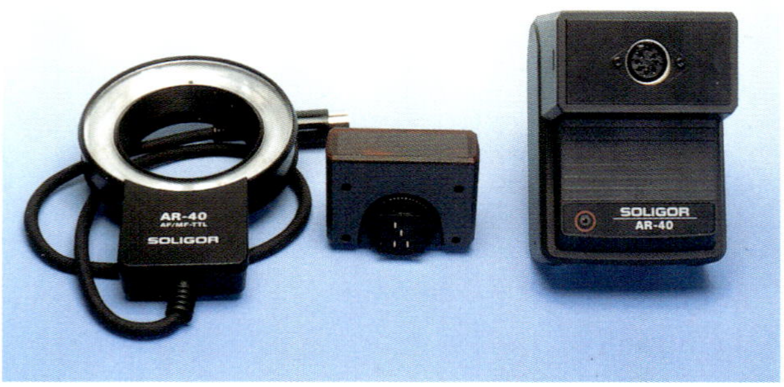

Fig. 2.2 Soligor AR-40 AF ring flash.

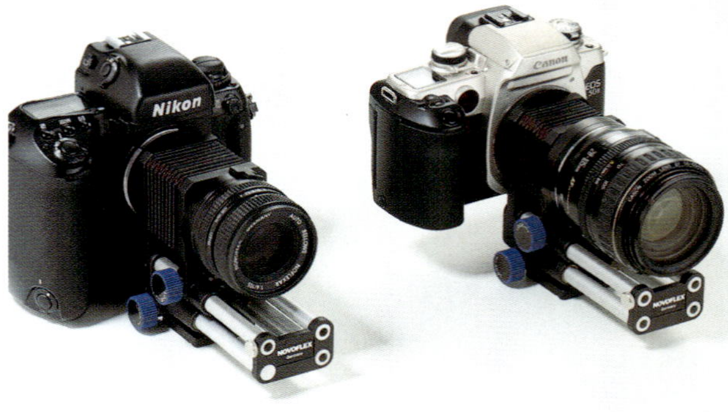

Fig. 2.3 The Novoflex automatic bellows is suitable for practically every SLR (Photo: Novoflex).

2.2 Basic Systems

2.2.1 Soligor Dental Camera System

Camera body
Soligor SA 300 camera body

Lens
100mm f/3.5 macro lens which permits a magnificaton ratio of 1:1. Using an achromat close-up lens can achieve a magnification ratio of 2:1.

Flash unit
The Soligor AR-40 AF/MF-TTL ring flash is available which has TTL metering (Fig. 2.2). Overall, a cost-effective, simple camera system.

2.2.2 Novoflex system

Has been used successfully for decades in the United Kingdom and the United States. Basis of the Novoflex system is the automatic bellows unit combined with a short mount lens (Fig. 2.3).

Camera body
No special camera body is specified, since the bellows unit can be adapted for practically all lens mounts. Thus existing camera bodies can be used.

Lenses
The combination of the automatic bellows unit with the Novoflex 1:4/105mm lens head. This achieves reproduction ratios of infinity to 1:1.3.

Flash units
The Novoflex Macro flash set (guide number 20) can be used as single flash or as a bilateral flash. A macro flash with TTL metering (see below) is also available (Auto Duo Flash).

2.2.3 Wolgensinger system

The system originally described by Wolgensigner can be put together using components from many manufacturers.

Camera body
Any SLR camera is suitable.

Lenses
Wolgensinger recommends a 50mm or 55mm macro lens in combination with a 2x teleconverter. This permits a magnification range of infinity to 1:1.

Flash units
Two flash units mounted on brackets. Flash exposure is regulated via aperture (first create flash bracketing series!)

2.3 Medical Systems

2.3.1 Medical Nikkor 120mm

The proven Nikon Medical Lens is currently not being sold in the European Union since it does not comply with the European Weak Current Regulation. Outside the European Union, such as in Switzerland, the lens is still sold (Fig. 2.4).

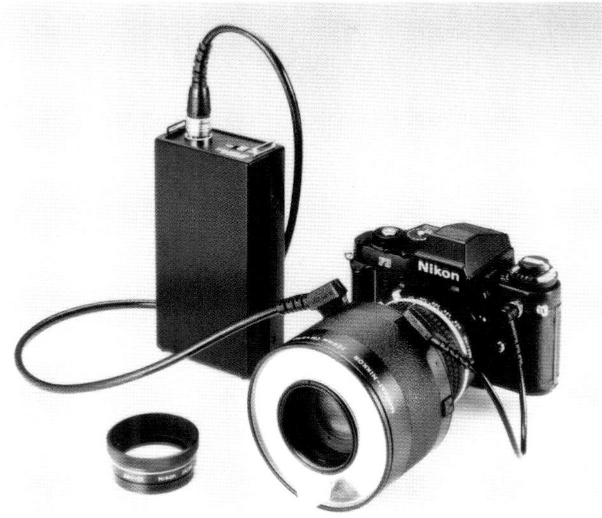

Fig. 2.4 The Nikon medical lens, which has been proven for years, is currently not available in the European Community.

Camera body
Any Nikon SLR which has an X flash synchronization setting can be used.

Lens
The f/4.0 120mm Medical Nikkor lens is a special lens allowing infinitely adjustable reproduction ratio settings between 1:11 and 1:1. A close-up lens, available as an accessory, permits magnification ratios to 2:1. The lens length remains constant when the reproduction ratio is changed (internal focusing).
The long focal length of 120mm is ideal for dental photography. The subject-to-camera distance at a magnification ratio of 1:11 is 160cm; 28cm at a magnification ratio of 1:2 and even 17cm at 1:1.
As is the case with all medical lenses, the f/stops of f/4 to f/32 are automatically set by setting the magnification. The lens can mark the magnification in the lower right corner of the image without having a data back. This reproduction ratio is displayed in the viewfinder as soon as the flash is charged.

Flash unit
The amount of light of the integrated ring flash is automatically controlled by the aperture, which is set along with the magnifcation ratio. The flash is either mains-powered or via an external battery connected to the lens. This makes the entire system somewhat clumsy to use.

Recommended accessories
The camera should have a grid focusing screen and a data back.

2.3.2 Yashica Dental Eye III

Currently this 35mm format camera is the lightest and easiest dental photo system.

Camera body
The special camera body has a permanently fixed lens, which cannot be detached. Controls are kept to a minimum to avoid incorrect settings. Camera and flash are powered by a lithium battery in the camera base. Thus there is no need for external cables (Fig. 2.5). The winder and automatic film rewind mechanism are integrated.
The only controls are a switch to turn the system on, a button for exposure compensation and a

switch to shut off the central flash or the entire flash system.
Standard fitting includes a data back and a grid focusing screen which greatly facilitates camera positioning.

Lens
The 100mm medical lens permits reproduction ratios of 1:15 to 1:1 (with the 2:1 close-up lens supplied as an accessory). The working distances and depth of field values are found in Table 2.1.

Flash unit
The ring flash integrated into the lens has a guide number of 12. Flash exposure is controlled by the aperture, which is automatically coupled to the magnification ratio. This is not a true ring flash: three flash tubes are fitted at 12:00, 16:00 and 8:00 o'clock. The flash can be completely turned off, for instance, for copying X-rays. The middle flash can also be turned off, thereby slightly increasing the plasticity of the images (Fig. 2.6a and b). Putting a finger over one of the two lower flash tubes increases the plasticity even more. A mains unit is also available to power the camera.

Accessories
Accessories available include a metal photo mirror, a close-up lens and an eye cup.

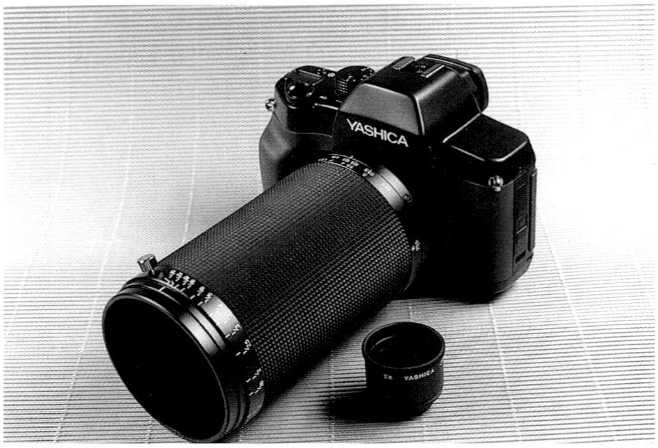

Fig. 2.5 The Yashica Dental Eye III, the currently lightest and easiest to use dental system.

Table 2.1 Working distance and associated depth of field.

Magnification Ratio	1:15	1:10	1:8	1:5	1:3	1:2	2:3	1:1
Working Distance (cm)	155	105	85	55	35.5	25.5	20.5	15.5
Depth of Field (mm)	204-109	139-73	110-62	70-41	43.5-27.5	30.5-20.5	23.5-17.5	17.5-13.5

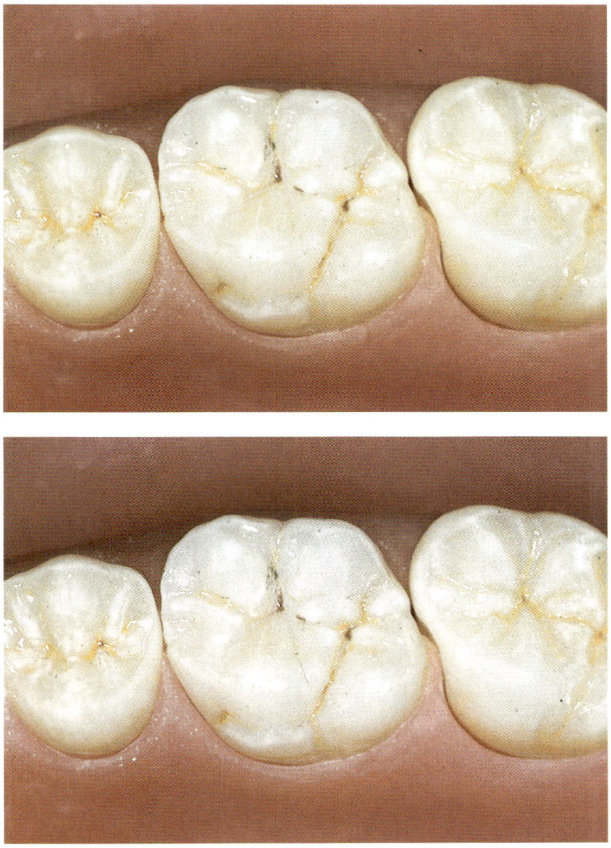

Fig. 2.6 Slight improvement of the plasticity in the image by switching off the upper flash reflector. In the case of (a) all reflectors switched on, in (b) the upper reflector is switched off.

2.4 Systems with TTL Flash Metering

2.4.1 Contax Dental System

The Contax Dental System is based on a development by the late dentist, Vonow, of Zurich. The equipment is produced and distributed by Dental-Foto-Technik A. Binz in Widen, CH. The system has recently been fundamentally redesigned using Nikon components. Since the old Contax system is still available on the secondhand market, it is described in its original form, followed by the Nikon Dental System.

Camera body
The Contax body (e.g. the 137 MD Quartz) with integrated winder was modified (Fig. 2.7).

Lens
A Zeiss f/2.8/60mm lens combined with a Kenko 2x Teleplus MC4 Teleconverter. This combination permits a reproduction ratio from infinity to 2:1.

Flash unit
Two high power, swivelling, side-mounted flash units, powered by battery. Small f/ stops are possible due to high output. Sidelighting results in very plastic illumination.

Accessories
Standard accessories are data back and grid focusing screen.

The Contax Dental System is not easy to use, but can achieve good results with experience.

Nikon variants of the Contax Dental System
The Modification VI Dental Flash system is designed for use with Nikon cameras. All current Nikon autofocus cameras are suitable. The camera body is used in conjunction with the 60mm Micro AF with a 2x teleconverter.

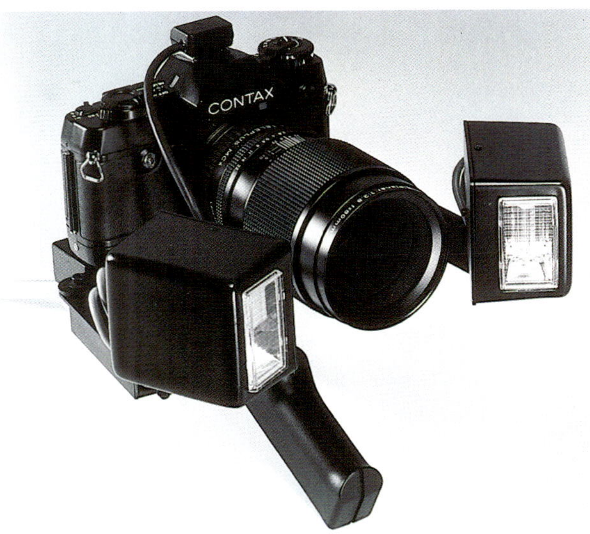

Fig. 2.7 The Contax Dental System.

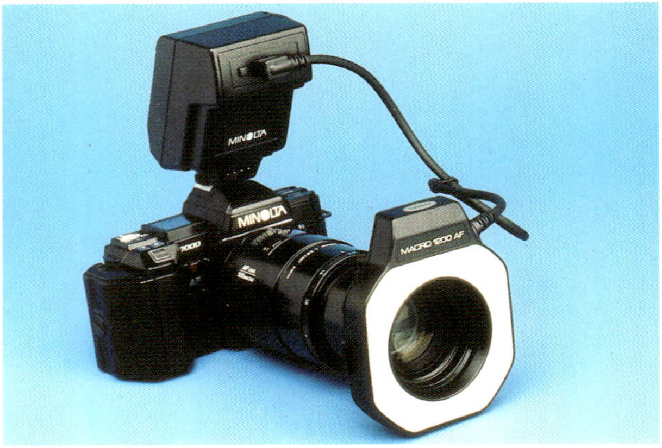

Fig. 2.8 Dental photography system of Minolta components.

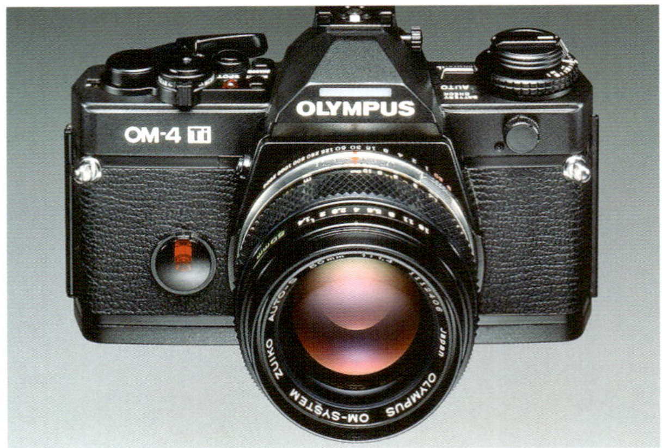

Fig. 2.9a Olympus OM4Ti camera body (Photo: Olympus).

2.4.2 Minolta system

Camera body
Dynax series (e.g. Dynax 505si, 800si or Dynax 7 or 9) camera bodies are recommended.

Lenses
Recommended are the AF Macro f2.8/50mm, AF Macro f/3.5/50mm or AF Macro f/2.8100mm (all have a magnification ratio of infinity to 1:1), also in combination with teleconverters (AF Apo Teleconverter II 2x) or close-up lenses (Fig. 2.8).

Flash unit
Minolta offers the 1200AF Macro Flash. This is a flash unit with four flash tubes operating either individually or together (guide number 12).
The Macro Flash was specially designed for close up photography and macro photography and for medical/scientific photography. It can be used with all Minolta Dynax SLR cameras as well as with older Minolta autofocus cameras. It has four individual flash tubes arranged in a square which can operate independently to avoid undesirable shadows or to achieve a particular pattern of shadows. The flash unit is attached in place of the lens hood directly on the lens. It is supplied with the FS-1100 hot shoe adapter, two adapters (filter sizes 49mm and 55mm) for attaching the flash unit to the lens; the control unit, the flash unit and a sturdy leather case.

Accessories
Integrated winder, data back, viewfinder.

2.4.3 Olympus dental system

Olympus has lost its leading role in medical photography systems, in part because of difficulties in ordering components through dealers. If this is the case, it may pay to try to obtain equipment from the Olympus microscope equipment section.

Camera bodies
The OM-4 Titan and OM-3 35mm cameras are still being produced (Fig. 2.9).

Lenses
The 80mm macro short mount lens with the auto macro tube is used, sometimes in combination with a close-up lens. This covers the reproduction ratios of 1:2 to 1:1.2 (2:1 with close-up lens). The com-

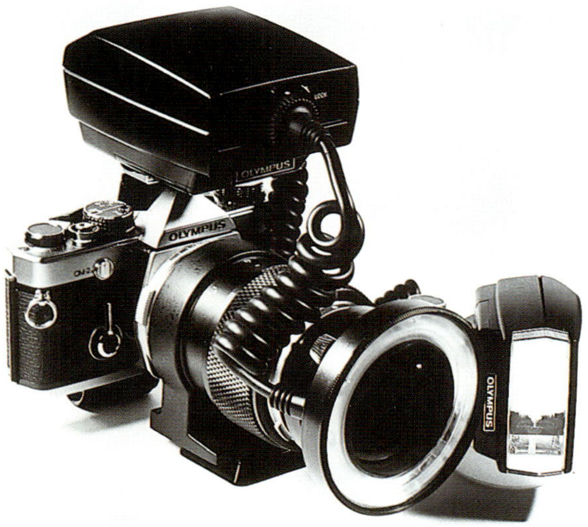

Fig. 2.9 Ring flash-point flash combination of Olympus components.

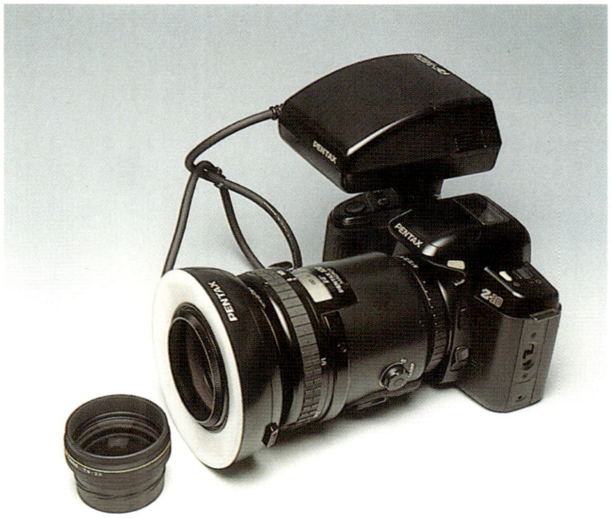

Fig. 2.10 Unfortunately now off the market and only available secondhand: the Pentax Dental System.

bination of the 135mm macro short mount lens with the auto macro tube permits a subject-to-camera distance of between infinity and 1:2.6.
The disadvantage is that lenses have to be changed at exactly those working distances which are most applicable to dental photography.

Flash units
Units available are either the T10 ring flash (guide number 10) or (better) the bilateral side flash T28 (guide number 28). The bilateral side flash can be mounted on the front of the lens and swiveled, but the tubes are quite far apart from the optical axis.

Accessories
Accessories include data back, focusing screen and motor/winder. Olympus systems have compact components, outstanding optical quality and a flexible flash system. However, Olympus' plans to produce high quality SLRs and accessories remain unclear.

2.4.4 Pentax

Up until a few years ago Pentax was marketing a very good and compact dental photo system; this is currently available only secondhand (Fig. 2.10). Nevertheless, it is possible to put together an equally good system using components.
The Pentax Z-1P body can be used, which has semi-professional equipment. The SMC-FA 100mm f/2.8 lens is recommended. This is a macro lens which can achieve a reproduction ratio of 1:1 (subject-to-camera distance at 1:1 30.6cm). If desired, the lens can be combined with a teleconverter (A-converter 2xL) in order to achieve a magnification ratio of 2:1.
The AF-140 C ring flash can be used. This has four flash tubes arranged in pairs which can also be fired in pairs. Guide number is 14.
The Lester Dine company offers a Pentax body with a Yuzo macroflash (see below).

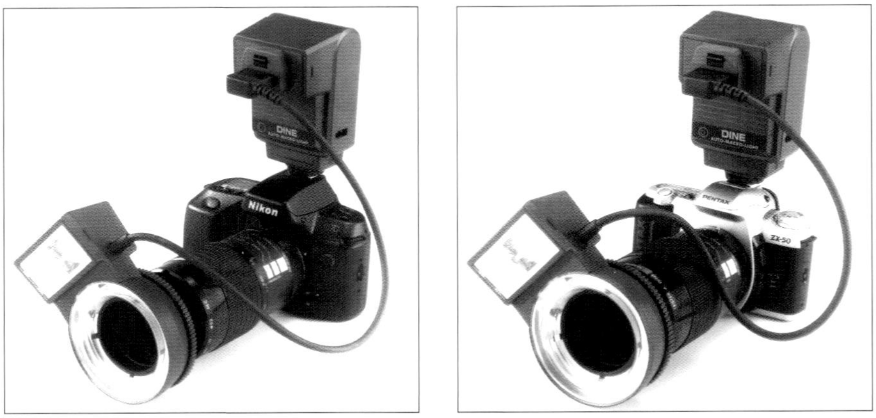

Fig. 2.11 Dental cameras from the US specialist company, Lester Dine. (a) based on a Nikon body, (b) based on a Pentax body.

2.4.5 Lester Dine system

The Dine company in the USA is the largest company which offers accessories and cameras for dental photography.

Camera bodies

Various camera bodies with TTL flash are available (Fig. 2.11a and b):

- Nikon N60 (F60)
- Pentax ZX 50

Lens

Dine recommends a 105mm macro lens which achieves a reproduction ratio of 1:1. The reproduction ratios which are most important for dental photography are marked on the lens. This helps to ensure conditions can be reproduced.

Yuzo macroflash

The real heart of the Lester Dine cameras is their Yuzo flashgun from the Japanese company. This is a ringflash/point flash combination with a guide number of 28 or 14 (ringflash). The ring and point flash can only be used alternatively; this is controlled by a switch on the back. Thus the ringflash can be switched on for use in intraoral photography or for extreme close-ups. The rotatable point flash is used in extraoral photography. This flash unit is also available in Germany. An adaptor allows the TTL system to be used with the most important SLR systems.

2.4.5 Nikon AF system

Nikon is one of the largest manufacturers of SLR-cameras providing the largest range of accessories. Combining Nikon components achieves systems which meet all requirements of dental photography.

Camera bodies

All camera bodies are suitable which have TTL flash control and which can accommodate interchangeable focusing screens (Fig. 2.12). For example, the F90x, F5, F100 and F80 are suitable.

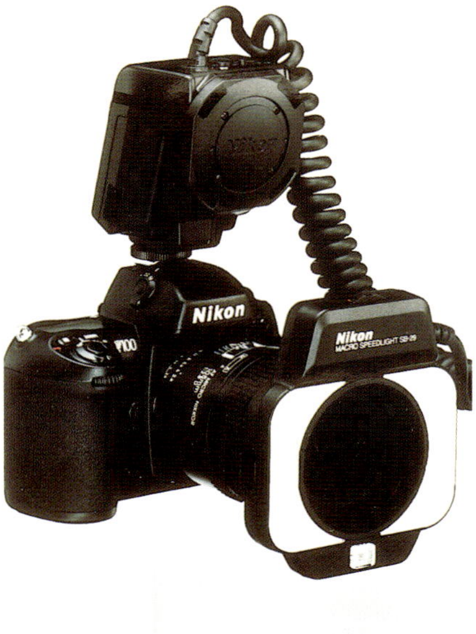

Fig. 2.12 Nikon dental photo system: modern SLR body, Micro Nikkor AF105mm lens and the new SB-29 macro flash.

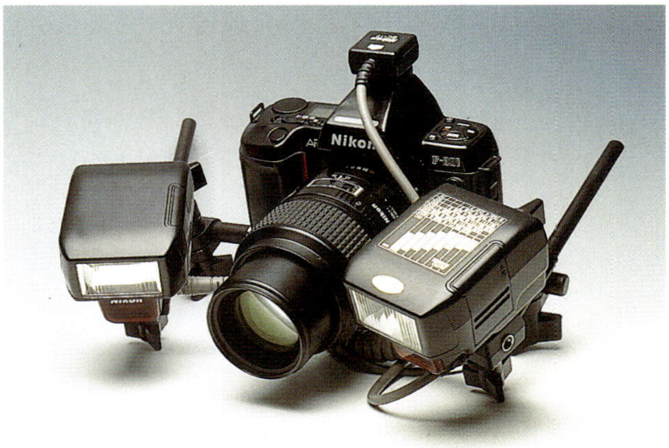

Fig. 2.13 In terms of quality, comparable to the Contax system: a side flash system with Nikon components.

Lenses
Macro lenses available are an AF Micro Nikkor 60 or 105mm lens. Both of these allow a maximum reproduction ratio of 1:1 without supplementary accessories. The combination with a TC 201 teleconverter increases reproduction ratios up to 2:1 with a double overall aperture. Alternatively, the 4T close-up lens in combination with the 105mm Micro Nikkor can be used.

Flashgun
The Nikon SB-29 Speedlight is a flashgun which has two flash tubes which are located at the 9:00 and 15:00 o'clock positions. The tubes can be fired individually to give the light a more directional character. Each flash tube can be set to 1/4 output. The flash can be rotated so that the flash reflectors can be at any position. Guide number is 11. The special feature of this unit is its preflash which fires for about 3 seconds at 40Hz and thus allows the light to be checked before the exposure is made.

Nikon bilateral flash system
Nikon components can be used to create a bilateral flash system (Fig. 2.13).
Two Nikon SB 23 Speedlights connected by an SC-18 unit. The SC-17 cable links this to the camera.
One alternative is to use the Novoflex Macroflash. Recently, Nikon bodies have been combined with the Mod. VI Dental Flash system which was originally used with the Contax Dental System (see Chapter 2.4.1).

2.4.6 Canon system
Other camera manufacturers offer systems comparable to those produced by Nikon. In the case of Canon, the EOS series camera bodies can be combined with the EF 100mm 1:2.8 macro lens or the EF 180mm 1:3.5L Macro USM (both achieve a reproduction ratio of 1:1), which can also be used in conjunction with a teleconverter, extension tubes or close-up lenses in order to achieve a greater reproduction ratio.

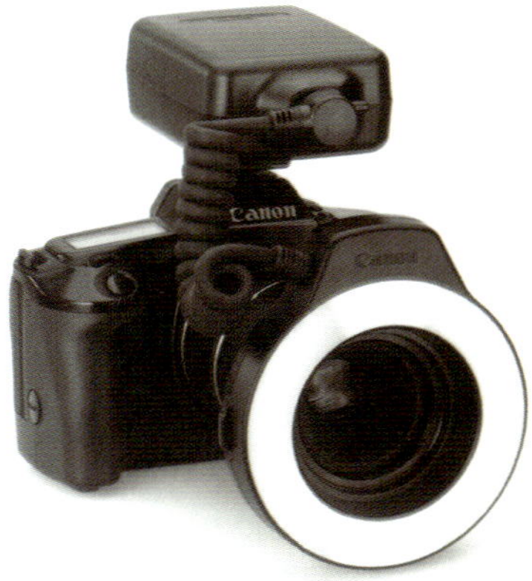

Fig. 2.14 Canon macro photo system with the ML-3 macro flash (Photo: Canon).

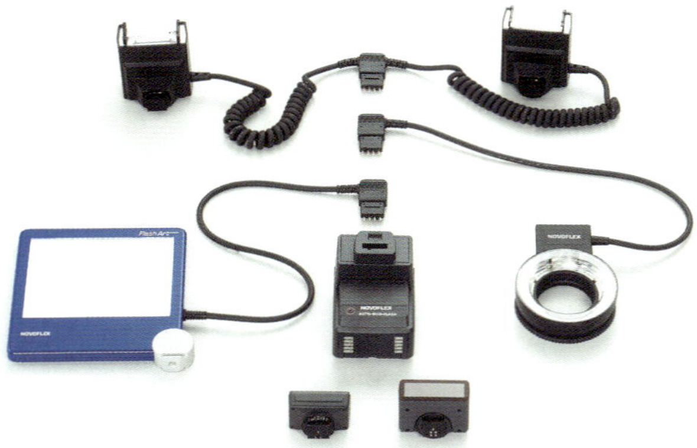

Fig. 2.15 Versatile flash system for all current SLRs: TTL flat flash panel, ring flash and Auto Duo Flash (Photo: Novoflex).

The Macro Ring Lite ML-3 (guide number 11) with two flash tubes is available (Fig. 2.14). The tubes of this ring flash can be fired individually or together.

2.5 Special Flash Units

2.5.1 Novoflex flash system

Novoflex offers a flash system with TTL control for all available SLRs. This system consists of a ringflash, a flash bracket system (Auto Duo Flash) and an innovative flat flash unit with a large flash area ("Flash Art"). The control unit for all three is identical and the cables are simply connected (Fig. 2.15).

This system allows all types of problems with flash photography for dental applications to be solved, using the ring or macro flash system for intraoral photography and the flat flash panel for portraits or object photography. Adapters connect the control unit with the camera's electronic systems.

2.5.2 Metz flash bracket system

Components produced by Metz can be used to achieve a flash bracket system similar to that of Novoflex; this system has TTL control (Fig. 2.16).

2.5.3 Soligor AR-40AF/MF-TTL ring flash

This ring flash system is suitable for all currently available camera types (Fig. 2.2). The control unit is obviously from the Yuzo company and its design is largely similar to that of the Lester Dine control units and that of the Novoflex Macro flash.

Settings are TTL, computer flash and manual. Guide number is 10.

Computer flash is possible with the "auto" setting. This setting is available in the control unit because the same body and electronic components are used for other flash units. However, computer flash is not suitable for close-up work, since the sensor is not located closely enough to the lens. This would result in incorrect exposures. Set at manual and at full power, an aperture of 1/16 is possible, which is particularly suitable for rapidly moving subjects. The AR-40 can be attached to lenses with front threads between 46mm and 62mm using various adapters. It is suitable for apertures of 50mm and over. Four minilights function as preflash. A mains adapter is available as an alternative power supply to four batteries.

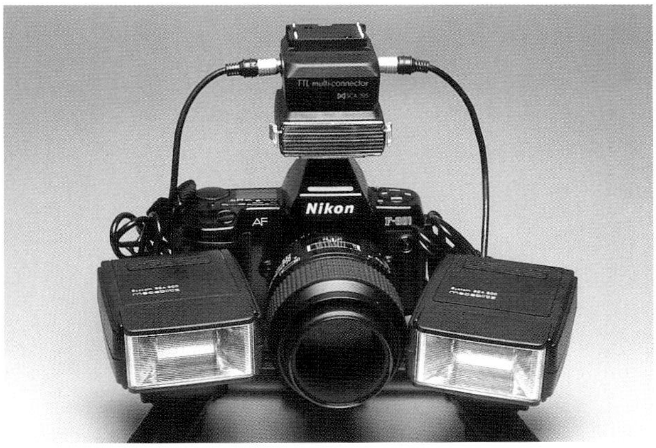

Fig. 2.16 A flash bracket system of Metz components is also available for the relevant camera systems.

2.6 Non-Proprietary Lenses

Macro lenses from other manufacturers are generally less expensive than original manufacturers' lenses and of similar optical quality. For dental photography the following are suitable:

- Tamron AF/MF SP 90mm f/2.8. Reproduction ratio 1:1. Available as an autofocus lens for Canon, Nikon D and Minolta.
- Tokina AT-X M AF 100mm f/2.8 Reproduction ratio to 1:1. Price around DM850.
- Soligor AF 100mm f/3.5 macro for Nikon; achieves reproduction ratio of 1:2 and 1:1 with the close-up lenses as part of package. Minimum focusing distance 43cm.
- Sigma AF 105mm f/2.8 Ex macro, rated of outstanding quality.

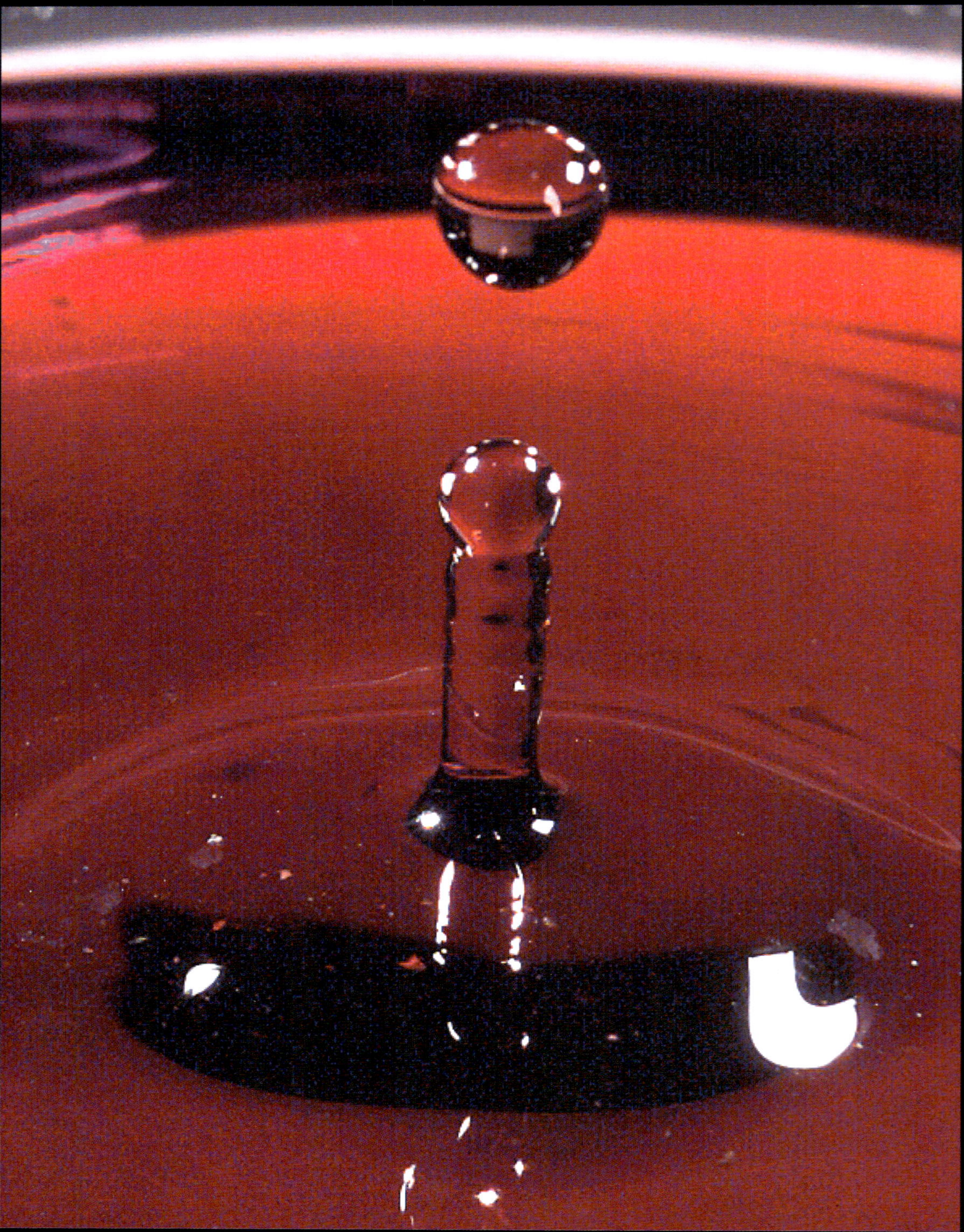

3 Perioral and Intraoral Photography

The main area for dental photography is making images of the mouth and the perioral region. The aim is to document the state and changes in state of the teeth, mucous membranes of the mouth and the perioral region under conditions which can be reproduced.
The main problems are the inaccessibility of oral structures, lighting within the mouth, framing the image and achieving conditions which can be reproduced.
The reproduction ratio required for this type of work is between 1:3 (perioral region) and 2:1 (upper middle incisors filling the frame, individual molar).
The following points are of interest:

- ✓ Aids to intraoral photography
- ✓ Visualization
- ✓ Standard views
- ✓ Photography of segmental views of teeth

➤ Objects such as this red wine appear colored because part of the white daylight (in this case the light from an electronic flash) is absorbed and other wavelengths, in this case, red, are reflected. (Photo taken with Kodak DCS 315, lit with two SB-23 units with power reduced 1/16th.)

3.1 Accessories for Intraoral Photography

In addition to the camera equipment, a number of aids for intraoral photography are necessary. They enable the subject, which is hidden behind lips, cheeks or the tongue, or which is not accessible for a direct view due to its position, to be made visible and photographed.

3.1.1 Lip and cheek retractors

Good intraoral images are not possible without the use of lip retractors. Opening the mouth cavity with the use of retractors is not only necessary in order to access the zone to be photographed, but also to achieve optimum illumination.
The most commonly used lip holders are those made of clear plastic; these are available in a variety of sizes (Fig. 3.1). They are the most comfortable for the patient and, if photographed, do not interfere with the image, since they allow the underlying structures to shine through. They also have the advantage that their size and shape can be altered.
It is recommended that one or two pairs be modified by separating a handle or cutting off one end. This allows mirror photography to be done more easily. Retractors made of wire are also in use which have a larger or smaller bend at either end (Fig. 3.2). The disadvantage here is that the center of the lips is not held and that the highly pol-

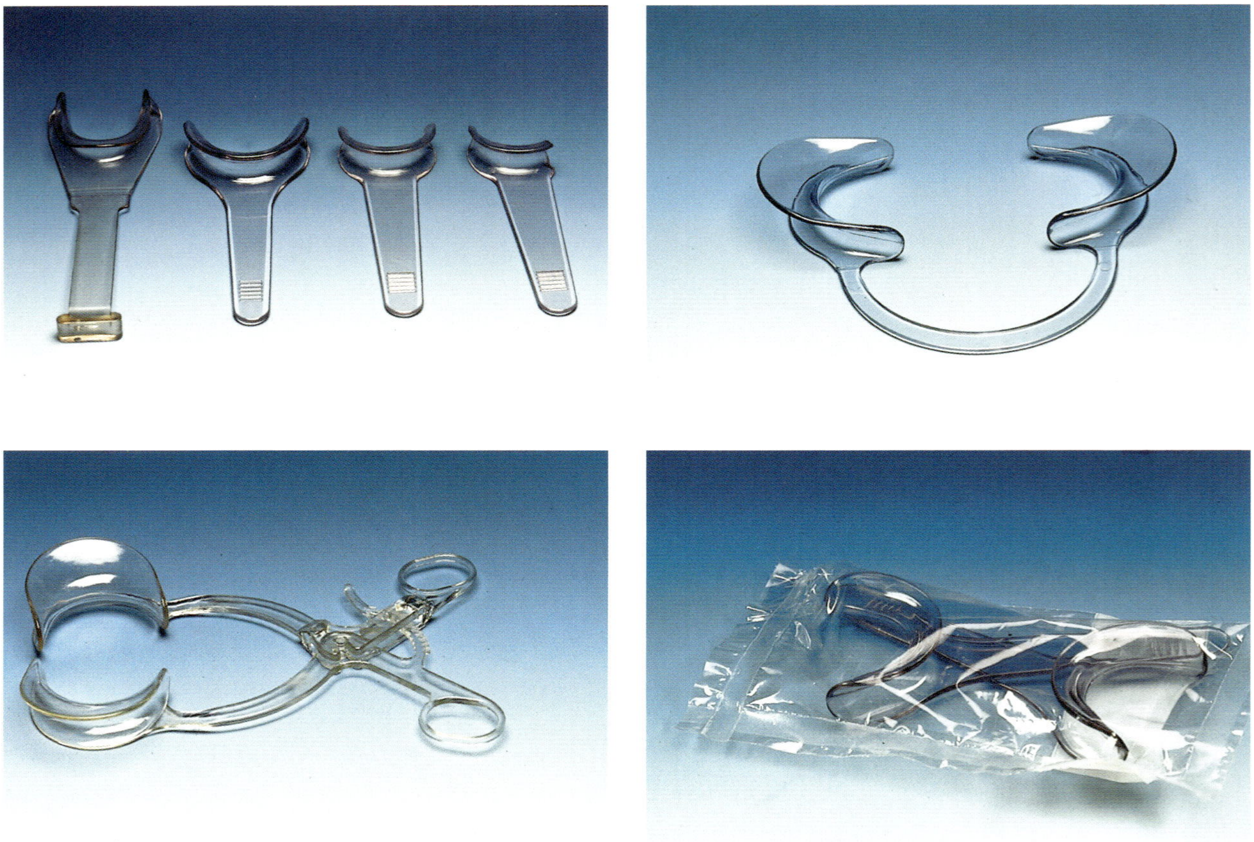

Fig. 3.1 Retractors are available in many forms and made of different materials. The most useful are individual retractors made of plastic. It is sensible to modify individual lip and cheek holders by trimming one of the curved ends (a) right retractor. (b) and (c) are self-expanding retractors which are used if not enough assistants are available to help. Plastic retractors can be chemically sterilized and prepacked hygienically (d).

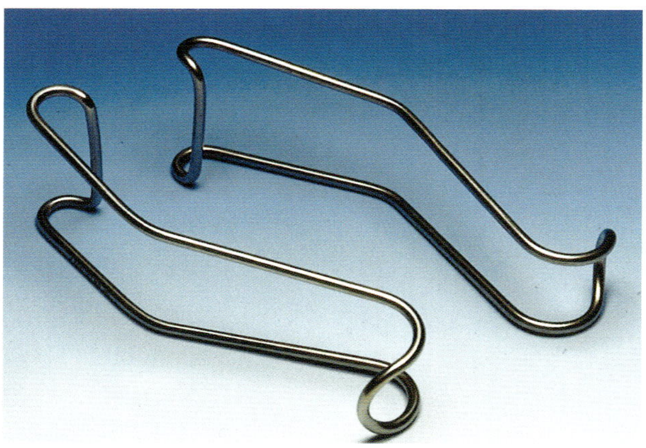

Fig. 3.2 Metal retractors can be easily sterilized in an autoclave.

ished metal can cause reflections. Making the surface more matte (blasted with aluminum oxide) can reduce the amount of reflections. Such wire retractors are recommended for photography with a long buccal mirror since the mirror can be inserted more easily between the upper and lower bends of the wire than by using plastic lip holders. Self expanding wire retractors are also in use and available in a variety of sizes.

Lip retractors made of metal (not wire) are not recommended, since the reflections from them can not be controlled and spoil the image. They also can cause incorrect exposures when using computer flash, because the flash sensor can be "fooled" by the strong reflections. These metal retractors are also difficult to modify.

Lip holders are generally used in pairs. As a rule, the largest lip holder possible should be used to open the mouth as wide as possible. The size depends not only on the size of the mouth cavity, but also on the tone of the lips.

Creme should be applied to dry and cracked lips beforehand to avoid lesions. The lip holder is moistened, inserted over the lower lip and carefully turned into the corner of the mouth. In so doing, no pressure should be exerted on the gingiva. See Chapter 3.3 and 3.4 for handling of lip retractors in various photographic situations.

3.1.2 Dental photo mirrors

Intraoral mirrors permit the indirect photography of areas of the mouth which are not directly accessible and, if correctly placed, alleviate the problem of depth of field (Fig. 3.3).

There are two types of photographic mirrors. Metal mirrors are inexpensive, robust and can be sterilized in an autoclave without any problem (Fig. 3.4). Optically they are inferior to glass mirrors, especially on the edges. Metal-film plated glass mirrors are more fragile and expensive, but yield far more brilliant mirror images and are therefore to be preferred (Fig. 3.5 and 3.6). A set of coated mirrors consisting of two palatal mirrors in varying sizes and a buccal mirror (Manufacturer: Evaporated Metal Films Corp.). This set permits overall views of the upper and lower jaws and buccal and oral partial views.

A set of mirrors developed in Professor Rateitschak's Department of Periodontology is

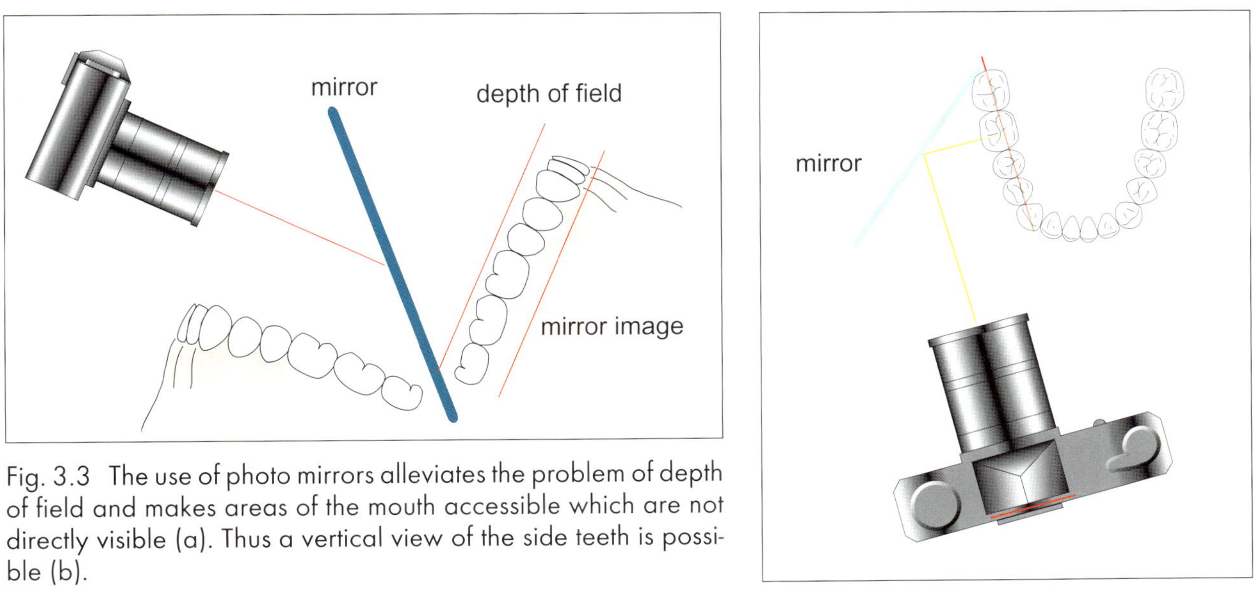

Fig. 3.3 The use of photo mirrors alleviates the problem of depth of field and makes areas of the mouth accessible which are not directly visible (a). Thus a vertical view of the side teeth is possible (b).

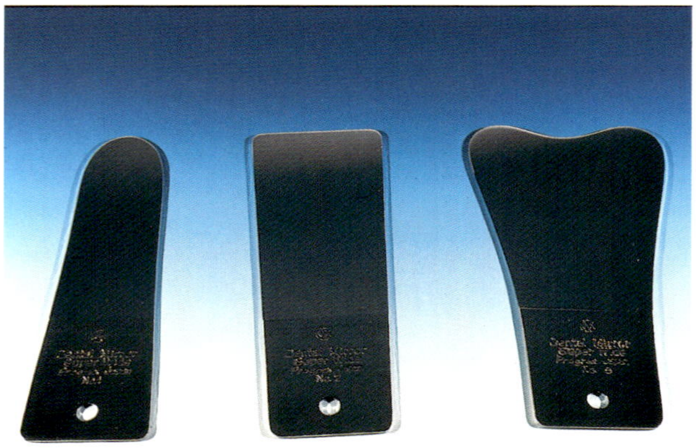

Fig. 3.4 Metal mirrors are robust but do not provide an image as bright as when using glass mirrors.

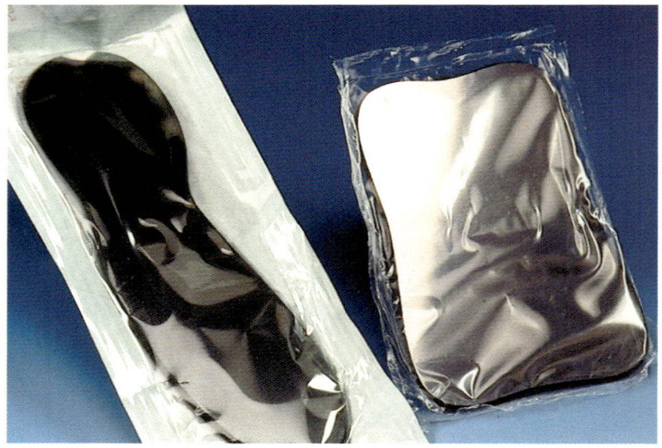

Fig. 3.5 Metal-film plated glass mirrors for lateral and occlusal views.

also commercially available. These are coated glass mirrors with a plastic handle affixed to the back in the manner of a cake knife. The plastic handles make them easier to manipulate (Manufacturer: Filtrop, Lichtenstein).

Rear-surfaced glass mirrors produce a double image depending on the angle of the mirror and the thickness of the glass. The main mirror image is produced by the back of the mirror, and the secondary mirror image is produced by the glass surface. This often makes the image appear to have camera shake (Fig. 3.8). Thus they are not recommended to our purpose.

Coated glass mirrors should be cleaned and disinfected carefully to avoid damaging the delicate metal coating. Soap and water or alcohol are suitable for cleaning before chemical sterilization.

Some points must be kept in mind in order to achieve good images using mirrors.

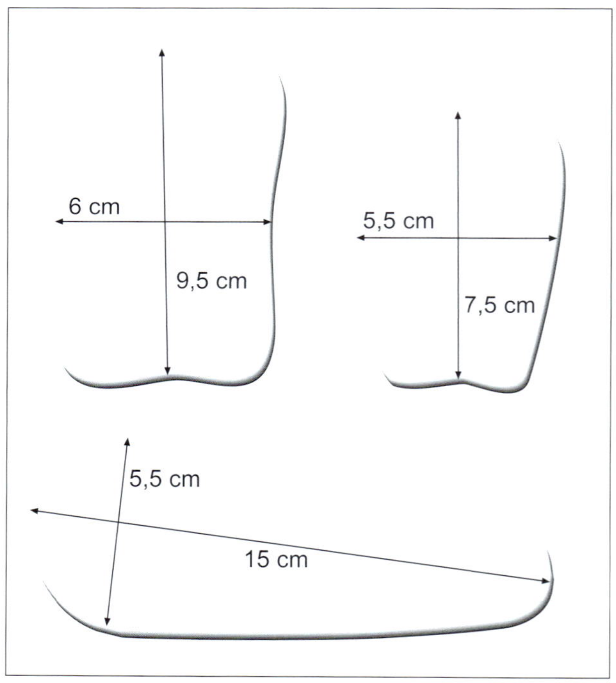

Fig. 3.6 Set of photo mirrors of plated glass, consisting of a buccal mirror and two different size occlusal mirrors.

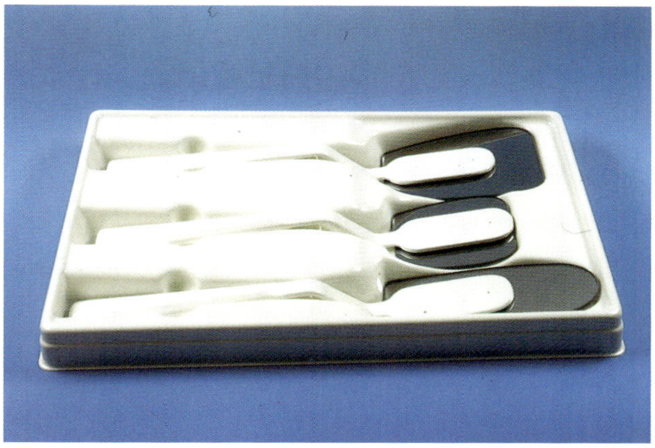

Fig. 3.7 Glass mirrors with glued on handles can facilitate intraoral photography in many cases.

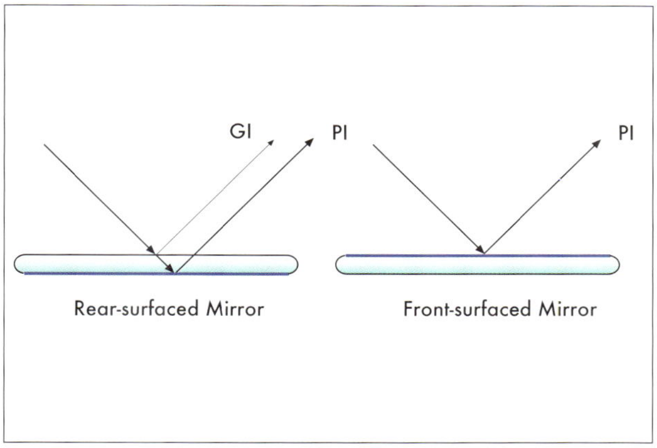

Fig. 3.8 Rear-surfaced mirrors provide a primary image (PI) from the back reflective surface, but also a secondary image from reflection off the front glass surface ("ghost image" = GI). Such mirrors are inexpensive, but not suitable for our purposes.

- ✓ The image should be framed if possible so that only the mirror image of the teeth is on the film. The slide can then be reversed and then resembles a photograph which was taken directly. Surrounding structures or edges of the mirror should be hardly visible or not at all visible.
- ✓ The fingers holding the mirror should be as far to the front as possible so that they too are not in the photograph. Here mirrors with handles are an advantage.
- ✓ Fogging on the mirror's surface can be prevented if an assistant warms the mirror first or directs air at it. Anti-condensation liquids can also be used.
- ✓ The patient is instructed to breathe in through the mouth and out through the nose during photography.

For suggestions on use of the mirrors for the various standard views, see below.

3.1.3 Black background

In images, particularly those taken of the front teeth, structures in back often are disturbing. This can be rectified by placing a black background made in the dental practice in back of the teeth (Fig. 3.9). Black plexiglass is most suitable for this purpose (available from do-it-yourself or hobby stores). This should be cut to size and rubbed with fine sandpaper to achieve a matte surface. Black cardboard or black plastic is also suitable, although less so for use near the side teeth. The black background makes the front teeth appear in isolation (Fig. 3.10). A black background is to be particularly recommended if the translucent regions of the teeth are to be shown.

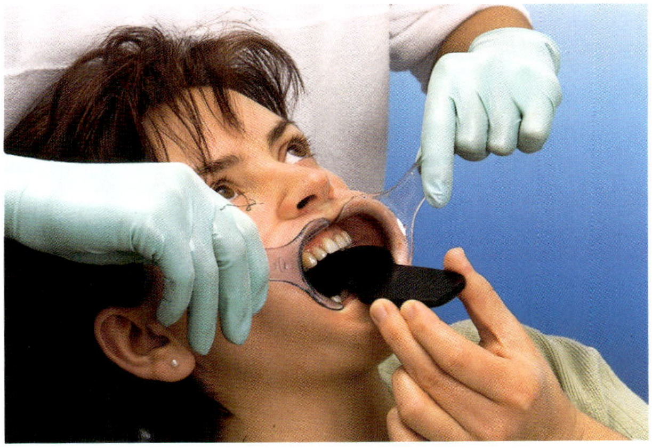

Fig. 3.9 A black plexiglas background produced in the practice is held in back of the teeth to "isolate" these.

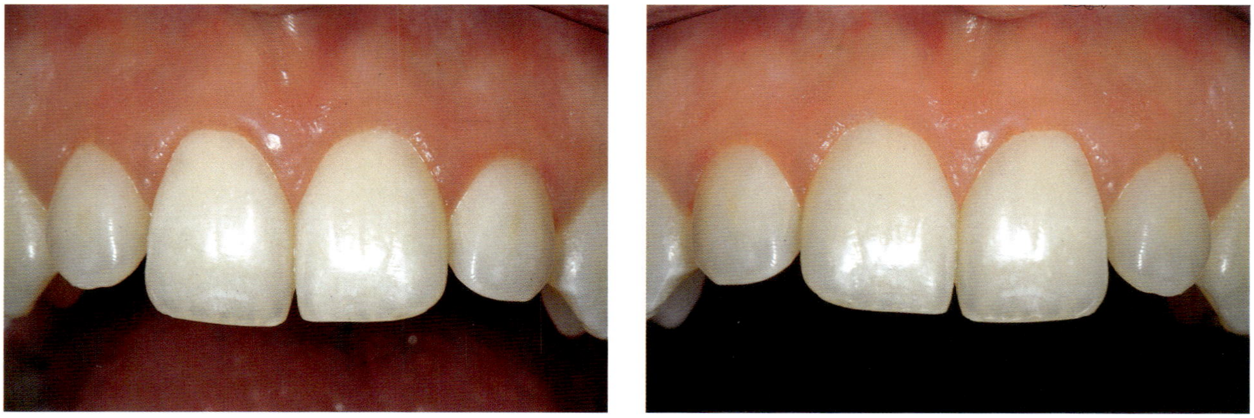

Fig. 3.10 Isolating the teeth (b) can improve image quality compared with not isolated teeth (a).

3.1.4 Other accessory equipment for intraoral photography

In many photographs the tongue must be restrained. This can be done using a plastic or glass spatula or the handle of a cheek holder. Disposable plastic spoons are also suitable; these can be used to hold back the lips of children.
Dental mirrors should be used for mirror photography only as an exception, and even then only if front coated mirrors are used.
For the most part, the metal holder around the glass is disturbing in the image. However, they are very suitable for holding the tongue or lips, especially when photographing lesions in the lip area. Making the metal surface matte reduces the reflections from the polished metal surfaces if the manufacturer has not already done this. In many instances the lips or cheeks can be held back with fingers (gloves). This should be done in such a way that the fingers do not appear in the photograph.
Gauze strips not only remove disturbing secretions and saliva, but are also handy for fixation of the tongue.
Air syringes or aspirators should also be mentioned; these allow an assistant to remove disturbing saliva bubbles etc.

3.2 Visualization

A widely held misconception is that what we see corresponds to reality. We have the idea that the "world outside" is projected from somewhere in the back of our heads. Naturally visual perception is a far more complex process which communicates many physiological and psychological influences; this process has by no means been completely researched.
Before pressing the shutter release, it is very important – not just in dental photography – to carefully consider a number of points. Visualization comprises the mental framing of the image before it is taken and the careful assessment of the image in the viewfinder. If an image is made without this visualization the resulting photograph can be disappointing. Only after the image is made, for instance, does the operator discover that the occlusion plane runs diagonally through the image, or he finds hairs of the moustache hanging down or even tartar which was not noticed during focusing, simply due to having "eyes only for the subject". However, if visualization becomes a habit, photographs will rapidly improve.

Points which must be checked before pressing the shutter are:

- ✓ Composition and framing of image
- ✓ Orientation of image
- ✓ Cosmetic issues
- ✓ Point of sharpest focus

3.2.1 Composition and framing of image

In terms of composition of the image, the rule of thumb is: the most important aspects in the center, the least important on the edges or eliminated altogether, e.g. the nose, which is included in palatal photographs, can sometimes ruin the whole effect of the image (Fig. 3.11). Such things are easy to eliminate if the viewfinder is deliberately checked.

3.2.2 Orientation of image

In general the photographer should get used to taking the image in the correct axis. This means:

- ✓ The optical axis should run through the occlusal plane. Photographing from below distorts the perspective of the incisors.
- ✓ In lateral views, try to photograph perpendicular to lateral teeth (with the aid of a mirror).
- ✓ Occlusal views should be as near perpendicular to the camera as possible (also with the aid of a mirror)
- ✓ Occlusal plane should be parallel to horizontal frame of the photograph.

See Figures 3.12 to 3.14.

The correct orientation is an important factor in producing reproducible images. Subsequent images should not be identical to the initial image, but should be taken from the same angle and at the same reproduction ratio. This means that the viewer does not have to reorientate him or herself when looking at a series of images.
Furthermore, the correct orientation of an image is important for physiological reasons in perception. Things which are horizontal – in keeping with the arrangement of our eyes – are easier for us to see than things which are diagonal or upside down.

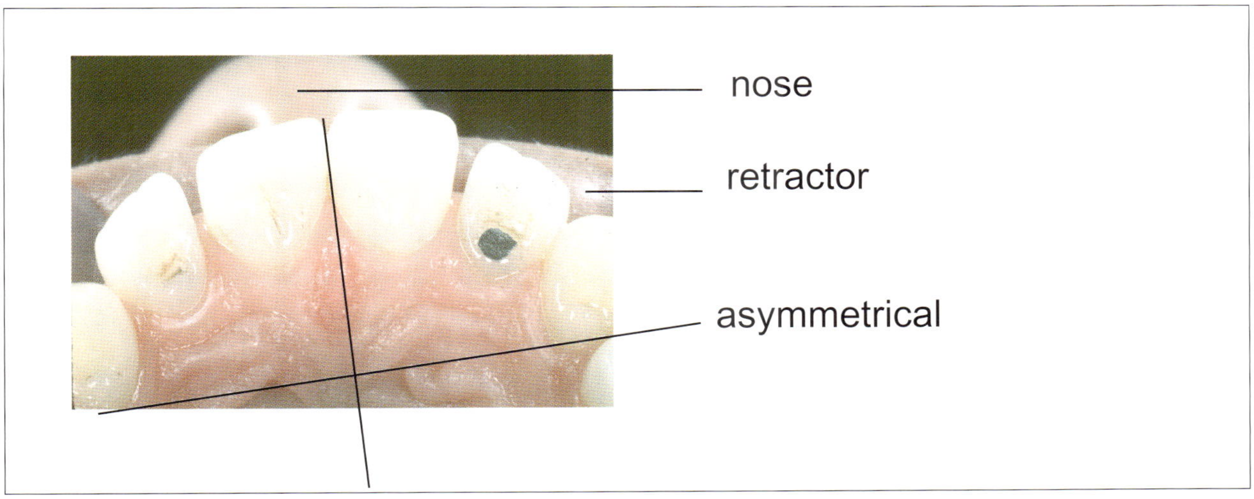

Fig. 3.11 Frequent errors: nose visible, cheek holders and asymmetrical composition of the image.

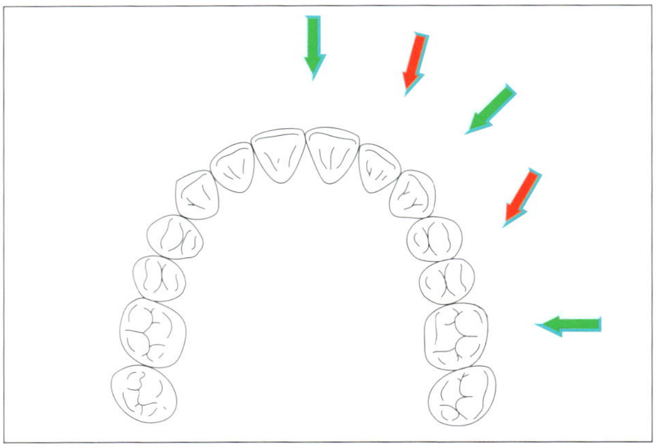

Fig. 3.12 The optical axis should be achieved in intraoral photography so that it is either directly from the front, lateral or at an angle of 45 degrees to the dental arch (green arrows). Non-defined alignment of the optical axis leads to images which can not be reproduced (red arrows).

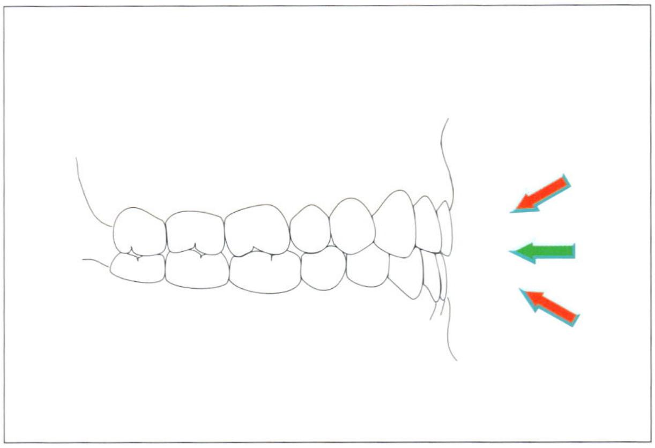

Fig. 3.13 Viewed from the side, the optical axis should be a continuation of the occlusal plane (green arrow) and should not be aligned with the teeth from above or below (red arrows).

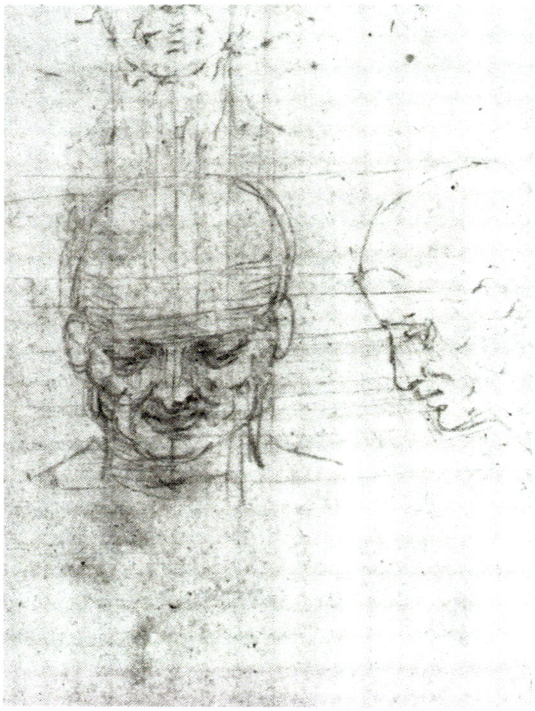

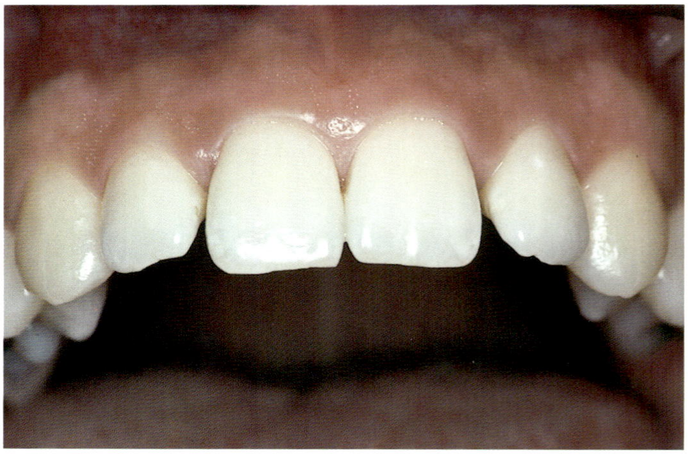

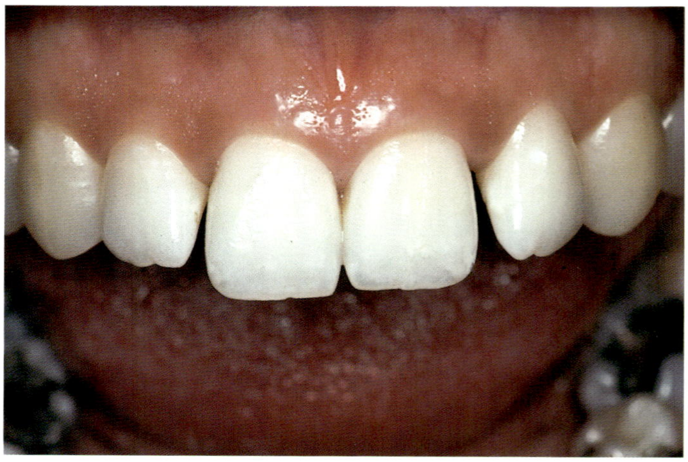

Fig. 3.14 Leonardo da Vinci already knew about the effect of the viewing angle on perspective (a). If one photographs from "below" into the dental arch, there is shortening of the perspective (b) and conversely, the front teeth appear longer (c).

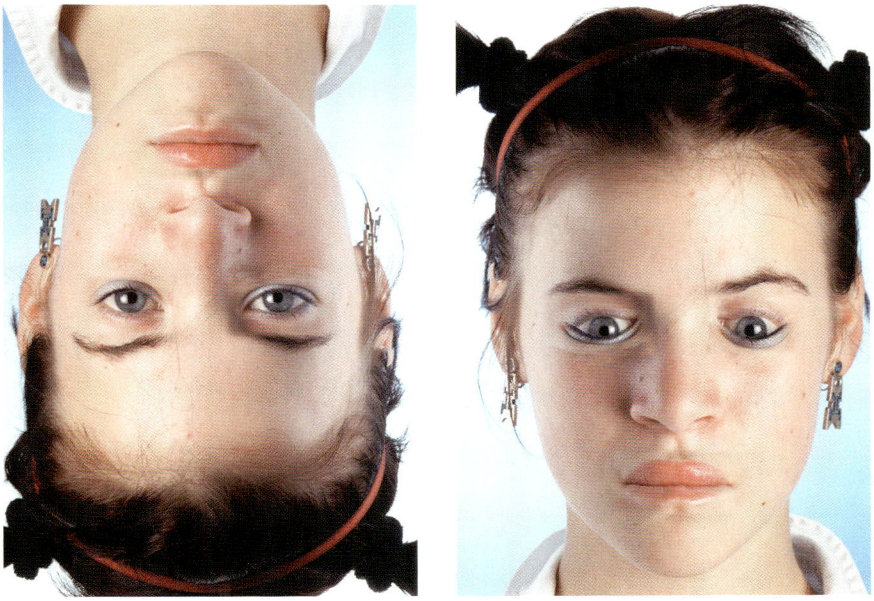

Fig. 3.15 The mouth and eyes were manipulated in this image. The distortions of this manipulation can not be detected if the image is upside down (a). If the image is in the correct position the manipulation can be seen (b).

3.2.3 Cosmetic issues

Tartar or disturbing plaque coatings should be removed before the image is taken if they are not the subject of the photograph. Plaque and tartar not only can reduce the impact of an image, but also can reduce its brilliance, which arises in part from reflections from clean teeth.

3.2.4 Point of sharpest focus

The problems of depth of field were already discussed in the framework of technical considerations. The entire dentition can only be photographed completely in sharp focus if the focal plane is positioned carefully. Therefore, do not focus on the front of the set of teeth. In a frontal view, the point of focus should be around the canines.

The person looking through the viewfinder is responsible for the end result of the image. He or she must take care that the above points are kept in mind, that no cheek holder creeps into the image, that the mirror shows no fogging and is correctly positioned.

3.3 Standard Views

Reproducible conditions for photography are sensible because they not only save time, but also achieve consistent results. For these reasons it makes sense to take the basic intraoral views in a standardized approach.

The basic intraoral views can differ for an orthodontist and periodontist. It is important to continue to follow the same standardized procedure once chosen.

General guidelines

Psychologically speaking, the oral cavity is a taboo area in people. In a way, photographing this area makes this public. Even though most patients are relaxed about this, some reactions by patients are due to this reason. Therefore it is not only important to ask the patient's permission to do this (generally granted), but also to communicate to him or her why this is being done. This helps create a relaxed and quiet atmosphere which is advantageous, since dental photography can be stressful and uncomfortable for a patient.

The patient should sit, leaning back slightly, in the chair. The height of the chair should be adjusted so that the patient's head is somewhat lower than the head of the photographer. Awkward positions over the patient can be avoided by asking the patient to turn or tilt his or her head.

Format, position and framing
All standard views are done in horizontal format. A stable position for the photographer is important, since the camera is handheld and not placed on a tripod. The upper arms are held against the upper part of the body, with the left hand supporting the front of the lens. The eye is not pressed directly against the eyecup, but slightly in back of it. The other eye should be open (Fig. 3.16). The photographer's leg should be supported by the outside edge of the patient's chair in order to find a secure, comfortable position.
Select the magnification ratio according to the desired frame and focus by moving the camera back and forth – not by turning the focusing ring! The magnification ratio frequently has to be adjusted slightly in order to fill the frame with the standard view. Fewer corrections are necessary with increasing experience.
A grid focusing screen is helpful in framing the image and orienting the camera. The middle of the image is placed on the central crosshair, then a check is made to see if the occlusal plane is horizontal. Finally, the edges of the viewfinder are checked to ensure that there are no disturbing details (nose, retractors, edges of mirror, etc) or whether the positions of the retractors and mirror have to be altered. If necessary, the focus plane is moved from the front point of the object somewhat in the distal direction in order to maximize the depth of field.
Several photographs should be made of the same subject, since in close-up photography even small changes in position can negatively affect the image. If both photographs are perfect, then a second "copy slide" is immediately available.

Lighting
Since focusing at close range in the dark oral cavity is very difficult, the operating light is used for illumination. However, it should only be directed at the edges of the mouth. Using a maximum amount

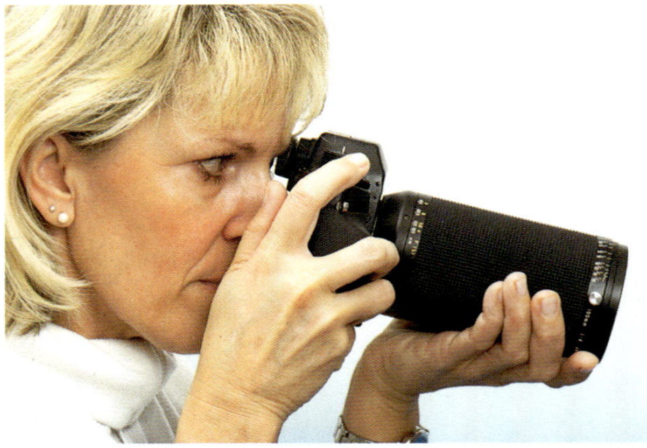

Fig. 3.16 Relaxed and secure camera position.

of supplementary lighting of the oral cavity would result in overexposure when using cameras such as medical cameras, which do not have TTL flash. Cameras with TTL flash measure the light reflected from the subject. This would not create overexposure, but this would cause a slight reddish yellow color shift, since the operating light generally has a halogen bulb which has a lower color temperature.

3.3.1 Frontal view (anterior-posterior)

Two variants are possible here, depending on the application of the image. These differ in their magnification ratios and framing. The procedure for taking these images is practically the same.

Variation 1: Overview of the entire dentition
The overview is preferred in particular for general purposes and orthodontics (Fig. 3.17).
The center of the image is the contact point of the

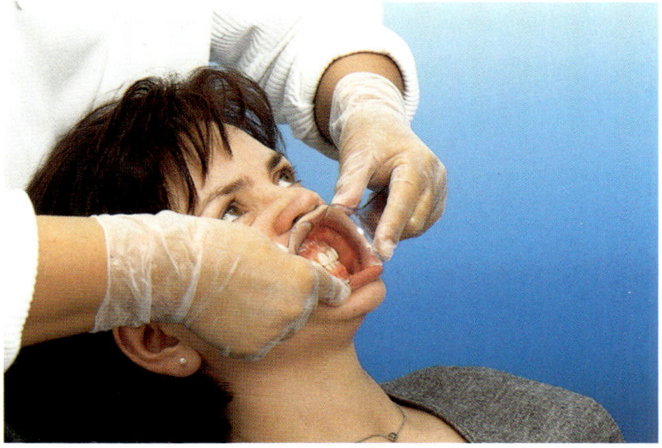

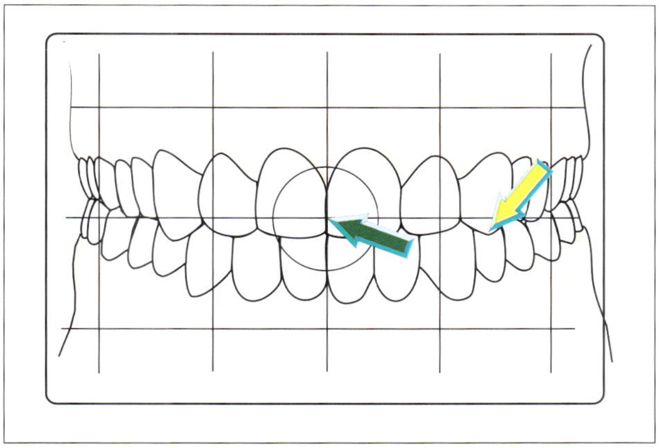

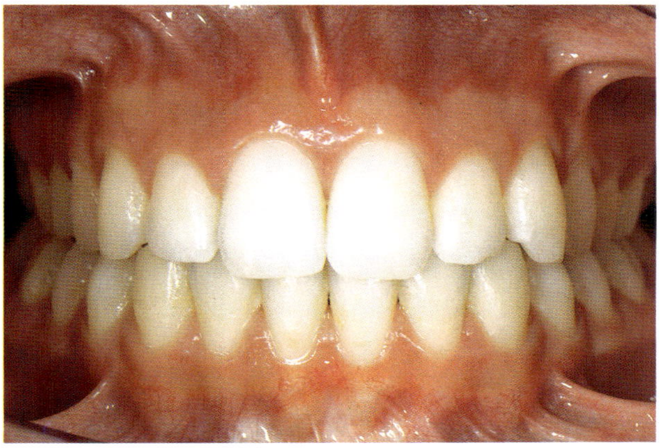

Fig. 3.17 Frontal view of the dental arch. Position of retractors (a), diagram of composition (b) and result (c).

upper central incisors. The reproduction ratio is about 1:1.8. The edges of the photograph are in the vestibulum oris.

Variation 2: Frontal view of the front teeth

This segmental view is generally selected in periodontology, but also for restaurative dentistry (Fig. 3.18).

The center of the image is placed on the contact point of the upper central incisors. The magnification ratio is about 1:1.2.

The side edges of the photograph are on the distal edge of the canines.

The retractors are inserted symmetrically and applied outward as much as possible, with the handles pulled forward slightly. This opens the buccal corridor, that is, the cheeks no longer lie against the buccal surfaces of the molars. Finally, the lips are tensioned by moving the retractors in parallel to the front. This prevents the middle of the lips "hanging" in the middle of the photograph. Pressure from the thumb or index finger is applied on the cheek retractors to prevent them from slipping when the lips are tensioned.

In both variants the center of the image is the contact point of the upper central incisors. To maximize the depth of field, focus on the canines (variant 1, overview) or on the mesial contour of the lateral incisors (variant 2, detail view)

Care should be taken that the occlusal plane is parallel to the horizontal borders of the frame (check focusing screen) and, when viewed from the side, the occlusal plane should be a continuation of the optical axis.

Lighting is provided by ringflash, bilateral flash system or side flash located in the 12:00 o'clock position. In a normal bite, this produces a fine shadow contour below the upper incisors.

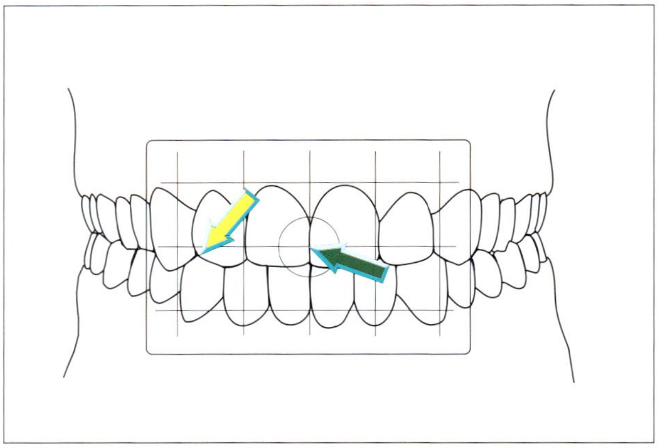

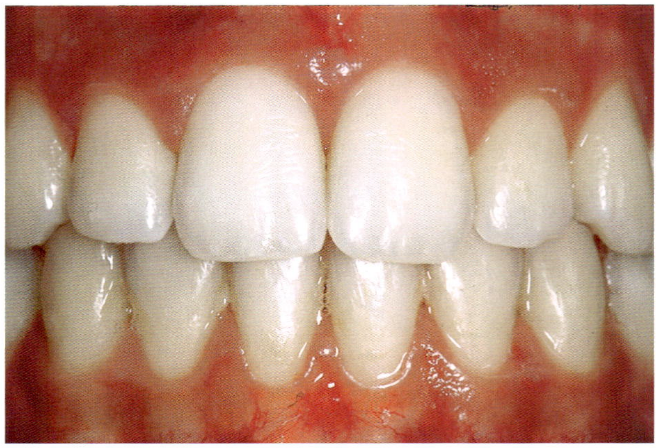

Fig. 3.18 Frontal view at greater magnification ratio. Diagram of composition (a) and result (b).

3.3.2 Oblique lateral view

This view is preferred over the purely lateral view since it can be done without using mirrors, making work much easier.

Two retractors are used. The side being photographed is uncovered toward the distal by maximum tension on one, while the second is used only to keep the lips apart (Fig. 3.19).

The reproduction ratio is about 1:1.5. The head is turned slightly away from the camera.

The center of the image is around the canine. The edges of the image are the lateral incisor on the side away from the camera and - depending on how far back the lips can be moved - the mesial contour of the second molar. Focus is on the first premolar.

The camera is positioned so that the occlusal plane is parallel to the horizontal edge of the photograph and in the center of the image.

For illumination a ringflash, a flash bracket system or a point flash can be used, which is positioned so that light "comes from the front teeth" (9:00 and 3:00 o'clock position).

3.3.3 Lateral views

Purely lateral views are used especially for periodontal and prosthetic documentation. Mirrors are always required. A sufficiently wide lateral mirror is inserted on the side to be photographed until the posterior border lies distally of the last tooth in the vestibule. It is turned to the outside as far as the cheeks and lips will stretch to allow this. Care should be taken that the edge of the mirror does not rest on the gingiva firmly since this can be very painful. To avoid this, the patient can be asked to hold the mirror, while the mirror position is gently manipulated by the photographer or assistant.

To prevent part of the final tooth near the end of the mirror being photographed directly along with the mirror image, the mirror should be moved outwardly and slightly parallel to itself. Mirrors with glued-on handles are particularly well suited to this. The mirror is turned so that the occlusion plane runs across the middle. A retractor is used loosely on the opposite side which holds the lips in position without stretching them.

If no sufficiently wide lateral mirror is available, then a narrow lateral mirror can be used in combination with a wire retractor. The camera and mirror are positioned so that the optical axis is as perpendicular as possible to the mirror image (Fig. 3.20). The occlusion plane runs horizontally in the

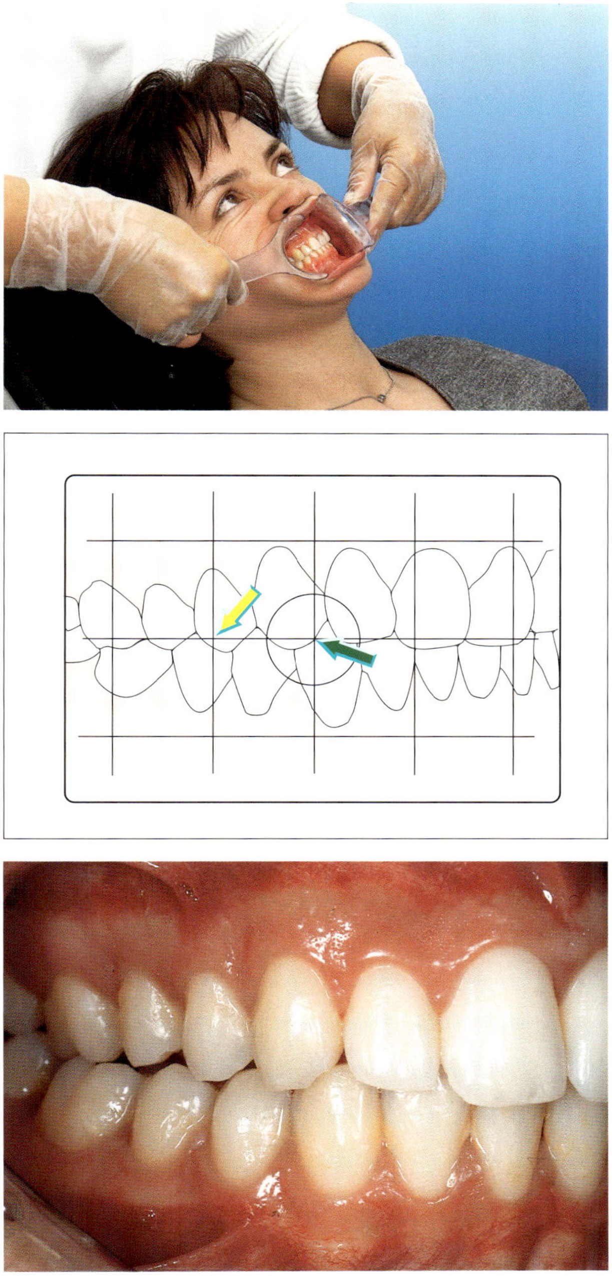

Fig. 3.19 Oblique lateral view. Position of retractors (a), diagram of composition (b) and result (c).

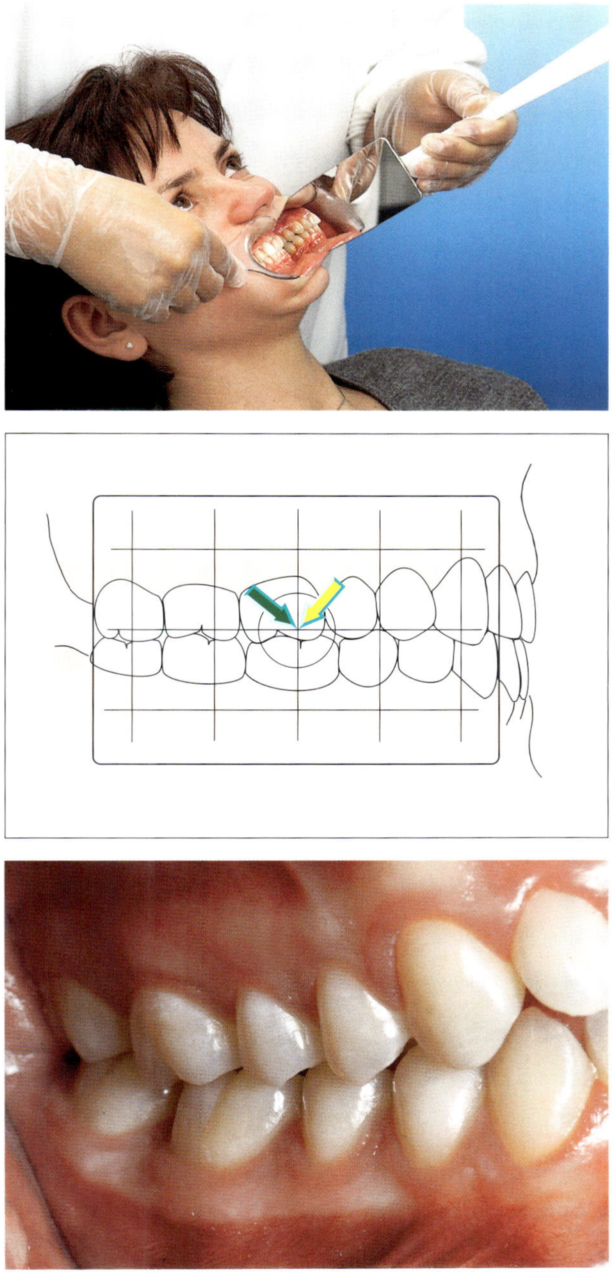

Fig. 3.20 Lateral views. Position of retractors and mirror (a), diagram of composition (b) and result (c).

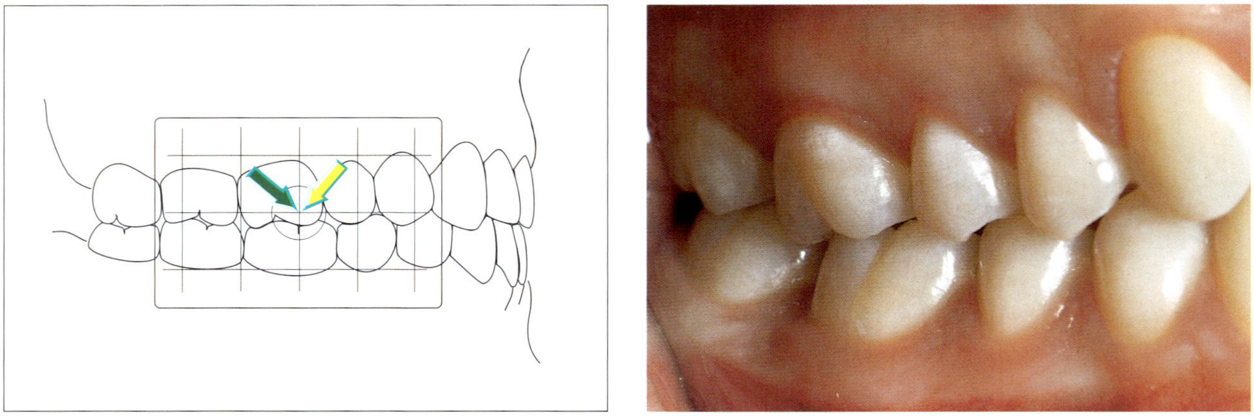

Fig. 3.21 Variant with larger reproduction ratio. Diagram of composition (a) and result (b).

middle. The center of the photograph and focus point are around the second premolars or the first molars, depending on the framing of the image. A reproduction ratio of 1:1 should be selected. This puts the side edges of the photograph mesial to the first premolar and distal to the second molar. If the canines are also to be photographed, a reproduction ratio of 1:2 should be selected (Fig. 3.21). As always when using mirrors, the mirror image should be in sharp focus. The edges of the mirror and adjacent structures are not photographed.
Lighting is provided by a ringflash or flash bracket system. If a single side flash is used it is positioned on the side oh the mirror (9:00 and 3:00 o'clock). This makes the side teeth appear particularly plastic.

3.3.4 Occlusal mandibular view

This is a photograph from an occlusal view of the entire dental arch of the lower jaw taken with the aid of a mirror (Fig. 3.22).
In order to have as much room as possible in the corners of the mouth for the mirror the retractors, which have been modified by being shortened on one side, hold the lower lip as far open as possible so that it is not visible in the mirror.

The palatal mirror is inserted with the broader end toward distal in the case of adults. The patient is asked to raise the tongue to the palate and to breathe through his or her nose. The mirror rests on the distal aspects of the last molars. It is turned upwards with the mouth wide open until it touches the incisal edges of the upper incisors. To prevent the parts of the last molars being photographed directly in addition to the mirror image, the mirror has to be shifted in parallel to itself toward the upper jaw.
The mirror and camera are positioned using the viewfinder so that the optical axis is exactly perpendicular to the mirror image of the occlusal plane of the dental arch.
The center of the image is at the intersection of the sagittal plane with the line crossing the second premolars which is positioned horizontally in the center of the image. Optimum focus is on the fissures of the lateral teeth. For adults a reproduction ratio of about 1:2 is preselected.
If only one sideflash is used this is employed in the 12:00 o'clock position.

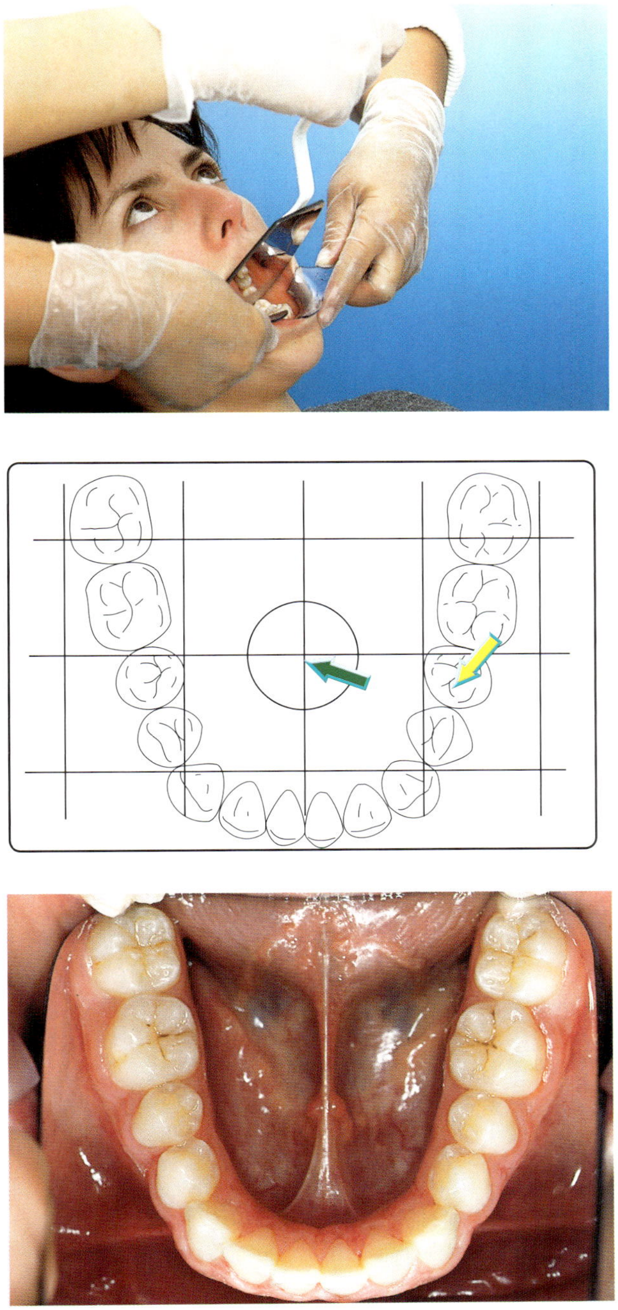

Fig. 3.22 Occlusal view of lower jaw. Position of retractors and mirror. Index finger holds the lower lip against the retractor (a). Diagram of composition (b) and result (c).

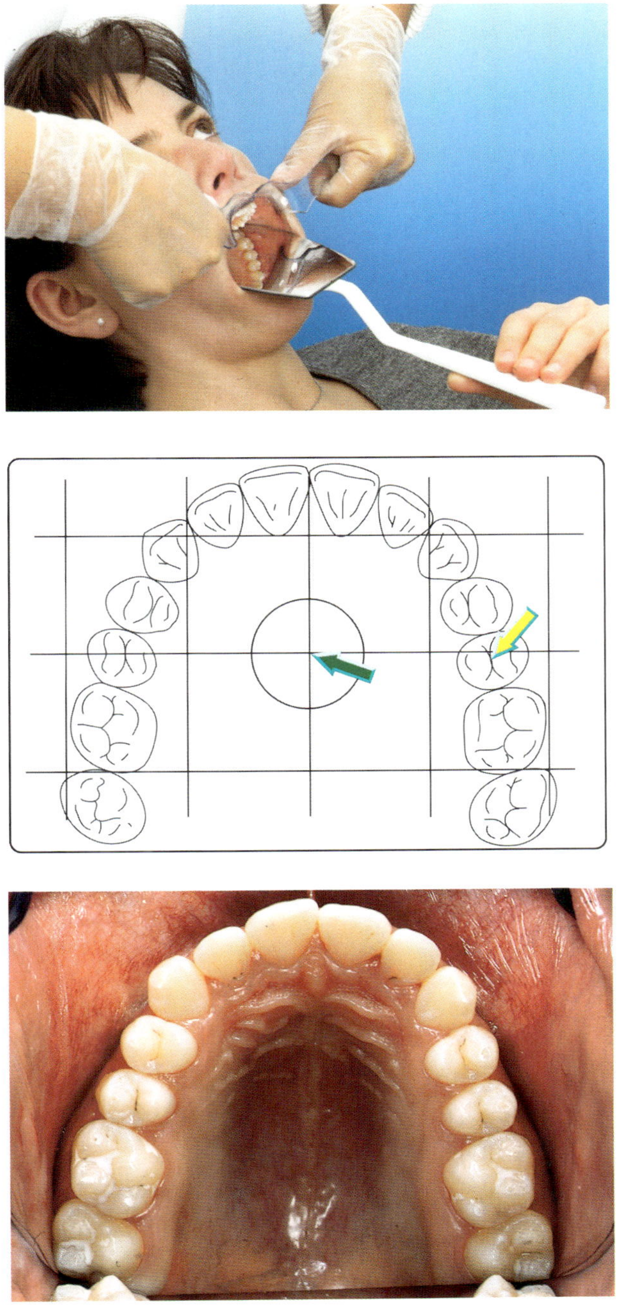

Fig. 3.23 Occlusal view of the upper jaw. Position of retractors and mirror (a). Thumbs hold the upper lip against retractor. Diagram of composition (b) and result (c).

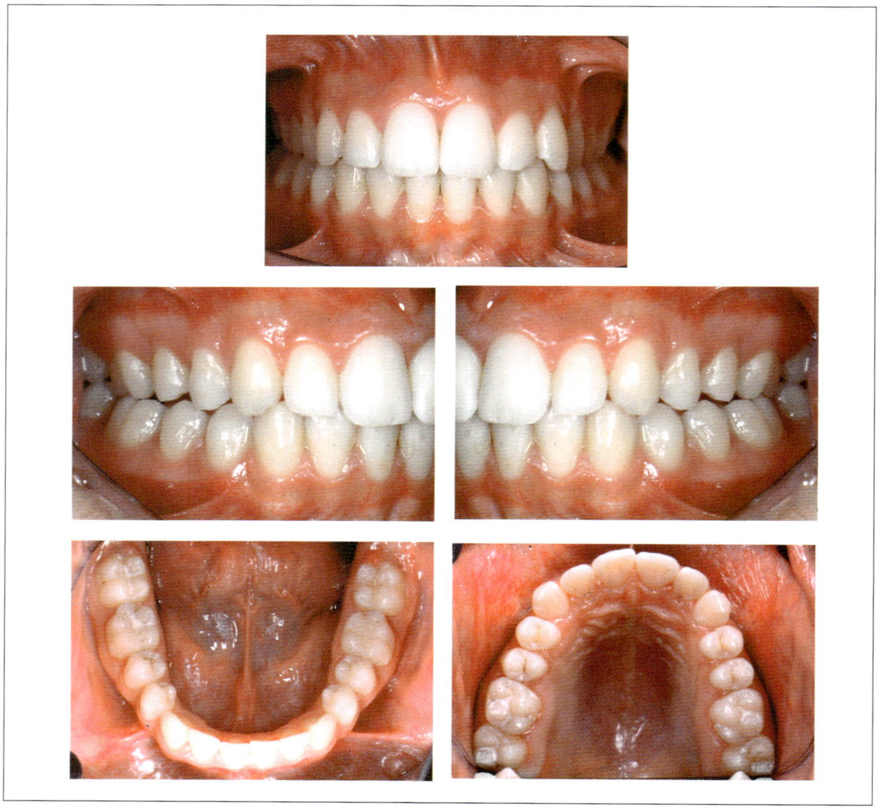

Fig. 3.24 Complete photostatus with oblique lateral views of the side teeth. Recommended for quick overview.

3.3.5 Occlusal maxillary view

The entire dental arch of the upper jaw can be photographed with the aid of a palatal mirror. This photograph is less difficult to take than that of the lower jaw. The palatal mirror rests on the distal aspect of the last molars and turned down as far as possible until it touches the lower incisors (Fig. 3.23). The upper lip is held as far out as possible using the retractors which have been shortened on one side, so that the lip is not longer visible on the mirror image. The patient is asked to breathe through the nose.

To avoid photographing parts of the last molars in direct view in addition to the mirror view, the mirror must be moved parallel to itself towards the lower jaw.

Using the viewfinder, the mirror and the camera are positioned so that the optical axis is exactly vertical to the mirror image of the occlusal plane of the dental arch.

The center of the photograph is at the cross-section of the sagittal plane with the connection line between the second premolars running horizontally in the middle of the image. Focus on the fissures of the side teeth. For adults a reproduction ratio of about 1:2 is preselected.

If only one sideflash is used this is turned to the 6:00 o'clock position.

Depending on the view selected, the above photographs produce different photostats consisting of five images each (Fig. 3.24 and 3.25).

Fig. 3.25 Complete photostatus with larger reproduction ratio, recommended, for example, for routine documentation in periodontology and prosthetics.

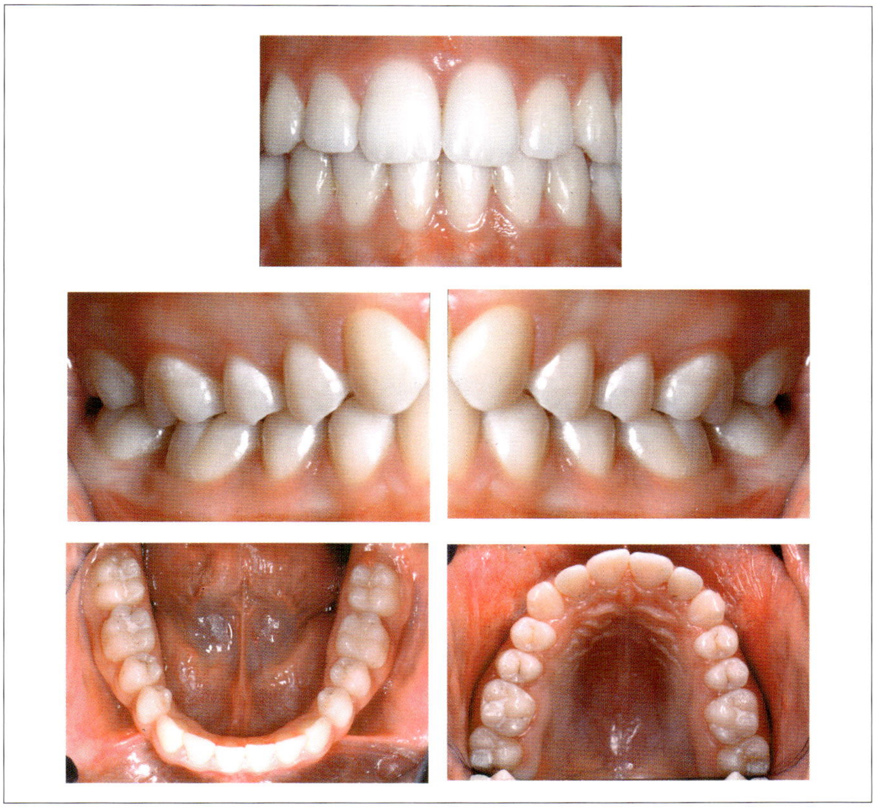

3.4 Supplemental Segmental Views

In addition to the standard views of the two dental arches segmental views are photographed to show details.
Here too, the basics should be adhered to in order to achieve reproducible images:

- Images with correct axis: perpendicular to the occlusal plane or row of teeth
- Occlusal plane always horizontal

3.4.1 Frontal view of jaw

Frontal views of the upper and lower jaw are especially useful for prosthetic and periodontal purposes.
The same procedure is used as with photographing a frontal view, differing only in that the patient has his or her mouth open. The center of the image is in the area of the interdental papillae of the upper or lower central incisors. Reproduction ratio should be about 1:1 (Fig. 3.26).
A black background is particularly useful for these photographs, as it isolates the front teeth.

3.4.2 Lateral view of the front teeth

This view is taken in particular to document the amount of overbite of the front teeth (prosthetic dentistry, orthodontic).
Both corners of the mouth are held back by lip retractors (Fig. 3.27). The recommended reproduction ratio is 1:1. This means that the side edges of the images are approximately between the first and second premolars on the one side, and in front of the incisors on the other side. The occlusal plane is horizontal. The same lighting is used as for a lateral view, that is, the main light is from the front teeth side.

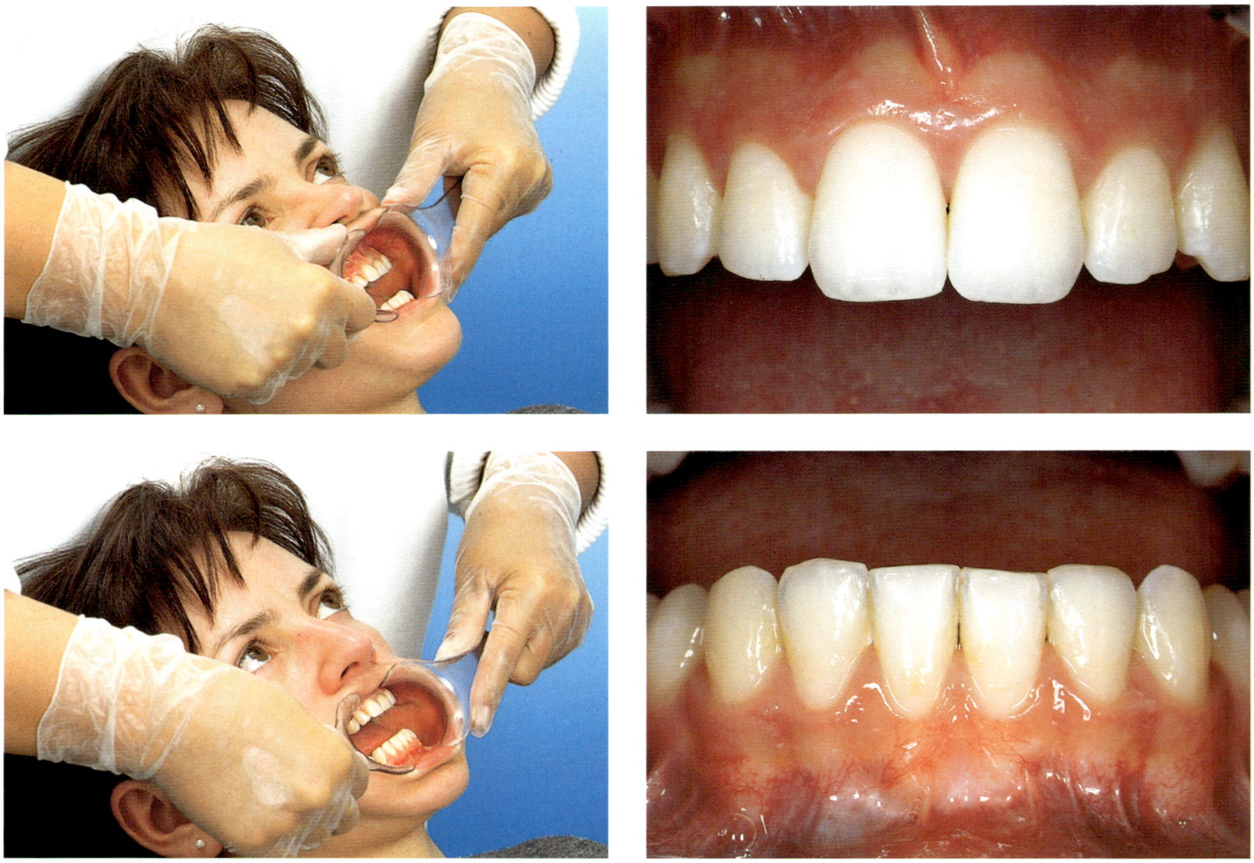

Fig. 3.26 Frontal view of the upper jaw-front. Position of retractors. The thumbs prevent lips from slipping out of retractor (a). Result (b). Analogous procedure for lower jaw (c and d).

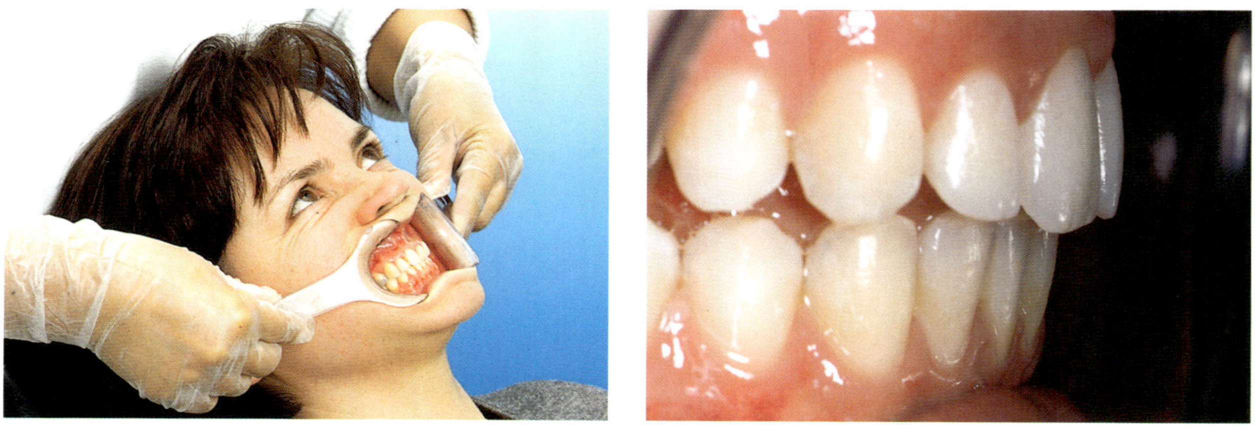

Fig. 3.27 Lateral view of front teeth. Position of retractors (a) and result (b).

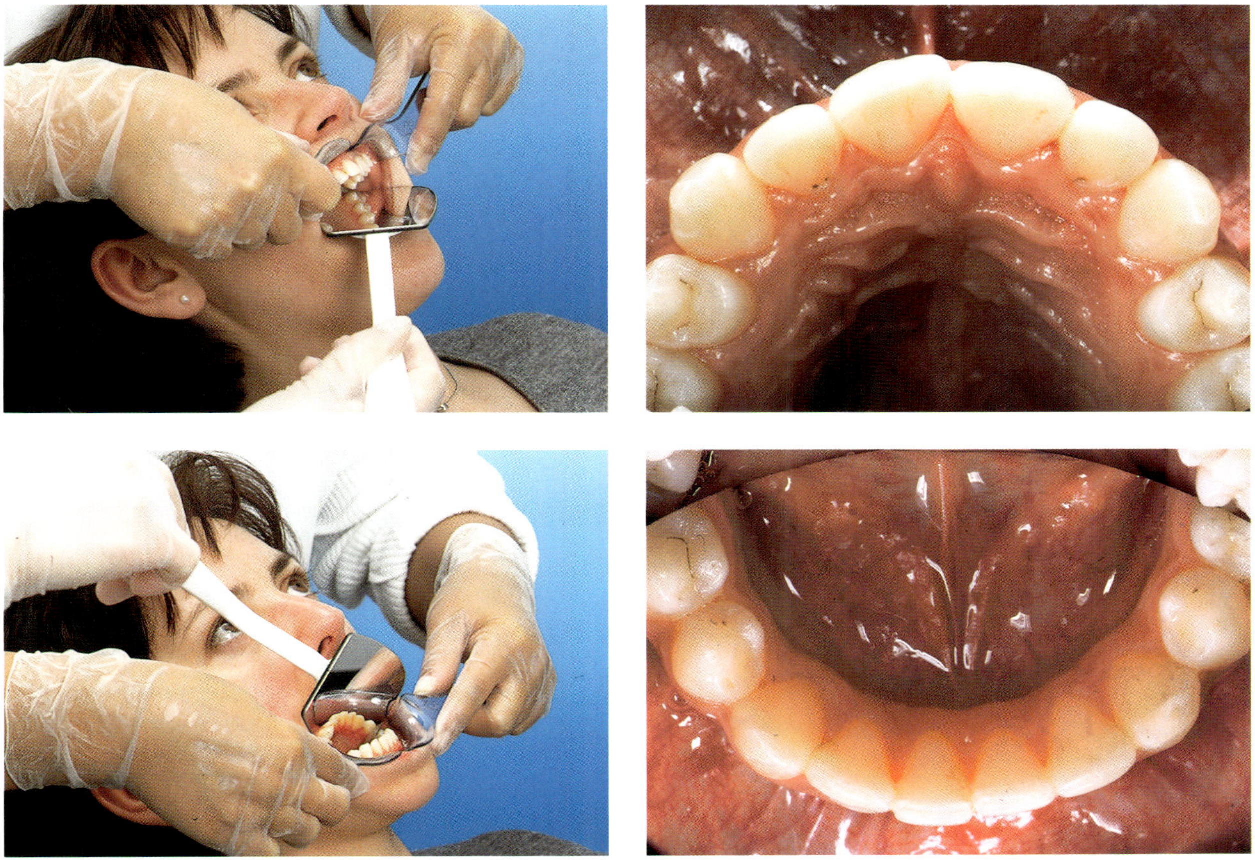

Fig. 3.28 Oral views of the front teeth groups. Position of mirror and retractors for upper jaw photograph (a) and result (b). Position of retractors and mirror for lower jaw view (c) and result (d).

3.4.3 Oral view of the front teeth

A photographic mirror is used to photograph the oral aspects of the front teeth. Use either a palatal mirror or the wider end of a lateral mirror. The patient should hold the tongue against the palate for photographs of the lower jaw.

The mirror and camera should be positioned so that the optical axis is vertical to the mirror image of the occlusal plane (Fig. 3.28). The reproduction ratio is between 1:1 and 1:2.

In this type of photograph it is especially important that the lips, cheeks, cheek holders, nose and other extraneous elements are not photographed as well.

3.4.4 Oral view of the side teeth

A buccal mirror is used to photograph the oral aspects of the premolars and molars. This mirror is placed distal to the final tooth to be photographed, inclined sideways and rotated along its longitudinal axis until it is possible to take the photograph (Fig. 3.29)

The reproduction ratio is 1:1 or greater. This brings the side edges of the image to mesial of the first premolar or the canine and distal of the second molar.

The mirror and camera are positioned so that the optical axis is vertical to the mirror image of the teeth.

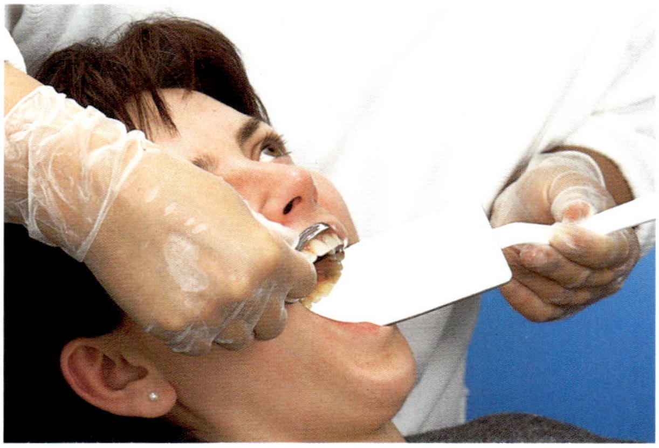

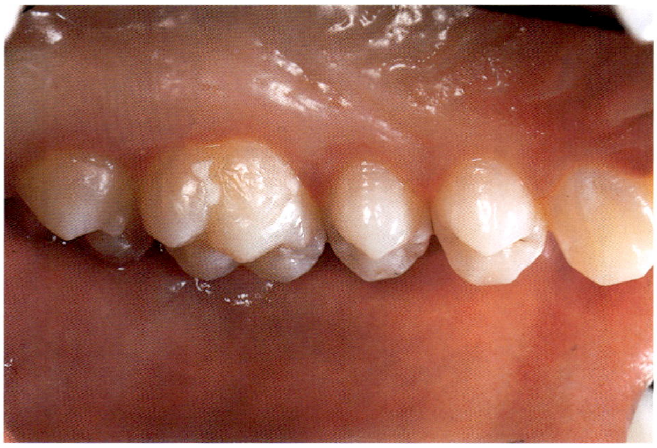

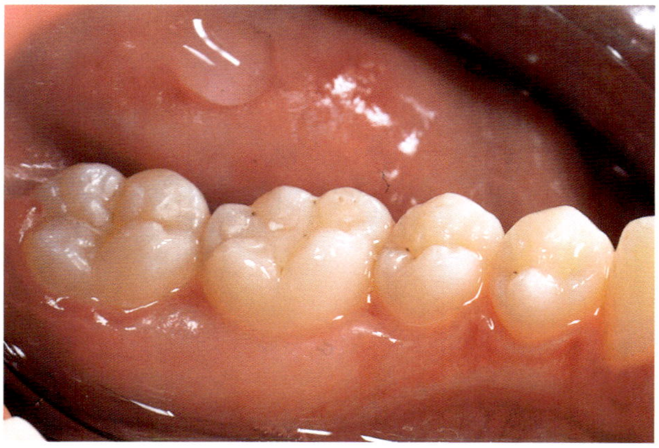

Fig. 3.29 Oral views of side teeth are produced with the buccal mirror which is introduced at an angle of about 45 degrees toward the side teeth (a). Result for upper jaw (b) and lower jaw (c).

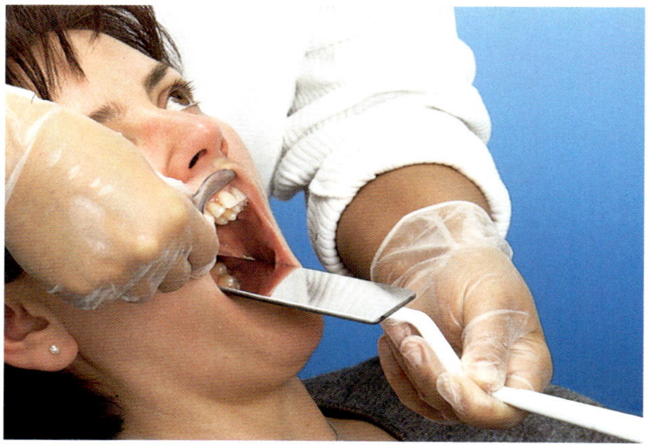

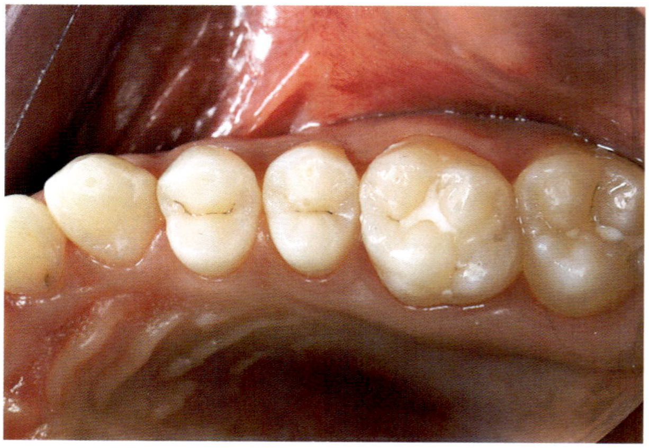

Fig. 3.30 Occlusal areas are also photographed with a buccal mirror. Position of mirror (a) and result (b).

3.4.5 Occlusal view of the side teeth

The procedure in this case is the same as for occlusal views. The lateral mirror is used instead of the palatal mirror. The mirror end rests on the distal aspect of the last tooth to be photographed and then turned as far as possible in the direction of the other jaw (Fig. 3.30).

The reproduction ratio is 1:1.

The optical axis is perpendicular to the mirror image of the occlusal plane of the row of teeth.

3.5 Reproducible Conditions – Making a Series of Photographs

If the aim is to show a course of treatment all photographs should be taken under the same conditions. This includes the reproduction ratio, direction of the photograph and the framing. This ensures that the person viewing the series does not have to reorientate him or herself with each new image (Fig. 3.31). If these photographs are made in one sitting this is not a problem: determine the point on which the crosshair of the focusing screen rests and leave other settings of the camera the same.

It is frequently not clear from the outset that one image can become part of a series. There are a number of ways of ensuring that these images are reproducible. In general, the basic instructions on setting up the camera should always be adhered to. A simple method is to file duplicates of the images (or second shots) in the patient's documents. These give an indication about the subsequent images which must be taken.

If certain standard views have been agreed upon in the dental practice these can also be noted in the records.

Front view			+
Lateral view left and right	┤	or	├
Upper jaw occlusal view			∩
Lower jaw occlusal view			∪
Side teeth upper jaw right	┘		
Side teeth upper jaw left			└
Side teeth lower jaw right	┐		
Side teeth lower jaw left			┌
Upper jaw frontal view			⊥
Lower jaw frontal view			⊤

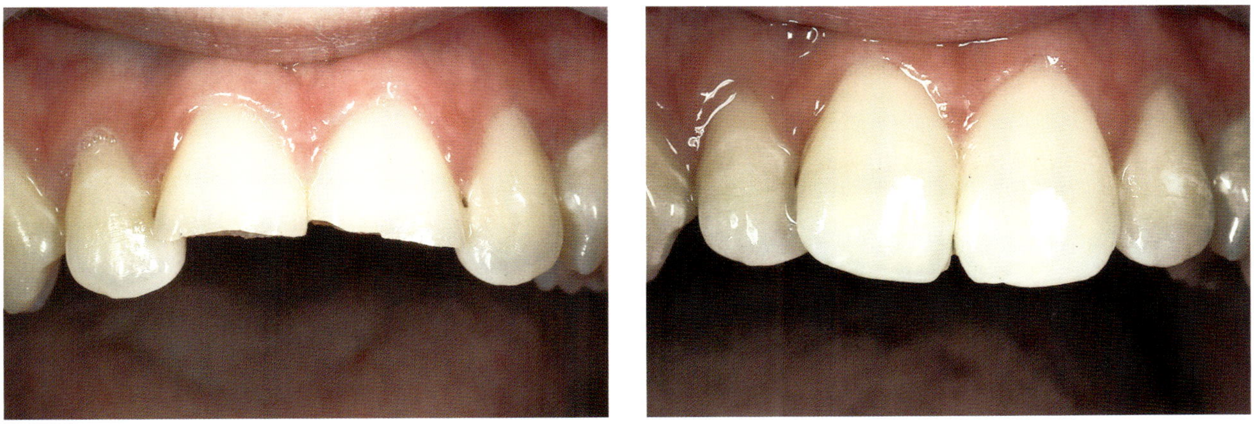

Fig. 3.31 When taking a series of images the basic position should not alter so that the viewer does not have to reorientate himself or herself with each new image. Front teeth after sports injury (a) and after reattachment of teeth fragments (b).

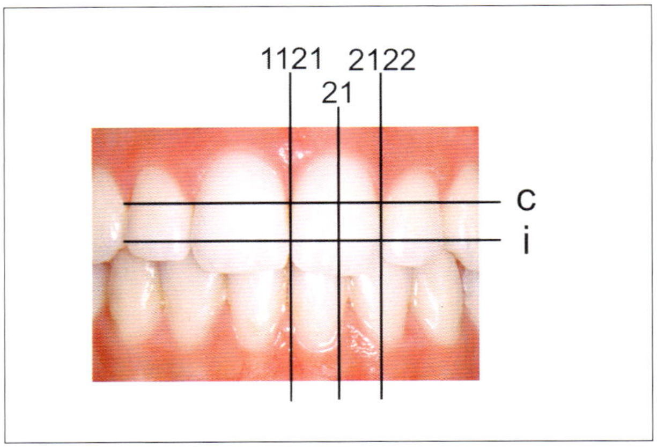

Fig. 3.32 The center of the image can be imagined as the intersection of two straight lines. The vertical lines either run through the middle of the tooth or through the neighboring contact points. The horizontal lines either run through the top of the papillae or the contact point in the incisal third.

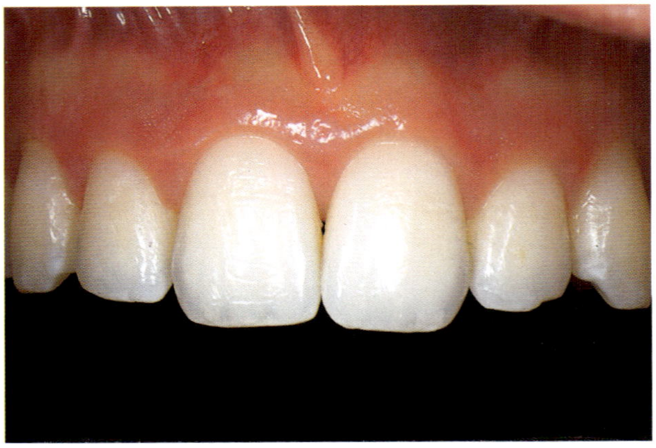

Fig. 3.33 A photograph from the front could be abbreviated 1121c 1:1b.

Another method is to note the key data used in photographing groups of teeth on the patient's card.
This data should provide information about the framing of the image, including:

✓ Position of the image center
✓ Magnification ratio
✓ Direction of camera

3.5.1 Position of the image center

The center of the image can be defined as the intersection of two lines, whose position can be reduced to only a few possibilities.
The verticals either run through the middle of a tooth or through the contact point of two teeth (Fig. 3.32). This can be written down as either tooth numbers or the numbers of the two teeth in question (e.g. 14 or 1121).
The horizontals run either at the level of the transition from the middle to the incisal third (abbreviation "i") or the transition from the middle to the cervical third (abbreviation "c")

A center of the image which lies on the contact point of the upper central incisors would thus be indicated as 1121i.

3.5.2 Magnification ratio

This is generally noted using the standard ratios, e.g. 1:2.

3.5.3 Direction of camera

The images should be taken in general from buccal, lingual/palatal or occlusal (abbreviations b, l, p, o).

In summary, the abbrevation 1121c 1:1 b characterizes a front view of the front teeth in a reproduction ratio of 1:1 (Fig. 3.33).
This method appears complicated at first sight, but is easy to use and has been proven in our practice.

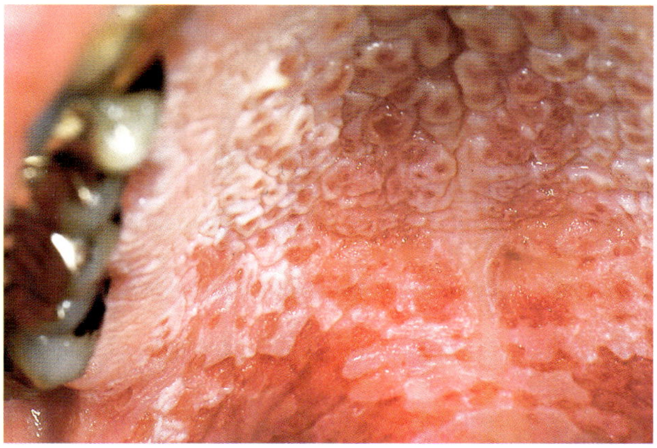

Fig. 3.34 Documenting changes of the oral mucosa is an important part of intraoral photography.

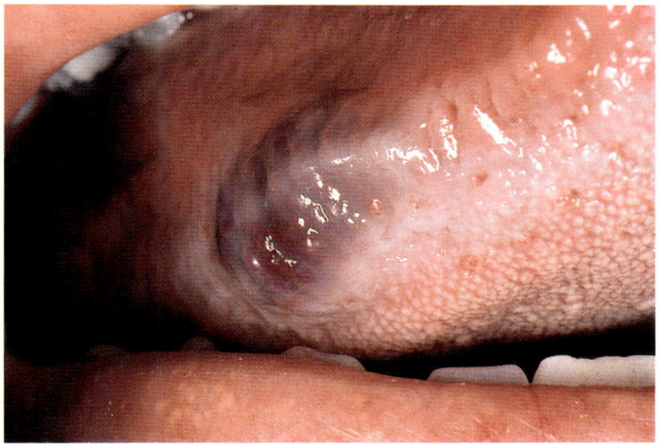

Fig. 3.35 Flat, texture lighting emphasizes the surface morphology of this haemangioma.

Always remember:

- ✓ Direction of the optical axis always perpendicular to the dental arch or to the tangent of the arch
- ✓ Occlusal plane parallel to horizontal edge of the photograph

3.6 Tips for Photographing Skin and Mucosa

Often it is the dentist who first is confronted with changes in the skin or oral mucosa (Fig. 3.34). He is the person who starts therapy or who at least paves the way for further therapy or diagnostic measures.

A camera should be available in the practice as a matter of course for stomatological treatment of the patient just as the X-ray system is for general dental treatment. Photographs of changes in the oral mucosa are especially important in diagnosis and in monitoring the progress of treatment.

It is important that the lesion is accessible to the camera. For this purpose, retractors, photo mirrors, dental mirrors, spatulas and gauze strips are useful.

The magnification ratio should be noted to allow comparison of size. It is recommended to keep the initial photograph in the patient's records.

Surface characteristics can be more clearly shown through suitable lighting. Light from a flat angle shows form and structure of a change (Fig. 3.35). Axial light (ring flash) gives good color rendition, but does not emphasize the morphology.

3.7 Photography of Surgical Procedures

Photography of oral surgery involves a number of points which are briefly discussed here.

Equipment
The same equipment is required as for clinical photography. It is especially important that no trailing cables compromise the sterility of the operating area. For the same reason a long subject-to-camera distance is required. If the operation area is in the mouth cavity, a ring flash is acceptable and less problematical to use.
Otherwise, a side flash or a flash bracket system produces more plastic results.

Image composition
If the person performing the operation is not the photographer, the photographer should be briefed on the significance and procedure of the operation.
It is important that the operating area and its surroundings are cleaned through thorough rinsing and aspiration and by changing the visible operation cloths (Fig. 3.36). Superfluous instruments should be removed in order to focus on important aspects.
If highly polished instruments are used they can lead to reflections and thus to incorrect exposures. Images can be spoiled if TTL flash units are used as the extremely bright reflections can affect the overall image brightness. This is not the case with medical lenses. If the surfaces of the instruments are made matte or the chrome surfaces turned this problem can be alleviated. Manufacturers produce most modern instruments with matte surfaces.
The image should be framed to correspond to the point of the view of the person performing the operation, thereby facilitating later orientation.
Scale can be indicated by placing objects of a known size in the photograph.
Detail views, which are difficult for the uninformed observer to grasp, can be supplemented with an overview.

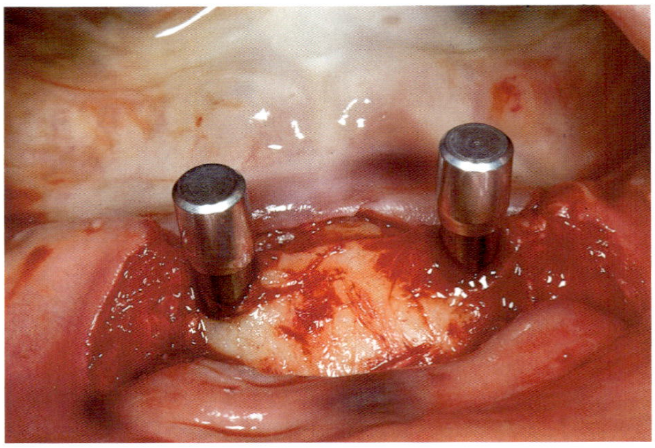

Fig. 3.36 In photographing during an operation it is important to keep the area as free of blood as possible.

3.8 Problem: Indicating Tooth Color for a Dental Technician

Exact rendering of the color of a tooth on a slide is a dream which would solve many a problem in prosthetic dentistry. Is it possible for the dental technician to select the tooth color in the dental laboratory only with the aid of a slide? To answer this question, we must examine the factors which influence color rendition on a slide. Important factors are:

- ✓ Camera technology
- ✓ Film
- ✓ Light (ambient light, electronic flash, examining light)

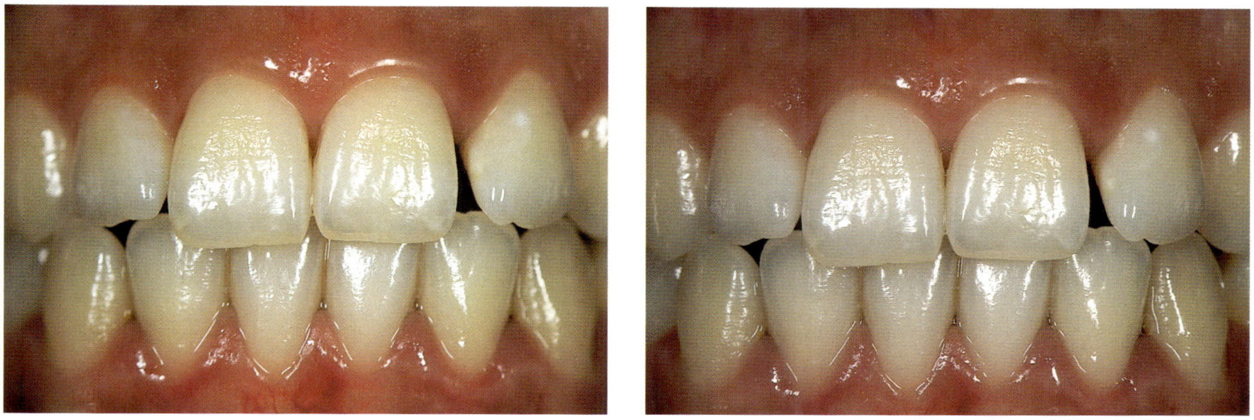

Fig. 3.37 Different rendition of brightness and color at different aperture settings. With open aperture (a) and smaller aperture (b).

3.8.1 Camera technology

Camera technology can play a role in color rendition. Accuracy of light metering differs up to 1/3 of a stop depending on the type of camera. The result is images which are a little bit too bright or too dark, which naturally influences color rendition (Fig. 3.37). These errors can be compensated by adjustments on the exposure correction control.

The type of measurement also influences image brightness. Different results are to be expected with center weighted or matrix metering, for example. The amount of white teeth to the overall image also plays a role. An image filled with white teeth taken with a camera having TTL flash will be too dark, since the white areas cause the camera's computer to miscalculate the overall image brightness.

The same is true for using a dark rubber dam (Fig. 3.38). This produces a bright image of the teeth and thus washes out their color. Tooth color can also be altered due to their drying out under the rubber dam.

3.8.2 Film

Each film has its own color characteristics – one is more colorful, the other cooler in its rendition of colors (Fig. 3.39). Even films from the same manufacturer can vary according to different emulsion batches. In order to achieve the greatest uniformity it is recommended that film for the entire year should be purchased at the same time – that is, film with the same emulsion number – and stored in the refrigerator. Development is another factor over which there is very little control. Quality laboratories which monitor development chemicals should be preferred to cheaper labs, since the demands on them are far less stringent.

3.8.3 Light

Light is naturally the most important factor in determining image color.

Ambient light

Every dentist is aware of the problems of lighting in selecting color. Daylight fluctuates strongly in color temperature and this of course also influences color rendition. Tooth color is generally selected by artificial light. These in turn vary according to the type of light tubes, their age, con-

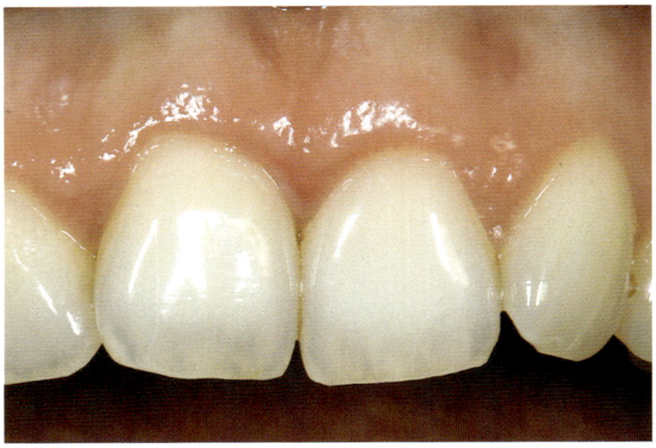

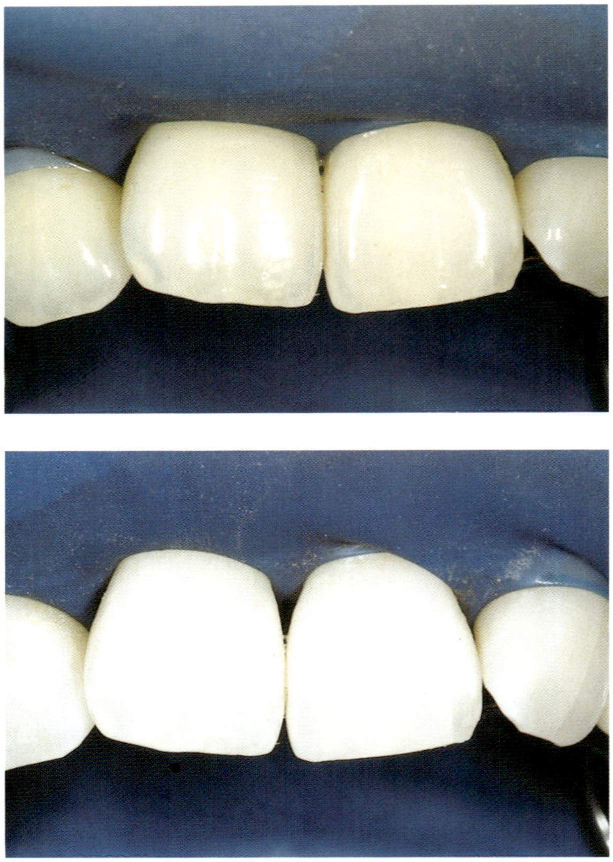

Fig. 3.38 Using a rubber dam can also influence brightness. Normal view (a), brighter rendition of front teeth after use of dark rubber dam due to automatic metering (b) and after teeth have dried out after 20 minutes (c).

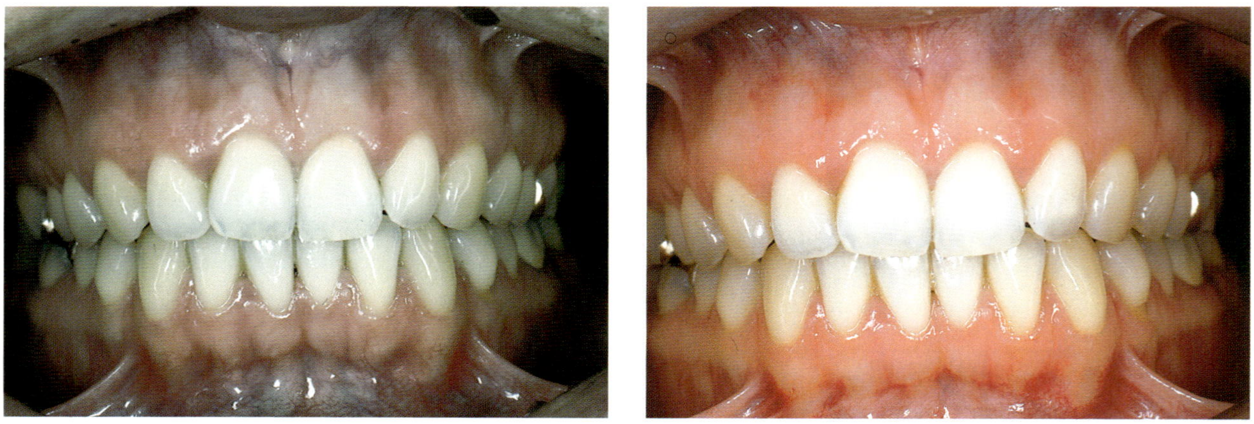

Fig. 3.39 Differing color rendition using different films. Kodachrome (a) and Ektachrome (b) compared.

densor voltage and the type of coatings on the tubes. The colors of the room also influence the light. A green wall creates a different color than a gray one. Things become even more complicated with the introduction of an operating light, especially if it is not daylight balanced. Here too, the age of the light source plays a role. All these factors naturally also influence color when using flash, since this creates mixed lighting. The proportion of mixed light from lamps in relation to flash depends on the type of flash control, and, in the case of TTL flash, also on the aperture. When using medical lenses try not to direct the operation light directly onto the row of teeth, otherwise this can cause overexposure. When using TTL flash a large aperture allows color temperature to be more strongly determined by the other light source. A smaller aperture almost eliminates the effects of the other light source (Fig. 3.40).

Flash

Flash itself of course also influences color rendition. Anyone using several flashguns is familiar with their wide variation in terms of color temperature. However, even the same flashgun can vary, depending, for instance, on the age of the tubes (Fig. 3.41). Even the instant in which the shutter release is depressed can play a role. If the shutter is pressed just after the flash ready light lights up dark images can frequently be the result, since the flash is not yet fully charged. It is better to wait an instant to achieve uniform results.

The direction of light also has an influence on color. Light from a low angle produces poorer color rendition than axial light. The direction of light depends not only on the position of the flash tubes but also on the subject-to-camera distance, that is, on the focal length used and the reproduction ratio.

Examining light

The final link in the chain is the examining light used by the technician to look at the finished slide. Looking at a slide on a daylight balanced lightbox produces different results from projecting the slide.

Polarizing filters

If polarizing filters are used when taking the picture, the color rendition is also affected.

Filters which completely eliminate reflections (cross polarizing filters in front of a ringflash and lens) lead to unnatural looking images (Fig. 3.42). A polarizing filter in front of a lens influences color especially if portions of the light (room lighting, operating light, flash) consist of polarized light (Fig. 3.43).

Routine use of polarizing filters is not recommended, since they reduce the light by two to three stops.

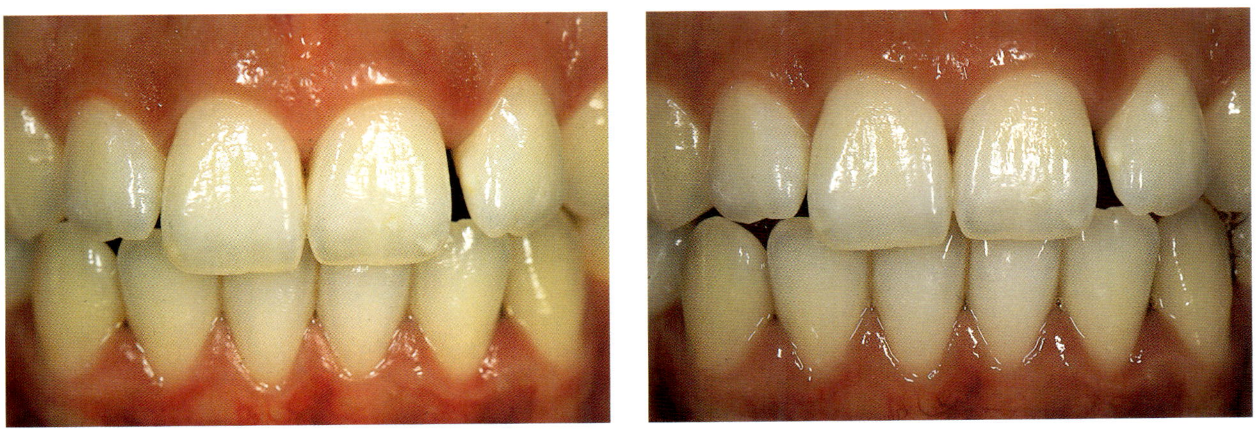

Fig. 3.40 Influence of operating lamp on color temperature is more evident with a larger aperture than with a smaller one. View (a) at f/5.6, view (b) at f/16.

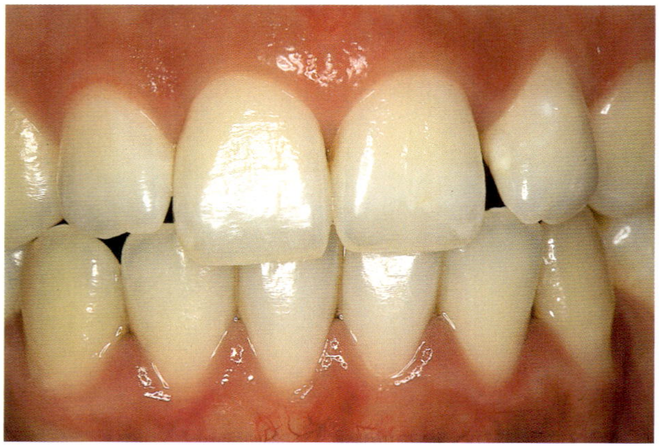

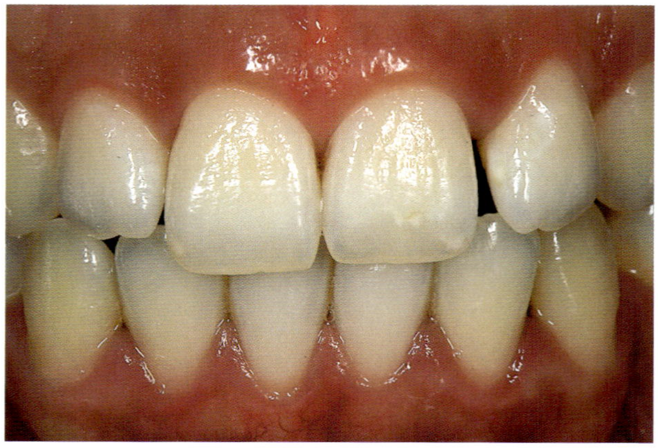

Fig. 3.41 Different flash units create varying color temperatures. View (a) with T10 ringflash, view (b) with Olympus T 28 side flash; other settings the same.

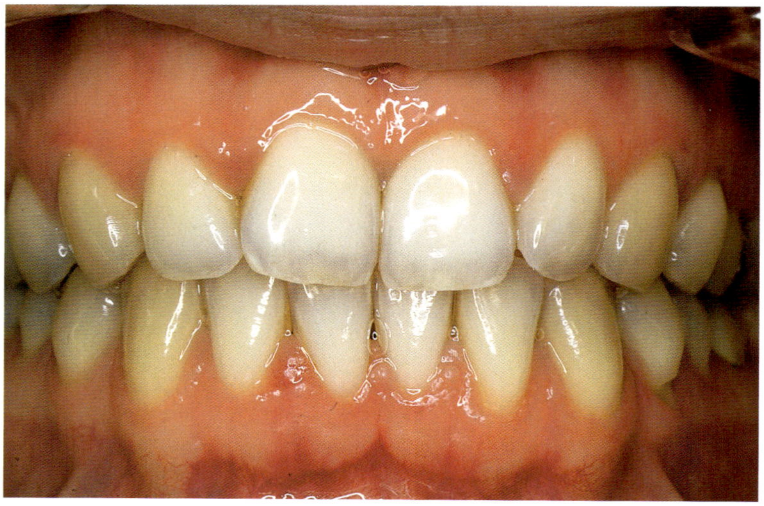

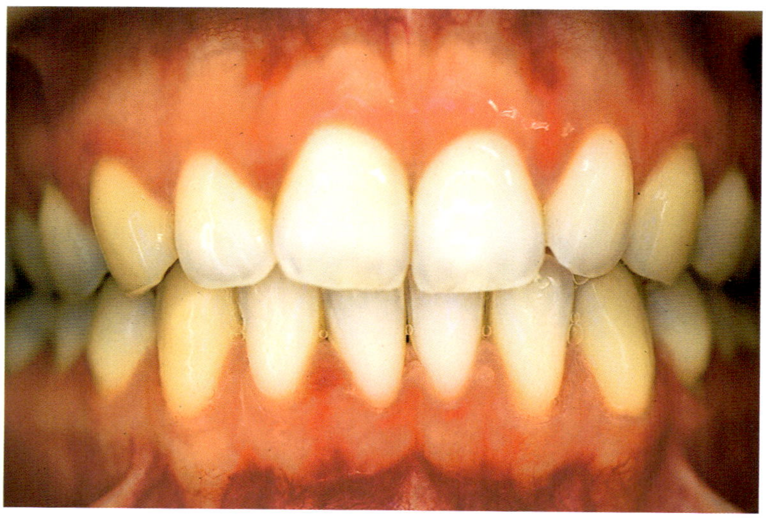

Fig. 3.42 Effect of a cross polarizing filter. (a) without polarizing filter. A cross polarizing filter (b) creates an image without reflections which appears strange.

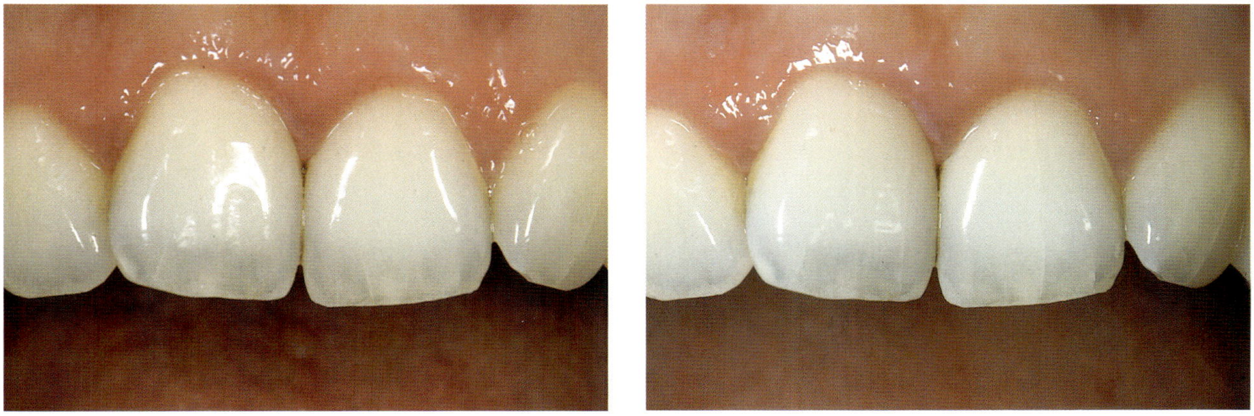

Fig. 3.43 If part of the light is polarized (here the operating lamp), using a polarizing filter improves color rendition. View without polarizing filter (a) in comparison to view with polarizing filter on lens (b).

Taking all these factors into consideration, it appears unrealistic to expect to determine the color of a tooth from a color slide. The photographer should aspire to achieve uniform conditions. This not only means using the same type of film with the same emulsion number, but also a certain consistency of lighting. The photographer should try to use daylight balanced room lighting and operation lights in order to minimize the effects of mixed lighting. Undesirable effects due to flash can be corrected using filters. It is helpful to produce photographs which show the tooth to be crowned with the color chart next to it.

In summary it can be stated that a photograph is very important information for the dental technician. However, the stage has not yet been reached when it is possible to send a slide and let the dental lab select the color.

3.9 Integrating Photography into the Dental Practice

Experience has shown that photography is only performed systematically in the dental practice if its routine is not greatly disturbed. Most practices generally operate under considerable time pressure. Since photography is time consuming, even when well organized, it must be ensured that it takes as little time as possible.

It is important to ensure that the camera and aids (mirrors/retractors) are at hand. If the camera first has to be "assembled" the image is generally not taken. Extra batteries and film should also be available.

As far as possible, photography should be delegated, which does present problems with special details which must be recorded.

Images which are sent to the dental technician should not be taken during the preparatory session, but during the appointment when the treatment plan is discussed with the patient. This also ensures that the film is developed in time and is ready when the slides are needed.

Images can be filed in a number of different ways. Image numbers can be entered using a databack.

Film		Camera	Lens	Accessories	Flash
No.	Date	Name	Diagnosis	M	Notes
01					
02					
03					
04					
05					
06					
07					
08					
09					
10					
11					
12					
13					
14					
15					
16					
17					
18					
19					
20					
21					
22					
23					
24					
25					
26					
27					
28					
29					
30					
31					
32					
33					
34					
35					
36					
37					
38					
39					

Fig. 3.44 A photography sheet can be used for important data. This allows images to be catalogued without any problems (M = Reproduction ratio [magnification]).

A more elegant solution is to enter the number on the unexposed strip between two frames. In many practices the initial step is to photograph the patient's record card with his or her name, thereby avoiding any confusion of images.

Another proven method is to produce the practice's own "photo sheets" which contain the most important image data, the diagnosis and patient name. Fig. 3.44 shows one such example.

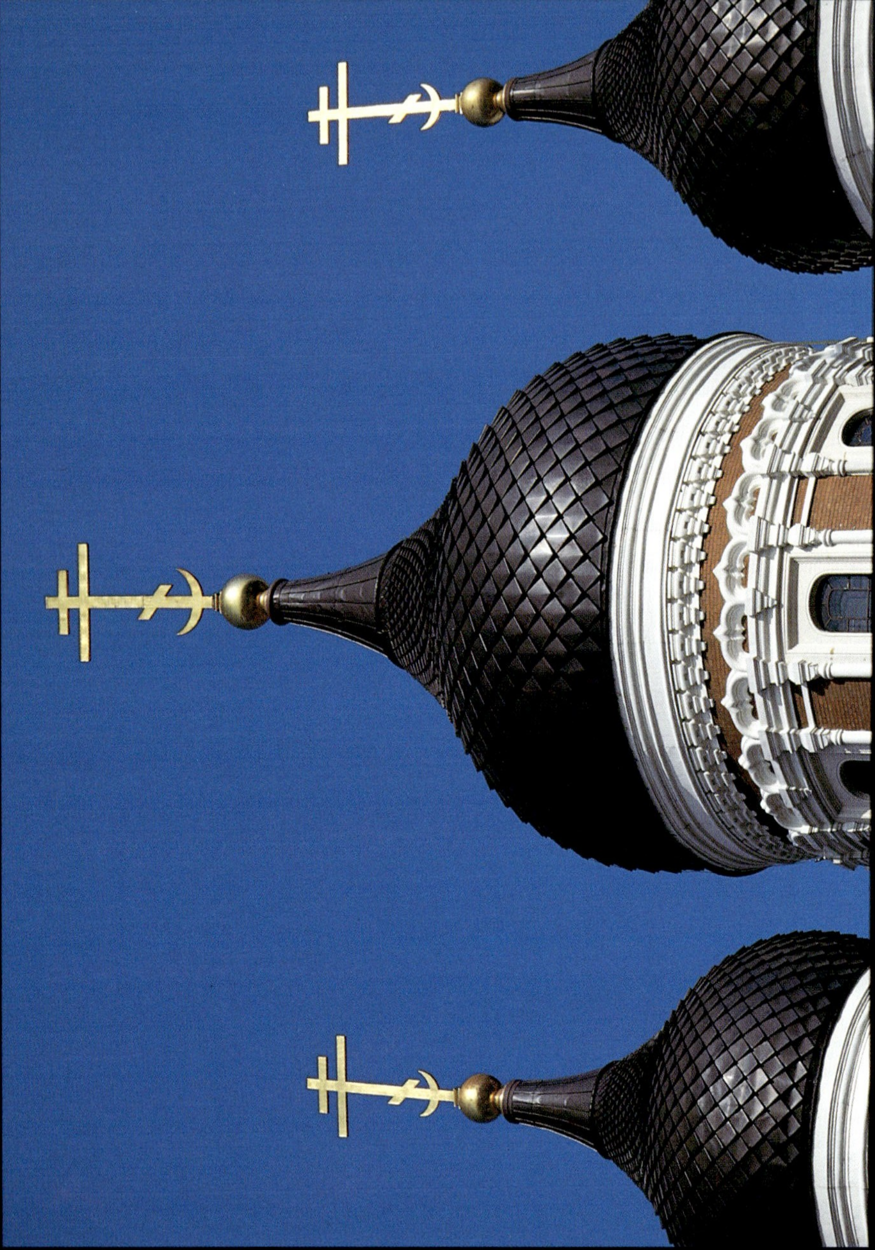

4 Portrait and Profile Photography

Dental portraits are predominantly for documentation. They are mainly used for orthodontics, surgery and prosthetic dentistry. If these images are to be used for documentation then the patient must be positioned in accordance with strict guidelines. If the images are to be used more to present an aesthetic impression of dental treatment there is more flexibility in positioning the patient.

Many light and color effects depend on light dispersion. If a light source strikes a barrier it is dispersed in all directions as would a jet of water hitting an obstruction. The type of dispersion depends for instance on the size of the particles causing the dispersion. If these are very small, that is, not larger than 10–20% of the light's wavelength, then violet and blue are scattered up to 16 times more than red. If the size of the particles is about the same as the wavelength, blue and violet are scattered only about four times more than red. If the particle size is much larger than the light's wavelength (1 µm and larger), then the scattering of the light no longer depends on the wavelength. The scattered light appears white to us.
The blue light of the sky is due to the scattering of light by the molecules in the atmosphere; their diameter is less than 0.0001 µm, that is, much smaller than the wavelength of the sunlight entering the atmosphere. It is the blue shimmering molecules of the atmosphere which gives us the impression of an illuminated vault above us.

4.1 Technical Considerations

4.1.1 Camera

The same camera can be used for portraits as is employed in intraoral photography.
It is especially important to use at least an 80mm lens in order to avoid distortions in the portrait (Fig. 4.1).
If portraits are taken frequently in the practice, then it is recommended that a specific area be set aside for this purpose. Patient and camera positions can be marked on the floor in order to ensure reproducible results. Rail systems with an adjustable arm fixed to the wall or ceiling can be useful for this purpose (Fig. 4.2).
Unlike in intraoral photography, the vertical format should be used to completely fill the frame.

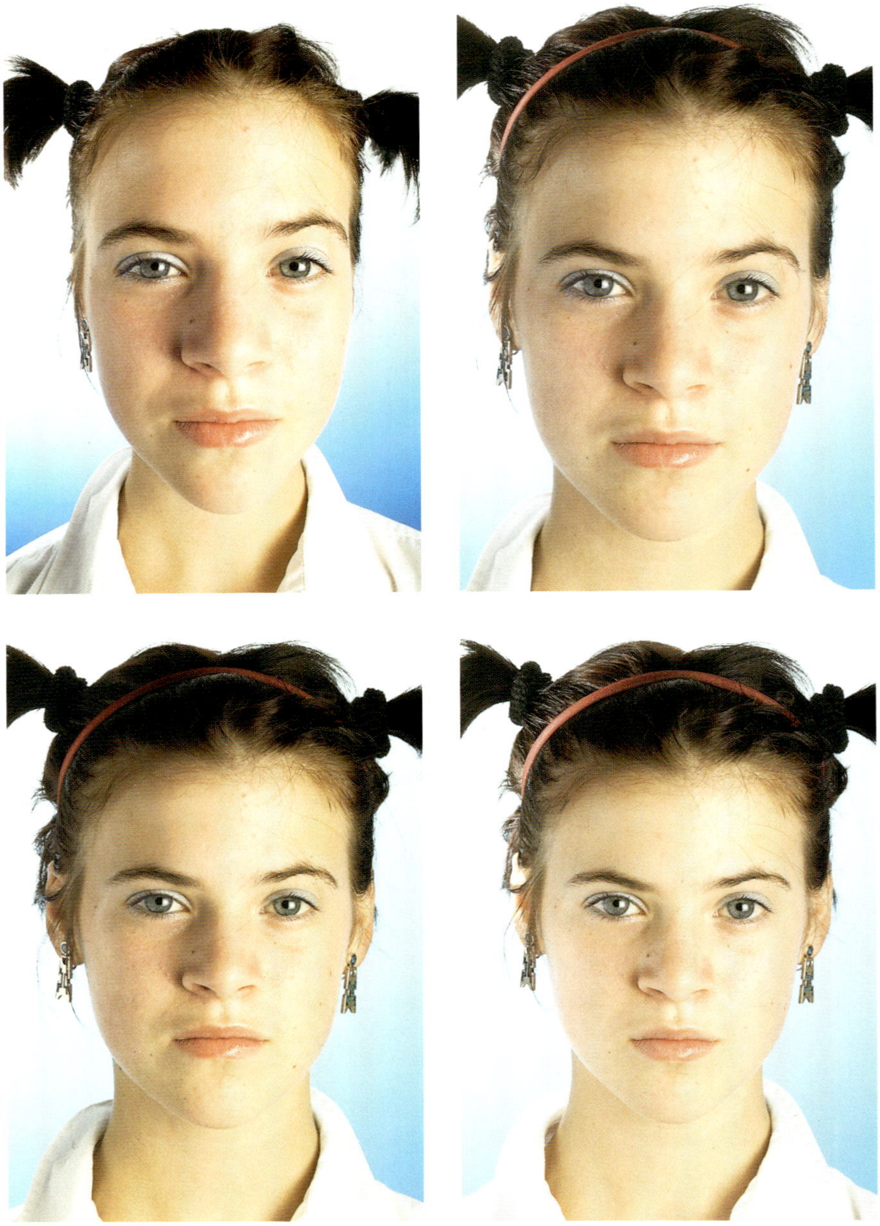

Fig. 4.1 Portraits with different perspectives using lenses with different focal lengths .28mm (a), 55mm (b), 105mm (c) and 200mm (d). The most natural appearance results from using a 105mm lens.

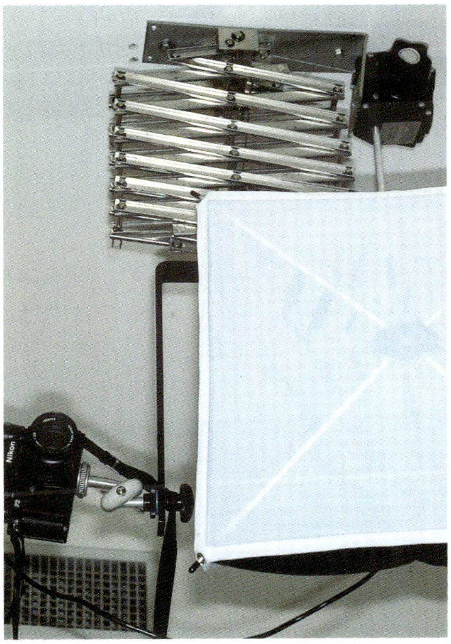

Fig. 4.2 A scissors arm allows the camera and flash to be hung from the ceiling, thus saving space.

4.1.2 Background

The background must allow a full assessment of the profile. It should be without structure and non-reflective. Gray or black decorative felt or cardboard have been proven useful for this purpose (Fig. 4.3). It must always be ensured that no objects of the practice appear in the image.
If a white background is desired (black and white photography) this must be illuminated separately by its own light source. In this case an exposure compensation (plus correction) may be necessary. When using black backgrounds there is the risk that dark-haired patients will not stand out sufficiently from the background.

4.1.3 Lighting

For the most part, flashguns used in intraoral photography are too weak and are therefore only a compromise.
Ring flashes should not be used at all, as they result in a completely flat reproduction of the face, and because of their low power and resulting large apertures, achieve images with too shallow a depth of field (Fig. 4.4).

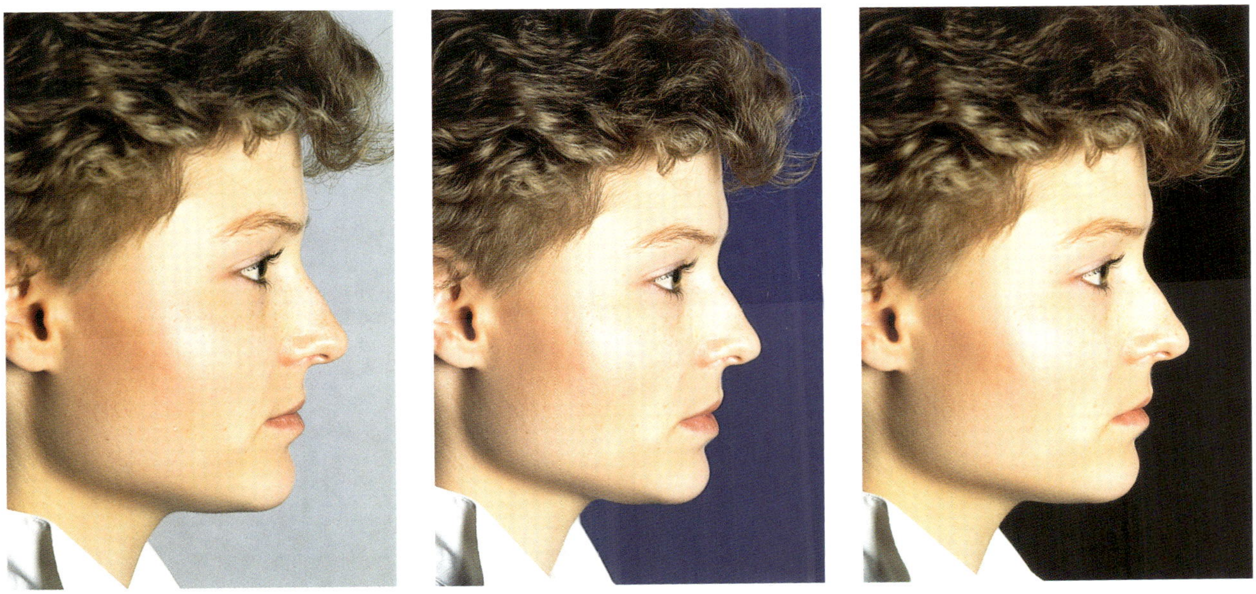

Fig. 4.3 Suitable background colors for portraits are gray (a), blue (b) and black (c).

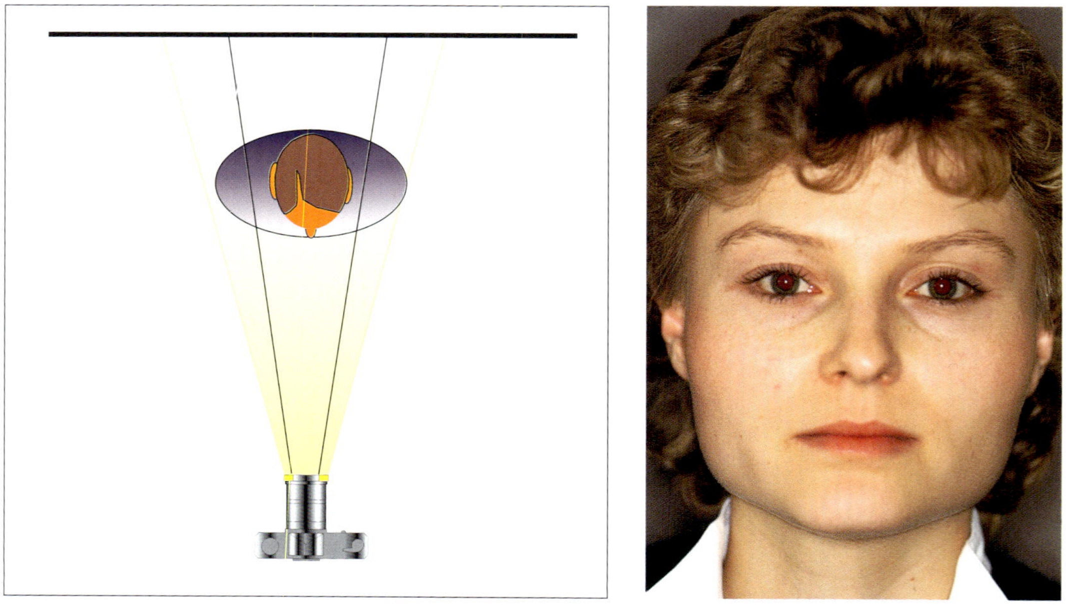

Fig. 4.4 Ringflash is not suitable for portrait photography. Diagram of lighting (a), result (b). The photo does not appear very plastic, has a shallow depth of field and exhibits "red eye".

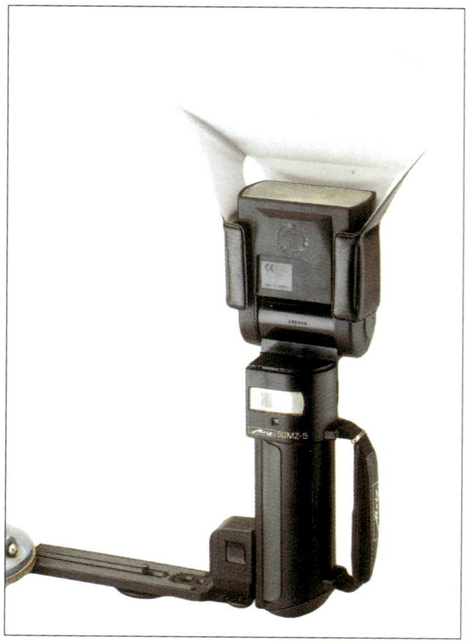

Fig. 4.5 Reflectors increase the size of the light from the flashgun, making the image softer and more pleasant (Photo: Metz).

Regardless of whether constant light sources (studio lights) or flashguns are used, the light source should be bright enough to allow apertures of between f/11 and f/22.
In order not to light the portrait too harshly the light source should be made larger, either by using a diffuser (soft box) or indirect flash by using a styrofoam sheet or a reflector (Fig. 4.5).
It is also possible to bounce the flash off a white wall or the ceiling, although this frequently results in images without much contrast.
In general it is sufficient to light the face with one light source. The side away from the light can be filled-in using a reflector. If the main light source is a flash it can be triggered via a cable. It is also possible to trigger the flash without a cable using a slave which is triggered by the camera's flash. If the flash is not TTL-controlled the correct aperture must be determined at the outset by a flash meter or by bracketing. Since the camera-to-pa-

tient distance and the flash-to-patient distance always remain constant then the setting determined can always be reused.
A second light source is required only if the background needs to be lit separately. This has the advantage of eliminating any shadow in the background and illuminating the background more brightly. A small secondary flash triggered by a slave cell is useful for this purpose.

4.2 Standard Views

Standard views are used to ensure reproducible images. The accurate positioning is achieved by using anthropological reference points (Fig. 4.6). The most important anthropological reference points are the tragion, orbitals, glabellars and nasion. These have corresponding points on the skin. The upper part of the tragus corresponds to the tragion and the orbital points are the width of the eyelid below an eye which is relaxed and looking straight ahead. The main reference points are the "Frankfurt horizontal" (tragion-orbital) and the orbital plane.
It is sensible to brief the patient shortly about the purpose of the photographs. Eyeglasses should be removed to avoid reflections. If the hair covers the ear it should be fixed back.

4.2.1 Frontal view (Norma frontalis)

The frontal view permits assessment of the proportions, form and symmetry of the face (Fig. 4.7). The head should be positioned so that the orbital plane and/or the bipupillar line is horizontal in relation to the horizontal plane of the photograph. A focusing screen with a grid is very useful for this. The patient should look directly at the camera in a relaxed manner. The camera should be about at the height of the middle of the face and in portrait format.
Space should be left on all sides between the face and the sides of the photograph. The upper edge

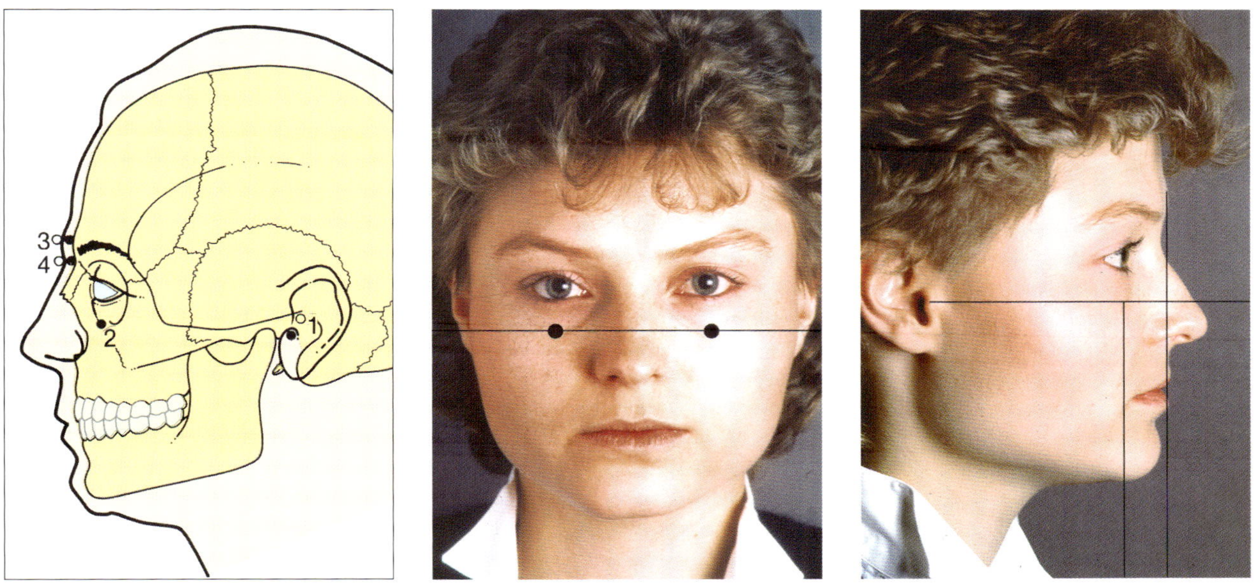

Fig. 4.6 The positioning of the head is done according to anthropological reference points. The diagram shows the tragion (1), orbitals (2) glabellars (3) and nasion (4). In a front view (b) positioning is done according to the horizontal connecting the orbital points or the bipupillar line. In a lateral view the Frankfurt horizontal is positioned horizontally (c).

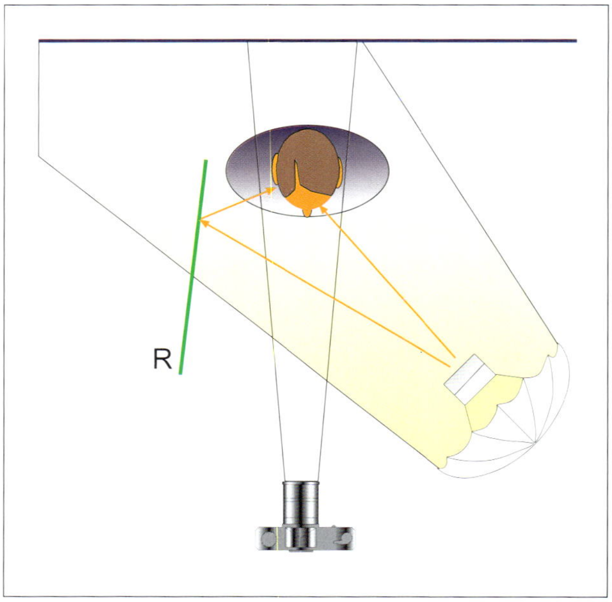

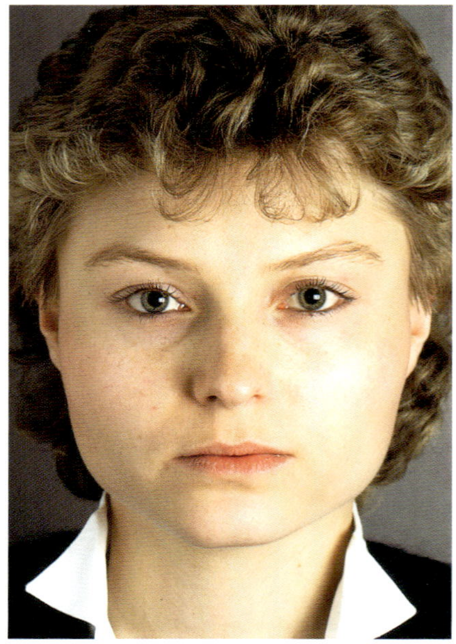

Fig. 4.7 Frontal view. Diagram of how the photo was taken (a) and the result (b).

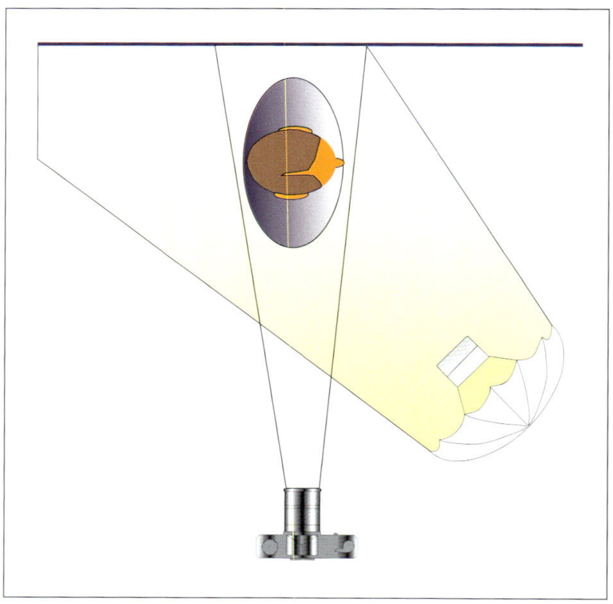

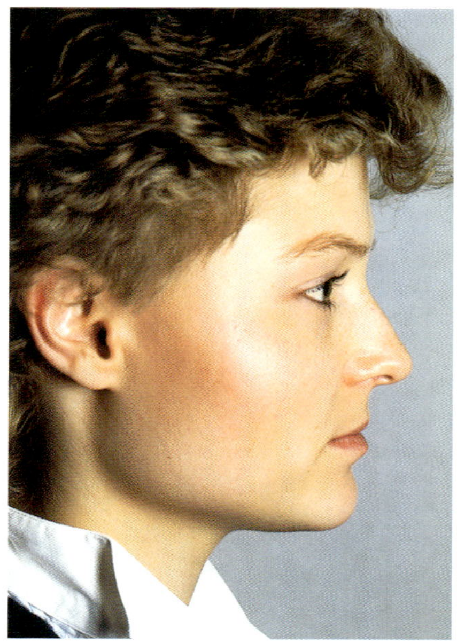

Fig. 4.8 Lateral view. Diagram of how the photo was taken (a) and the result (b).

Fig. 4.9 For reproduction reasons, the subject's head should be turned slightly in the direction of the camera to correctly show the contour of the face.

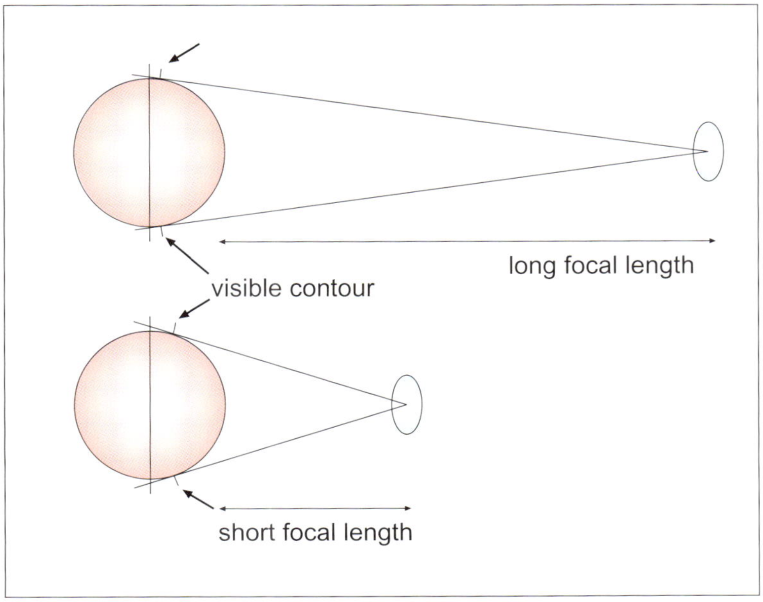

of the photograph should be just above the top of the head and the lower frame line around the larynx.
Focus on the patient's eyes.
Light should come diagonally from the front, leaving the patient's shadow out of view of the camera. The side away from the light is filled-in by a styrofoam sheet or a reflector.

4.2.2 Lateral view (norma lateralis)

Profile photographs allow assessment of the profile and the classification according to certain basic types of face (Fig. 4.8).
The patient's head should be positioned so that the Frankfurt plane is horizontal and parallel to the horizontal frame of the photograph. The patient should look straight ahead in a relaxed manner, keeping his or her jaw closed in a typical manner and the lips also relaxed.
A mark on the wall or mirror hung there can aid in this positioning.
For reproduction reasons it is recommended that the head should be turned slightly (3–5 degrees) toward the camera (Fig. 4.9).
The image should be framed so that the upper edge of the photograph is just above the part and the lower around the throat. Showing the back of the head is not necessary. The remaining free space should be in front of the profile. Focus on the patient's eye.
Lighting for lateral views should always fall on the patient's profile (light always from the point of the nose). This has the advantage of clearly showing the mandibular margin and keeping the patient's shadow out of the picture (Fig. 4.10). If the portrait is lit from the back of the head the angle of the jaw is not shown clearly and the nasal labial line will be unflatteringly lit (pouchy cheeks).

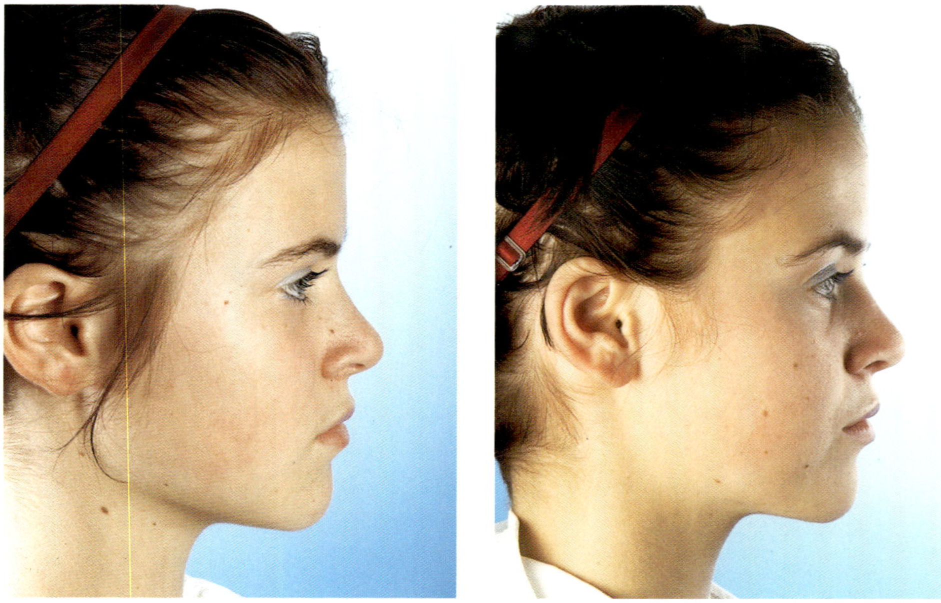

Fig. 4.10 With lateral photographs, it is important to always allow the light to fall on the profile from the "nose side". Thus the angle of the jaw is shown nicely (a). If the light comes from back of the head, the profile is shown unfavorably (b).

4.3 Additional Photographs

4.3.1 Photographing the target bite

In orthodontics it is often a therapeutic goal to change the position of the lower jaw. In order to assess the extent of the changes in the soft tissue profile in advance the patient assumes the lower jaw position which is desired. Such images also contribute in remotivating patients and their parents when their compliance decreases by once again visualizing the improvement in the profile.

4.3.2 Three quarters profile

Especially in surgery on the jaw and in prosthetics, portraits are taken from a three quarters position in which the sagittal plane of the patient and the optical axis of the camera are at approximately 45 degrees to each other (Fig. 4.11).
The other aspects are similar to the above.

Difficulties can arise in reproducing the head position of the patient for this shot. It is recommended that the patient turns his or her head away from the camera until the contour of the eye furthest away from the camera appears to touch the lateral visible contour of the orbita.

4.3.3 Head tilted back 45 degrees

Photographs are taken with the head inclined back 45 degrees especially in the case of patients with cleft palates, but also before plastic surgery in the nasal region; it is also usual to make an additional image with the patient's mouth open (Fig. 4.12).

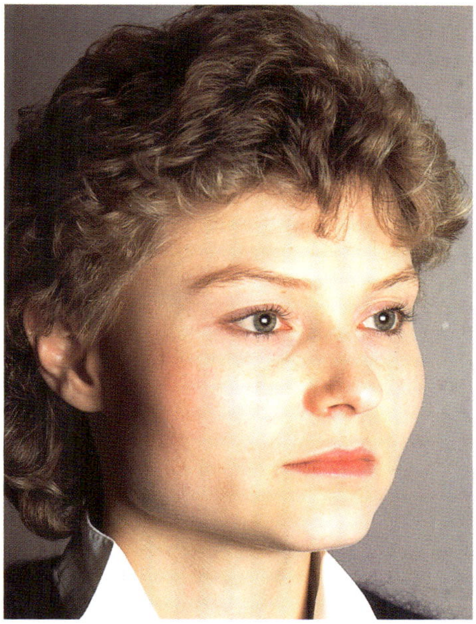

Fig. 4.11 Three quarters profile.

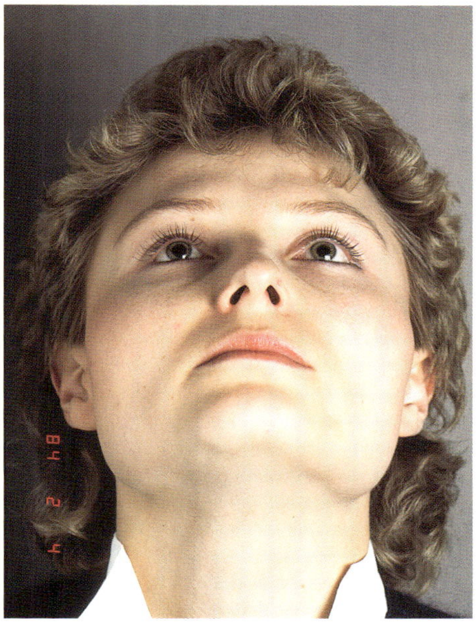

Fig. 4.12 Frontal view with head tilted back (45 degrees).

4.3.4 Esthetic purposes

Documenting the esthetic effect of reconstructions is an important task in dental photography. A three quarter view is often used for this purpose and the patient encouraged to smile. The photographer may need to encourage the patient to do this ("Smile!" "Say cheese!" "Please look up slightly!") since very few patients are relaxed and spontaneous in front of the camera (Fig. 4.13).
Computer simulation programs have largely replaced earlier methods of using photo montages and models to picture the effect of surgery on soft tissue morphology and the profile.

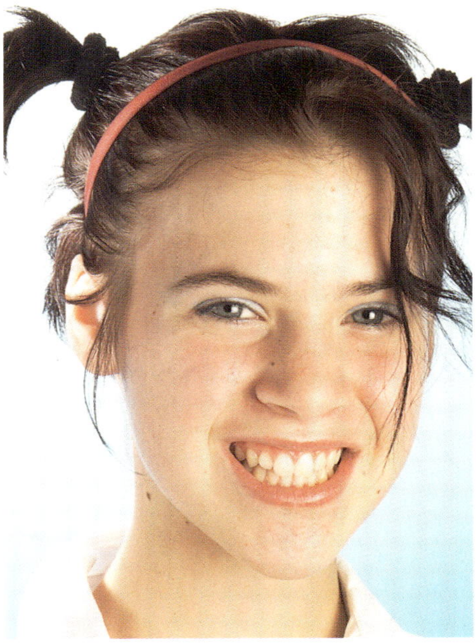

Fig. 4.13 Photographs to illustrate esthetic characteristics give subject and photographer more latitude.

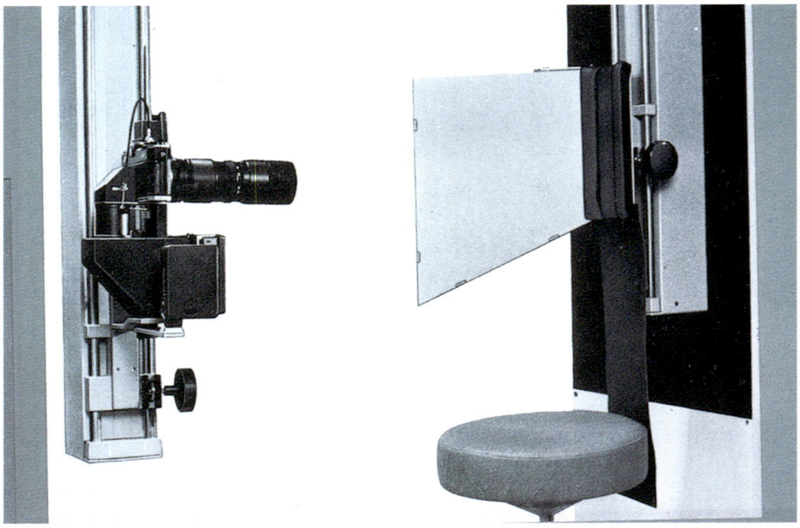

Fig. 4.14 Voss Photostat system.

4.4 Photographic Accessories

The appliances used to anchor the subject's head in the early days of photography due to the long exposures required have been largely been dispensed with. The Voss patient photostat system allows the head to be steadied far better and also photographed in frontal and lateral views through the use of a mirror (Fig. 4.14).

A self-made angled mirror (two folding mirrors with wooden frames) is recommended for documentation of the frontal and the two lateral views in one shot (Fig. 4.15). However, it usually takes longer to set up the mirror than it does to make three separate exposures.

If it is necessary to document dimensions exactly a millimeter scale can be included in the photograph; this is held up to the middle of the face in profile photographs.

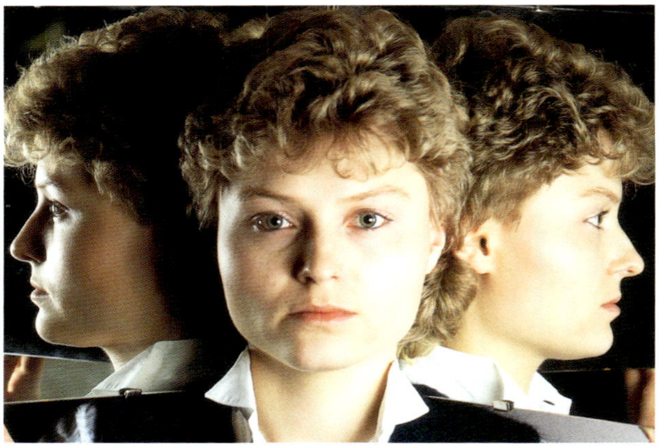

Fig. 4.15 An angled mirror allows frontal and both lateral views to be photographed simultaneously.

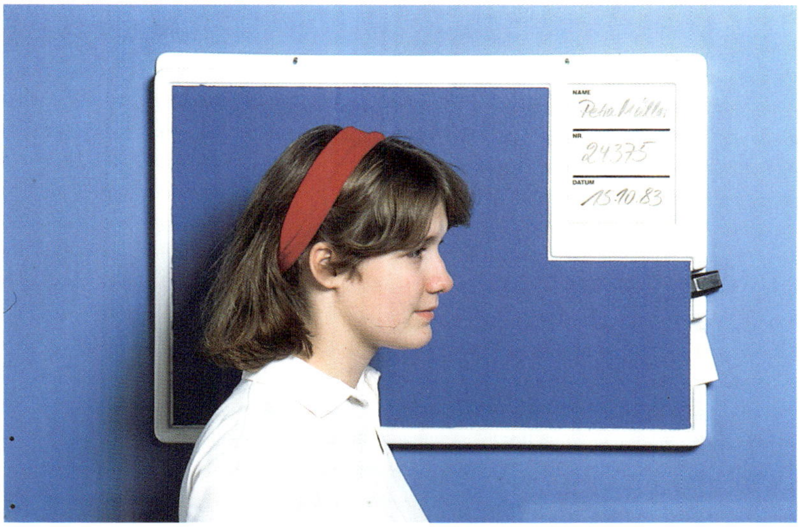

Fig. 4.16 The Hinz photo background (Photo: ZFV-Verlag [ZFV publishers]).

The photo background from Hinz is designed to document the patient's name, number and date of photograph; the photograph is taken in horizontal format (Fig. 4.16). A more elegant solution is to include the patient's number through the use of a data back, which also allows the film format to be better used for the portrait.

Checklist for portrait photography

- ✓ Camera is in vertical format
- ✓ Aperture f/11, f/16 or f/22
- ✓ Minimum focal length 100mm
- ✓ Camera level with the middle of the face
- ✓ Patient's head aligned (bipupillar plane or Frankfurt horizontal)
- ✓ Lights for profile photographs positioned on the nose side
- ✓ Focus on eyes

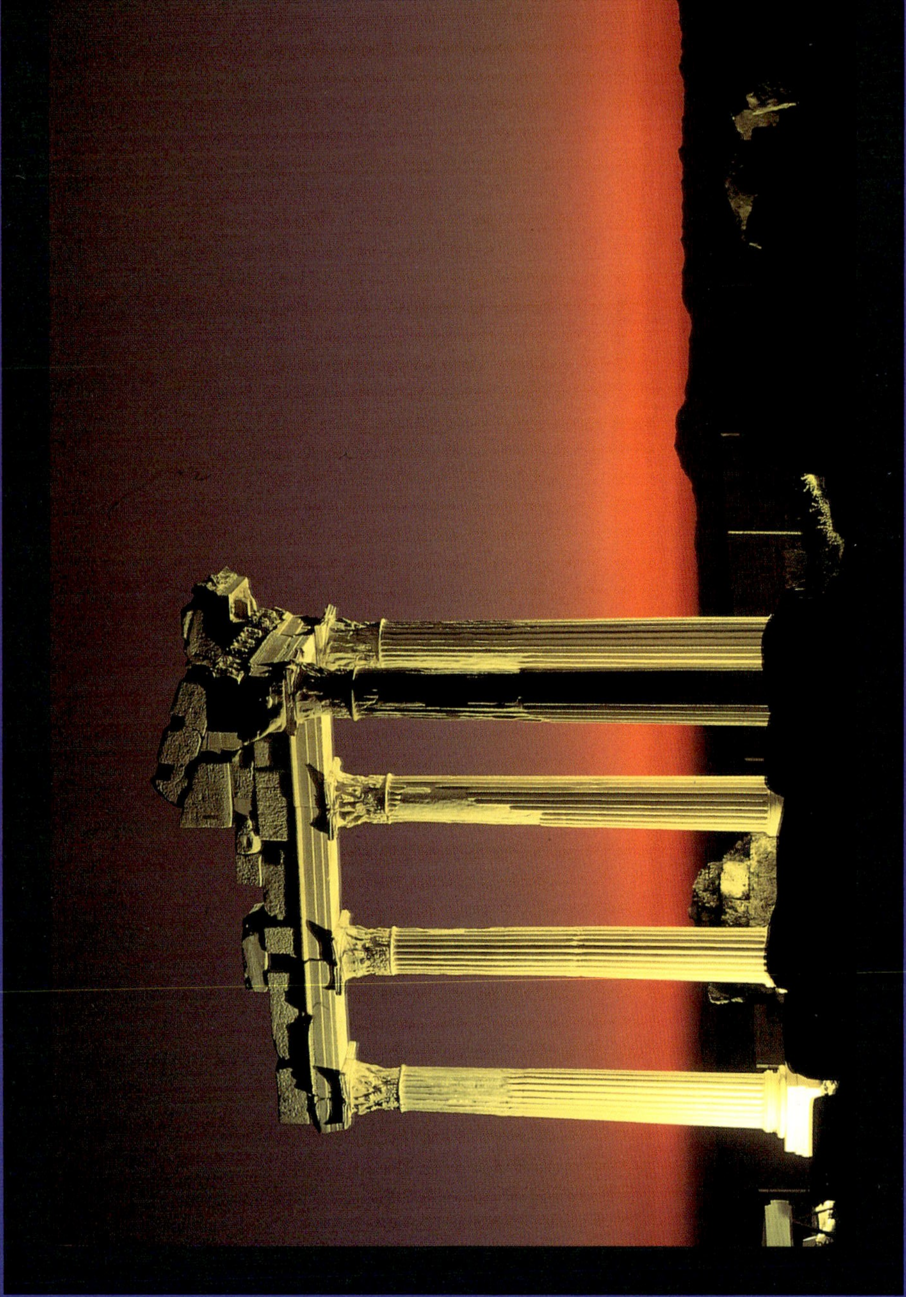

5 Photographing Objects for Dentistry and Dental Technology

Many objects which are commonplace in our day to day dental practice are worth photographing. These include dental instruments, models, teeth, gross specimens and other things. Many of these objects are very small, highly reflective and often have a very bright surface. These present problems in photography.
The purpose of photographing these is for documentation, patient information and producing illustrations for lectures and publications. As in the case with photography for other purposes, the goal is to present the maximum amount of information, fill the frame and create images with optimum perceptibility.

The red light of sunrise or sunset is due to the scattering of light. If the sunlight strikes the atmosphere at a shallow angle as is the case in the morning or evening, blue light is continuously scattered, not only due to contact with the molecules in the atmosphere, but also to droplets of water and dirt particles. The longer the light path the redder the light. The sun too appears red and not white. The reflection of the red light lends a reddish color to the clouds, dirt in the atmosphere and the entire landscape. Even after the sun sets its luminescence can still be seen in the sky; meteorologists term this purple light.

For these reasons, three points covered below are of special importance:

- ✓ Placement of the object
- ✓ Selection and arrangement of a suitable background
- ✓ Proper lighting of the object

5.1 Positioning of the Object

In contrast to clinical photography, object photography can be undertaken with a stabilized camera, that is, by using a tripod or copy stand. This has the advantage of allowing the image to be assessed at leisure in the viewfinder; in this instance also, a constant light source can be used (see below).
The objects should be placed so that even an uninformed observer can see and easily recognize them. This means, for instance, that they have a clear contour and are presented so that they are perceived in three dimensions (Fig 5.1). In most cases this is an oblique view from above. The objects should also be placed to make the best use of the depth of field. If possible, the object should be placed perpendicular to the optical axis. In order to increase perceptibility of the image the objects should be placed so that the axis of the object is parallel to the upper and lower edge of the photograph.

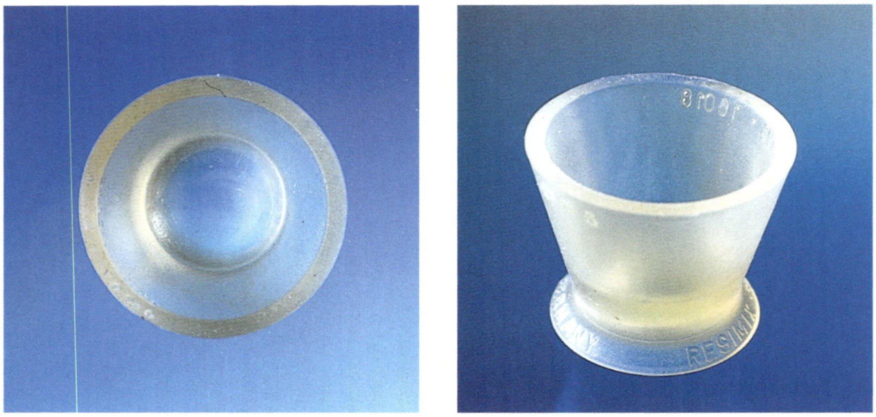

Fig. 5.1 This vertical shot does not provide the viewer with sufficient information (a). An angled view (b) is better and aids in recognition of the object.

Various means are available to help position the camera and objects to ensure the above considerations are met.

5.1.1 Camera stabilization

Copy stand

Purchase of a copy stand (e.g. Copylizer, Kaiser Fototechnik) is recommended if object photography is undertaken frequently (Fig. 5.2). Such systems are modular and can be expanded if required. A few points should be kept in mind when buying such a system:

✓ Sufficient stability
✓ Large enough baseboard
✓ Long enough vertical column
✓ Daylight balanced softlights

A baseboard with an integrated lightbox is recommended. The camera arm should allow the camera to be positioned in several axes. A useful feature is an object holder, a glass plate which can be moved vertically and inclined in two axes (see Fig. 5.13).

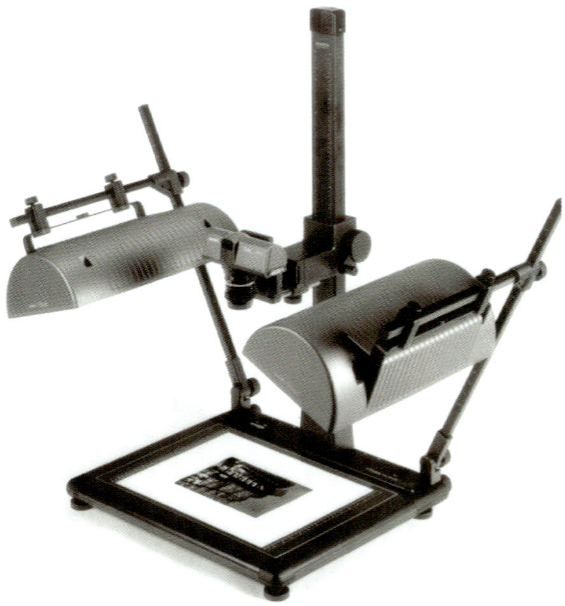

Fig. 5.2 The Copylizer from Kaiser Fototechnik is a professional copy system with an integrated light box in the copy stand (Photo: Kaiser).

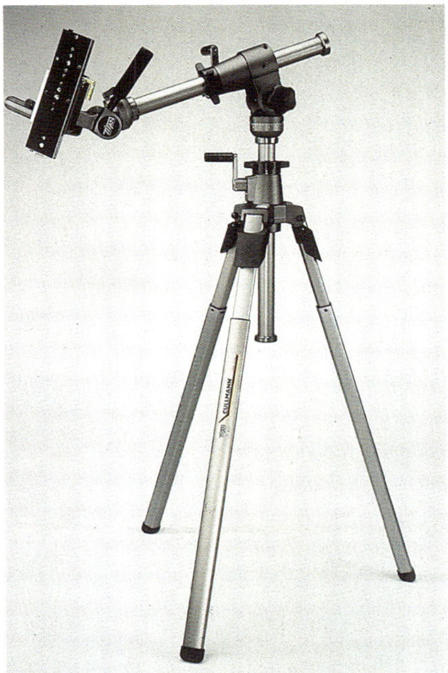

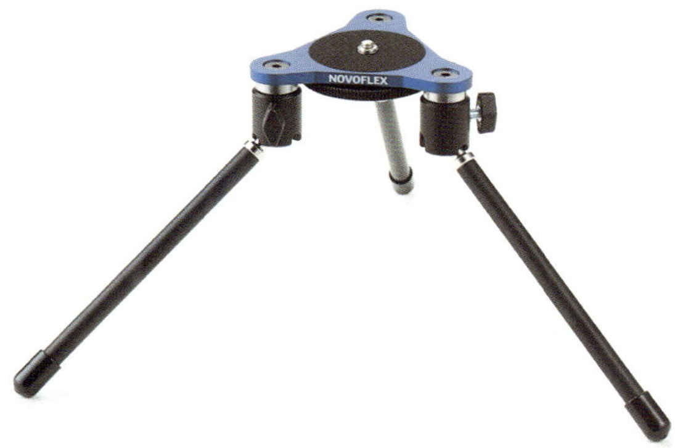

Fig. 5.3 (left). Stable tripod with a macro arm (Photo: Cullman).

Fig. 5.4 (above). It is especially important to check the stability of small tripods (Photo: Novoflex).

Tripods

A tripod allows more flexibility in camera positions than a copy stand (Fig. 5.3). Tripods which stand on the floor should have a macro arm, a horizontal arm which allows the camera to be moved by millimeters. Tripods today are made out of heavy metal or are stable systems of carbon fiber. Tripods, especially ones suitable for the worktop, should be checked for stability. (Fig. 5.4)

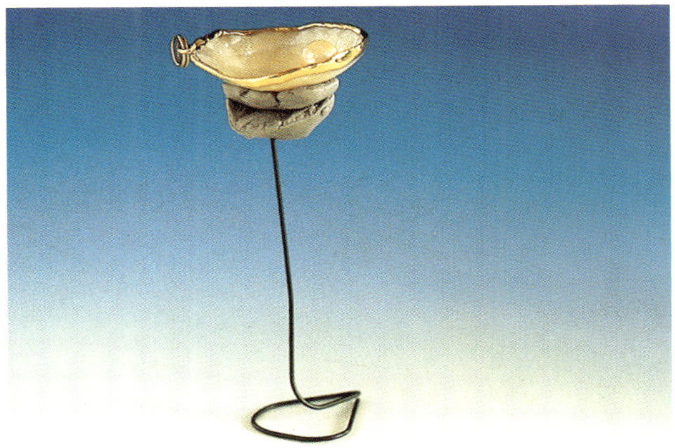

Fig. 5.5 Simple means – here wire and plasticine – can be used to hold small objects in position.

5.1.2 Holding the object

Adhesives are available from photography stores which aid in fixing an object in a particular position (Haftplast, Hama). Silicon impression material or soft wax as used in dentistry are also suitable (Fig. 5.5). Alligator clips as used in electronics are also inexpensive means of anchoring small objects. Rod sets, for example, from Novoflex, are also available from photographic suppliers. Matte black paint reduces reflections and the visibility of the means of fixing the object in the picture if a black background is used.

When photographing from the vertical a wire run through a cardboard can allow an object to be fixed so that it "floats" in front of the background. Spherical tables are used to allow objects to be rotated in all directions. Flash brackets or a model table of a parallelometer from a dental laboratory can also be used.

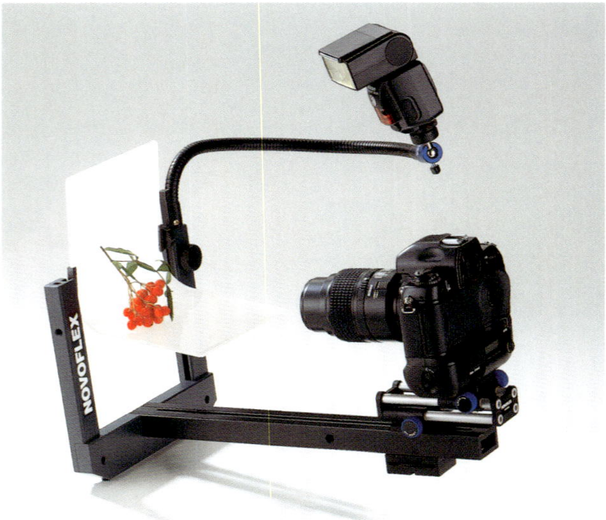

Fig. 5.6 Novoflex macro/copy stand (Photo: Novoflex).

Professional equipment suppliers offer shooting tables of various sizes, e.g. the Novoflex Macro/copy stand (Fig 5.6). The Top-Table system from Kaiser is a "classic" among these tables; it can be used for many purposes and allows objects to be photographed in isolation (see below).

5.2 Selecting and Arranging Suitable Backgrounds

The most important criterion for perception of an object is that it stands out from the background (Fig. 5.7). A suitable background isolates the subject and emphasizes its contours. In general, the most suitable ones are those which have a single color, are matte and without any structure.
The arrangement of the background depends on the camera direction (Fig. 5.8). When photographing vertically the base is also the background. When photographing horizontally, the base flows into the background. This should be set up to curve to avoid a disturbing horizontal line in the picture. This type of arrangement is used in the design of special tables for photography. It is also possible to produce individual arrangements using cardboard, plexiglas or velvet.

5.2.1 Isolating an object

It is generally advantageous to isolate an object optically. It gives the impression that the object is floating without a visible shadow and focuses the

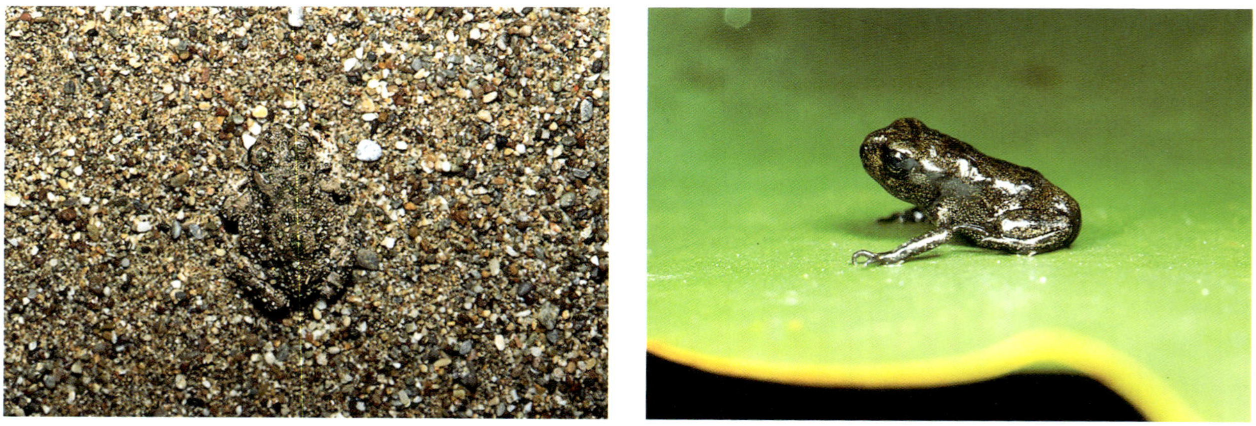

Fig. 5.7 Objects can be perceived only if they contrast with their background. If not they cannot be detected. This principle – known as mimicry in biology – is demonstrated here with a sand frog (a). The survival of animals which stand out from their backgrounds depends only on large numbers.

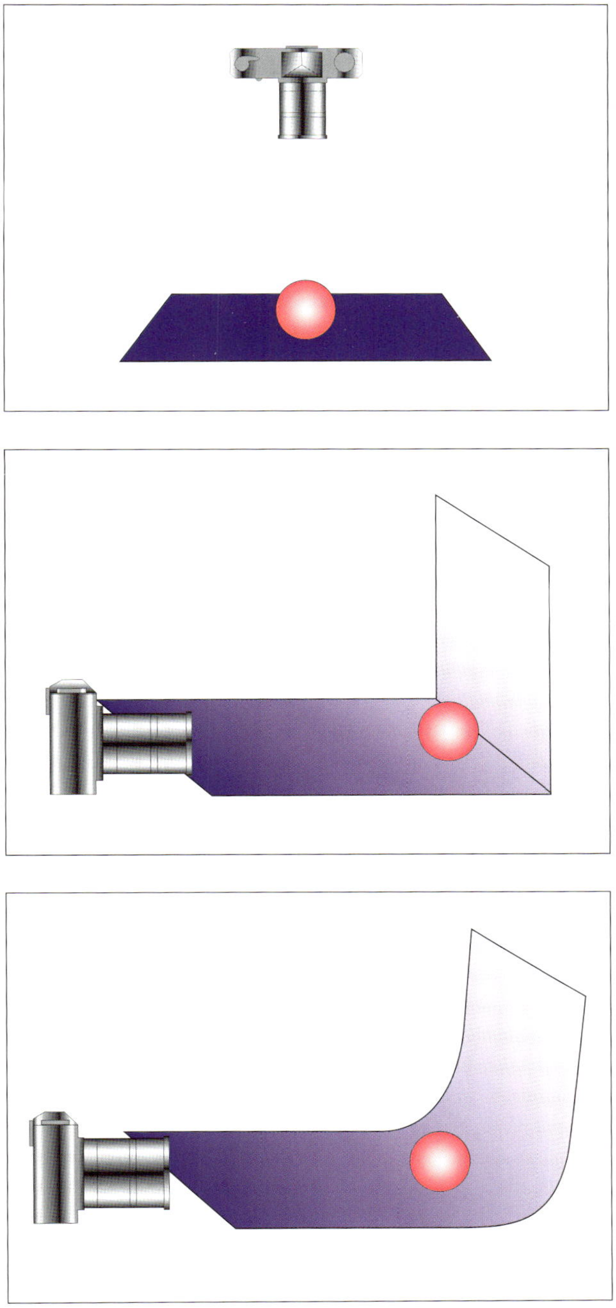

Fig. 5.8 With a vertical photograph (a), the base is also the background. In photographing horizontally a sharp division between background and base should be avoided (b), since this creates an irritating line in the photo. A curved surface is much better (c).

observer's attention completely on the object. In psychological terms this corresponds with the so-called figure-background relation. We perceive the content of the picture as the "figure" and the remainder as the "base". The better base and figure are separated the greater the impact the picture has and the simpler the perception.

This isolation is achieved by an appropriate combination of background arrangement, placement of the object and lighting.

When photographing horizontally, the object-background-distance is large enough and the main light is positioned so that the object's shadow is outside the viewing field of the camera (Fig. 5.9). The object is placed directly on the base.

With vertical shots the objects are isolated using a glass plate which is about 15 cm above the base (Fig. 5.10). If the lights are arranged properly the object's shadow is out of camera's viewing field. The main advantage of this type of isolation is that the base color does not affect the object's color, which is especially important in dental photography. This can be achieved using simple glass plates, a Jobo Variocopy table, the Kaiser copy stand object holder or the TopTable system, depending on the size of the object (Fig. 5.11 – 5.14).

The TopTable system consists of a curved opaque Perspex sheet on which objects are placed directly or on colored cardboard backgrounds. An additional table, with a clear Perspex sheet, can be mounted on top of the basic table. The objects placed on this combination seem to float above the surface of the table or the background attached to it. There is also a table with a flat crystal glass plate to go on top of the basic table. It is used for example for photographing objects which present hygienic problems such as pathological specimens. A strong holding frame helps hold colored or diffusion filters and lighting equipment.

Using glass plates to isolate objects presents problems with reflections. If the camera is vertical in relation to the glass plate it can be reflected in this (Fig. 5.15). This problem can be solved by fitting a black cardboard under the camera with a hole cut out for the lens.

Reflections from objects on the glass surface present a more severe problem (Fig. 5.16 and 5.17).

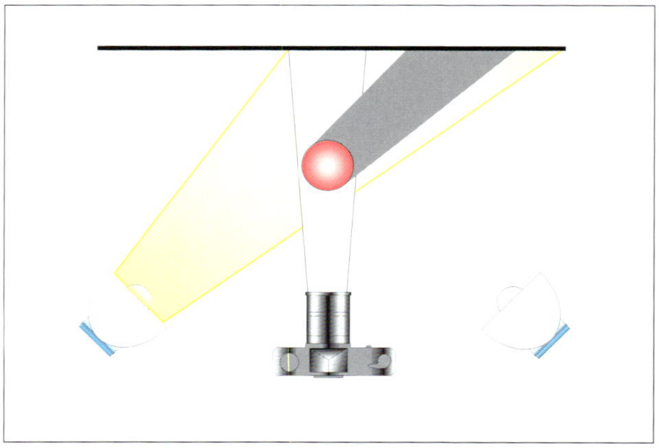

Fig. 5.9 Diagram showing how to isolate an object when photographing from a horizontal angle. The distance between the object and the background and position of the light source is set so that the object's shadow is outside the camera's view.

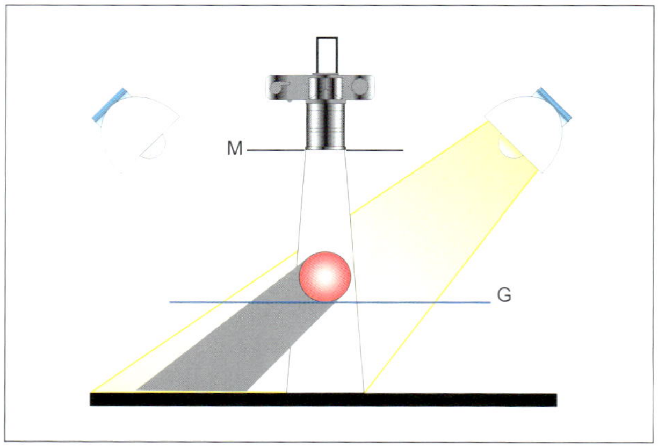

Fig. 5.10 When photographing from a vertical angle a glass support is used to isolate the object. Here too the position of the light source and the distance from the base are set so that the object's shadow lies outside the camera's view.

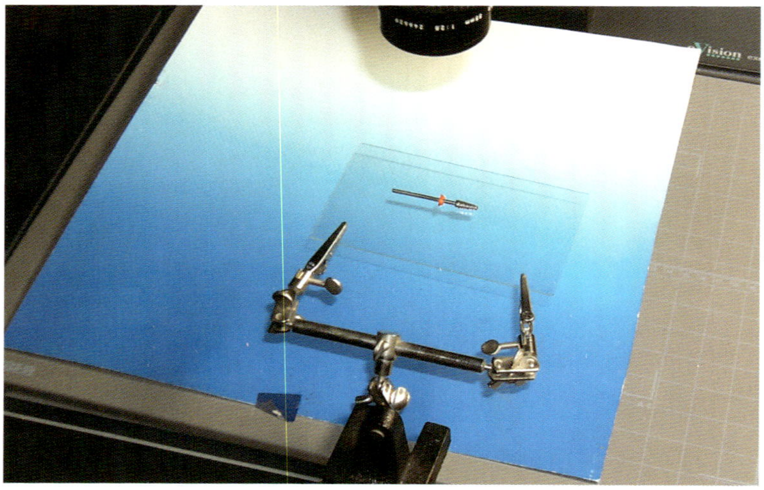

Fig. 5.11 Isolation of a small object using a simple glass plate.

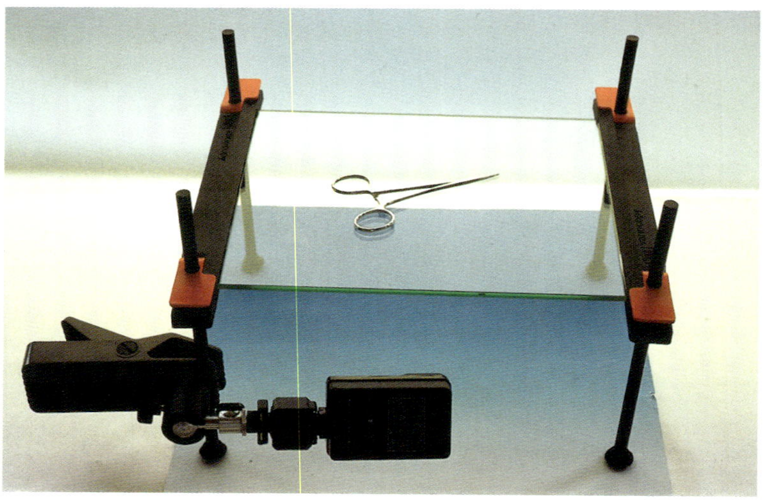

Fig. 5.12 The Jobo Variocopy table for trick photography can also be used to isolate an object.

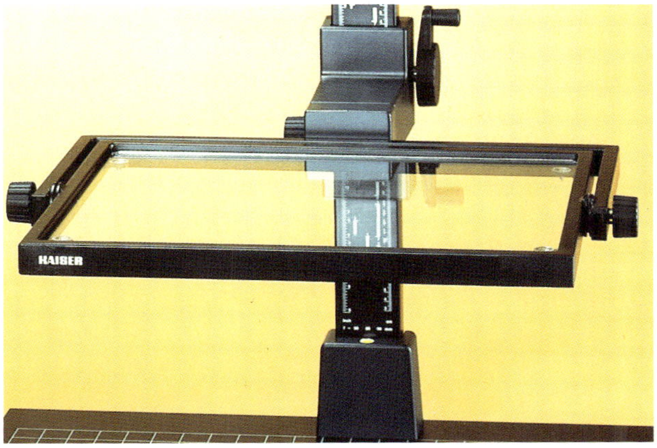

Fig. 5.13 Kaiser Fototechnik's copy stand system also includes a holder for objects. Attached to the column, it can be vertically adjusted and rotated in two axes (Photo: Kaiser).

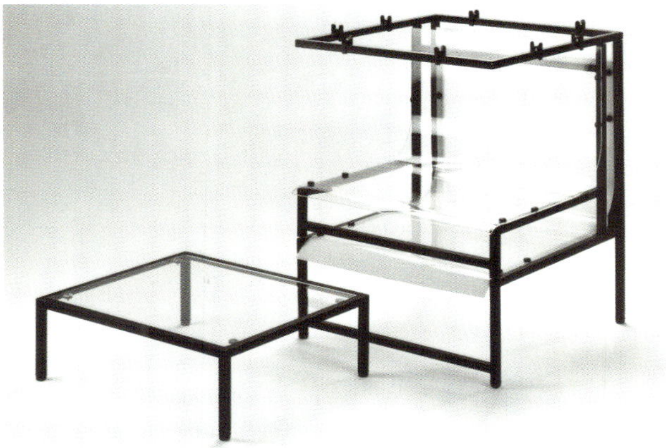

Fig. 5.14 The Kaiser TopTable system is a good aid if object photography is frequently done (Photo: Kaiser)

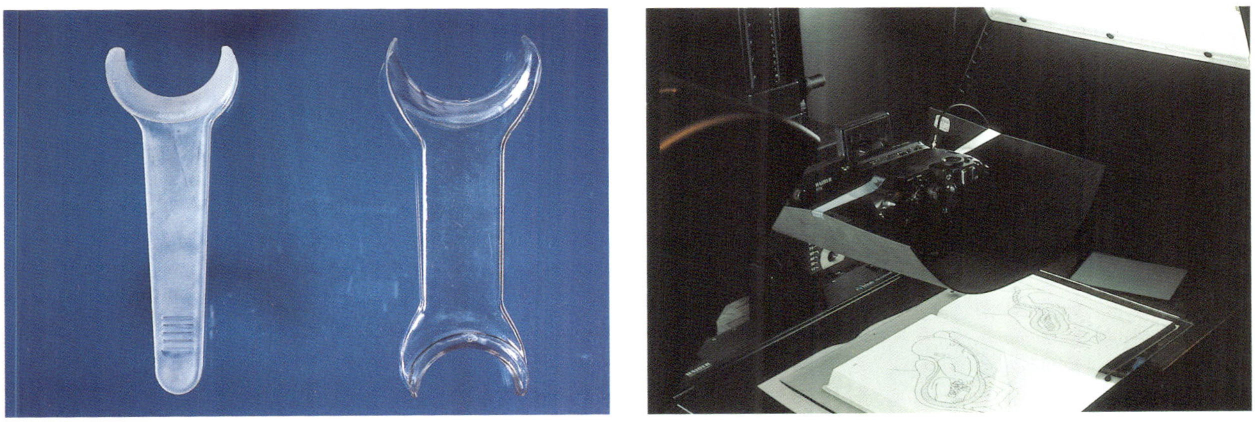

Fig. 5.15 A reflection of the camera is visible between the two objects (a). This reflection can be easily eliminated by placing a piece of black cardboard in front of the camera with an opening cut out for the lens (b).

Such reflections consist of polarized light unless caused by metal. Reflections from objects onto glass plates are eliminated by using a polarizing filter. This is fitted in front of the camera lens; the photographer looks through the viewfinder turning the filter until the reflections are eliminated. Sometimes it is necessary to change the angle of the optical axis to the glass plate to completely eliminate reflections.

5.2.2 Background color

There is no universal background which is suitable for all purposes. Selection of a particular background depends on many factors such as the color of the object and the purpose for which the photo is being made (print, projection, etc.).
In general it is better to restrict the number of backgrounds, making it easier to put together series of photographs without subjecting the observer to too many colors.

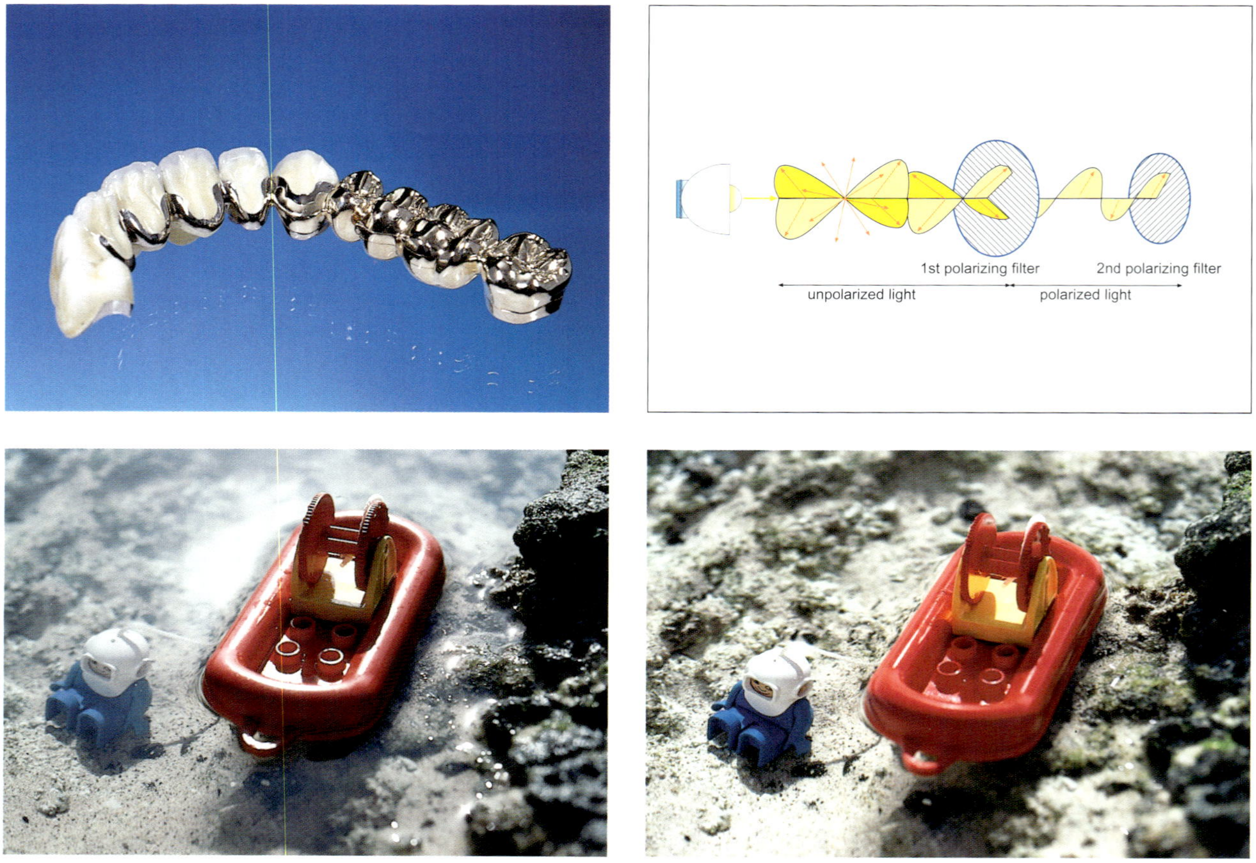

Fig. 5.16 Reflections from an object frequently ruin a photo (a). This problem can be solved by using a polarizing filter. Unpolarized light vibrates transversely in all planes around the beam axis. Using a polarizing filter restricts the vibrations to one plane: the light is polarized (b). A second polarizing filter with a "grid direction" perpendicular to this blocks this polarized light. Reflections from glass and the surface of water mostly consist of polarized light (c). These reflections can be eliminated by using a polarizing filter (d).

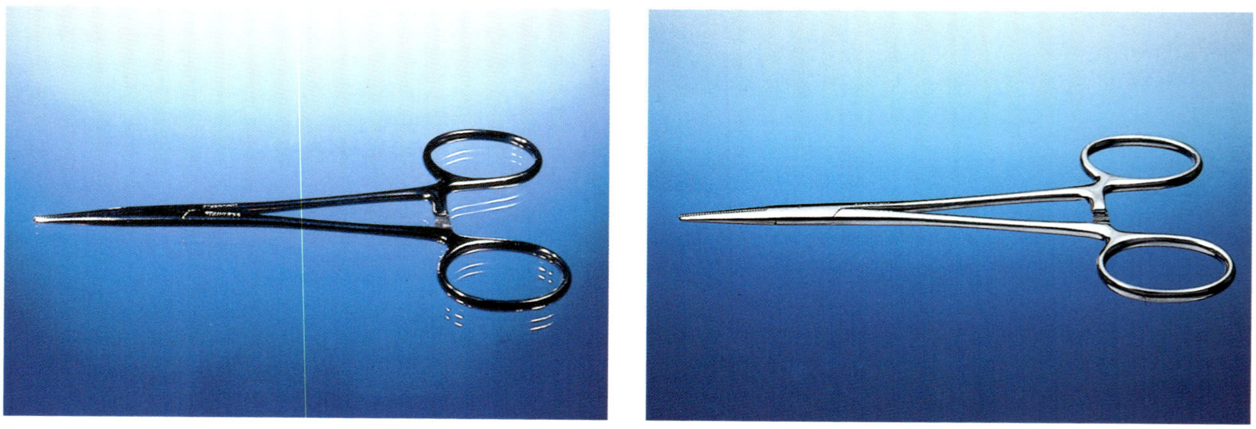

Fig. 5.17 Distinct reflections from the object on the glass plate (a). The same object, photographed using a polarizing filter and a light tent: the reflection has disappeared (b).

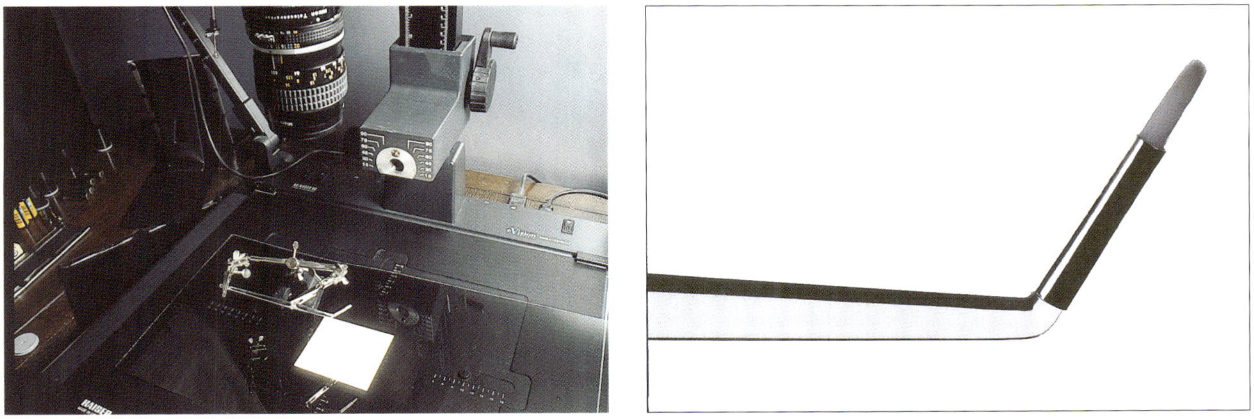

Fig. 5.18 Set up for achieving a white background (a) and the resulting image with "plus correction" for exposure (b).

White background

Especially objects which are dark can be photographed particularly well against a white background. White backgrounds are often used in black and white photography and reproduce best in printing.

White backgrounds can be problematical in slide projections because they tend to blind the observer. Especially when alternating with dark slides white backgrounds can lead to visual tiredness.

A white background is created either by placing the light source under the object (for example a light box) or simply by using white paper or styrofoam under the glass plate which is used to isolate the object (Fig. 5.18). This must be lighted separately to avoid creating a gray background. The brightness of the white background should be about 100% (= one f stop) greater than the brightness of the object. The object should not be placed directly on the white background to avoid "washing out" the object colors and structures.

It is important to mask off the area around the object which is out of the viewing field of the camera in order not to lose contrast in the photo through flare light entering the lens. Photographic suppliers offer special masks for this purpose, but black cardboard can also be used.

Other problems with using white backgrounds are covered below.

Black background

A black background not only creates a pseudo three dimensional reproduction of the object which appears to float on the background, but it also dramatically increases the luminous power of the object's colors. Fine nuances of color are rendered well, since the object's color is not affected by that of the background (Fig. 5.19). Another advantage of a black background is that it almost intrinsically eliminates shadows. Dust particles and fingerprints on slides are not seen under projection.

A black background is produced by using black cardboard or black velvet; the objects are placed on these or they are laid on the glass support which is used to isolate the object (see below). Placing small objects on a mirror creates a black background behind the object which is shown twice, in this case.

Black backgrounds can be problematical if the object's color does not contrast sufficiently with them. Showing a long series of slides with low brightness can tire the viewer.

Black backgrounds can also cause difficulties in exposure measurement. Since the camera does not "know" what it is photographing, the exposure is set so that it always creates average image brightness. A small bright object on a black background thus leads to overexposure of the object, since the overall brightness which is required to

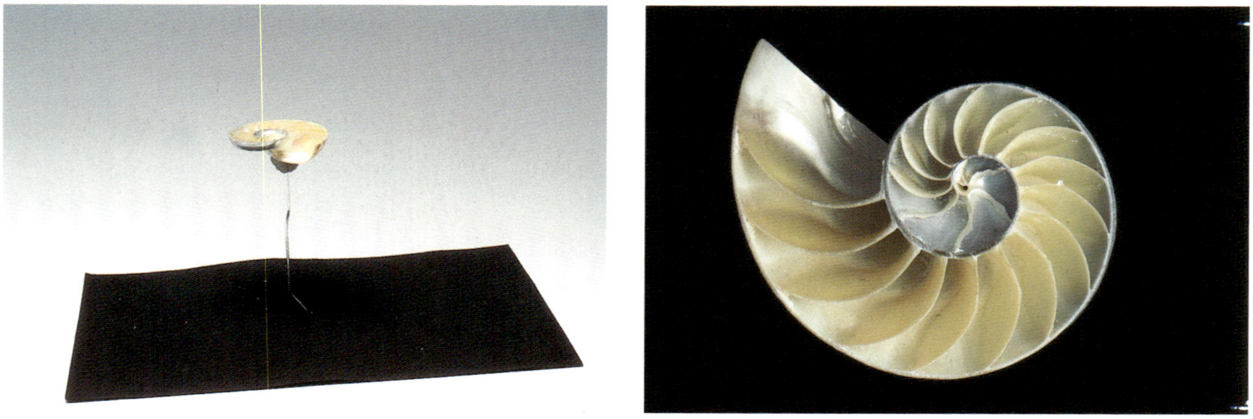

Fig. 5.19 A simple piece of black cardboard through which a wire is passed attached to the object to create a black background (a). The final image does not give any indication of the simplicity of the arrangement.

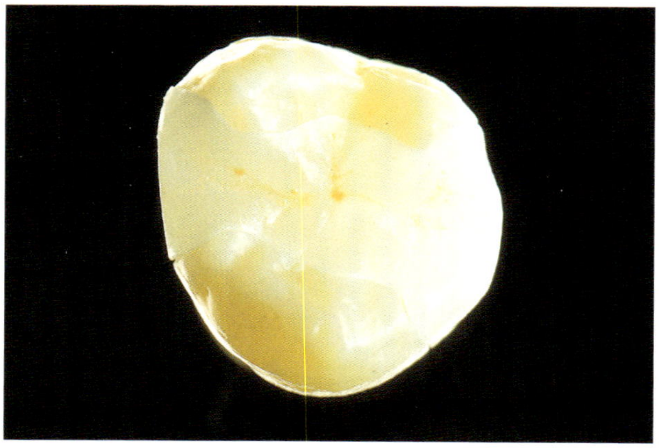

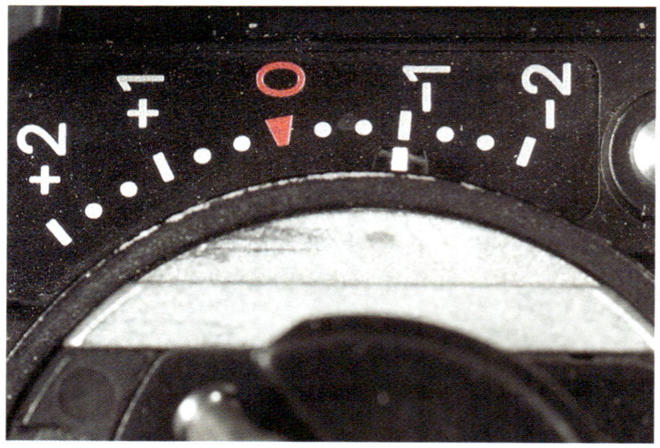

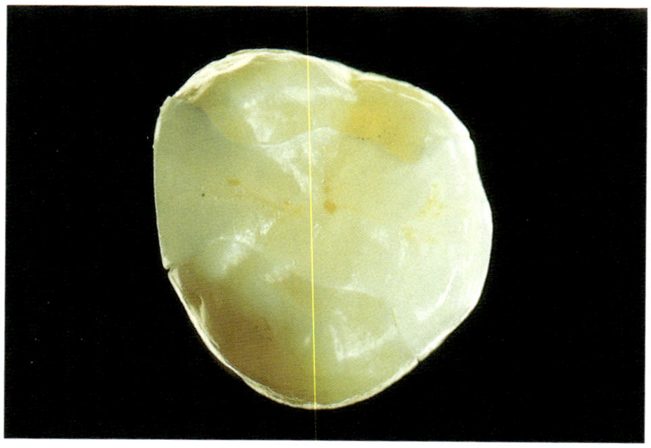

Fig. 5.20 Black backgrounds can cause objects to be overexposed (a). A minus correction (b) achieves correct exposure (c).

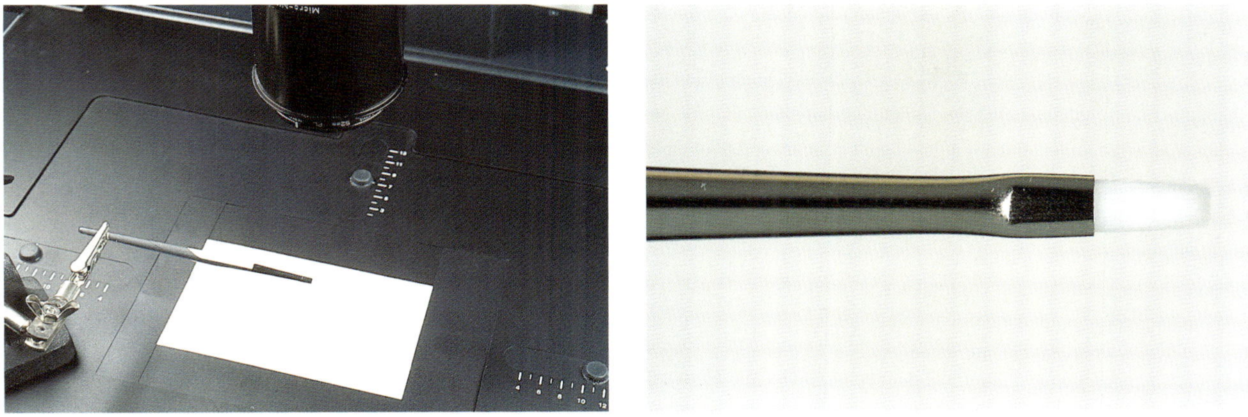

Fig. 5.21 A gray background can be created in the same way as a white one (a). The drop in brightness between the object and the background creates the bright gray color (b).

produce an average exposure has to come from this small object (Fig. 5.20). In this case it is helpful to use spot metering on the object or a "minus correction" by using the exposure compensation of the camera. The amount of correction depends on the size of the surface of the bright object in relation to the overall image area. In case of doubt, bracketing in 1/3 stops leads to the correct exposure.

A white background or a white object with a large surface can lead to exposure problems. A white plaster model or teeth which fill the frame require a "plus correction" to achieve correct exposure.

Gray background

If there is a universal background, then it is the gray one, since it does not cause problems in determining exposure. Gray also does not affect the color nuances of the object (Fig. 5.21).

A gray background is created using gray cardboard, upon which the object is placed. White paper placed at a suitable distance under an object can also result in a gray background due to the reduction in brightness. Illumination with polarized light also can be used to create a gray background (see below).

When printed in black and white, colored objects photographed against a gray background may not appear sufficiently isolated.

Colored backgrounds

Colored backgrounds take advantage of the visual attraction of colour, and focus the observer's attention to the image (Fig. 5.22). Special color boards are available from photographic suppliers; these are placed under the glass support which is used to isolate the object. It is advantageous to restrict the number of colors used to facilitate the putting together of slide series.

A number of factors are important in selecting colors:

- ✓ The background should isolate the object. Placing a yellowish gold object on a yellow background for instance makes little sense. This is especially important if the image is later to be reproduced in black and white (Fig. 5.23).
- ✓ Background and object colors should be harmonious. For example, a red object looks better on a blue background than on a green one (Fig. 5.24).
- ✓ The background color should not dominate the image, but it should also remain in the background visually. Sensory physiological factors play a role in this. Just as in the case with camera lenses, the human eye focuses different colors on different planes. Red, for instance, is not a background color, as it is optically perceived to be in front of the object (Fig. 5.25). Renaissance painters already knew and observed

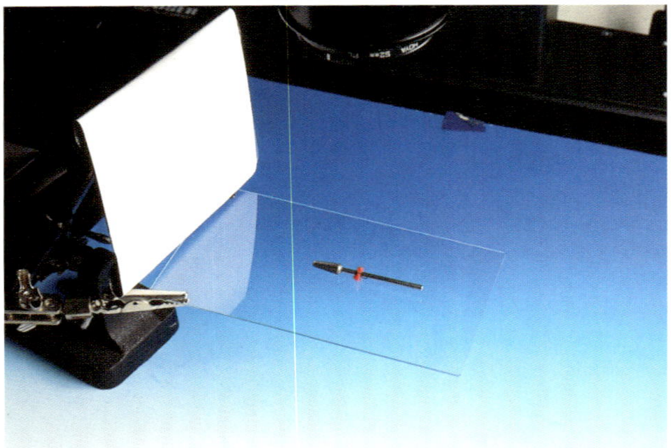

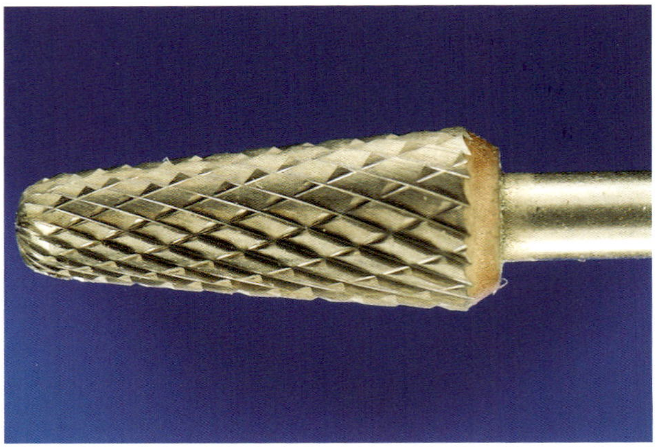

Fig. 5.22 Arrangement for a color background (a). The small field of view and the short exposure makes the background appear very dark and without gradation, although a graduated background was used (b).

this. In paintings of the Virgin Mary she was always clothed in a blue gown; the more "earthly" saints or their companions who were closer to us were always clothed in red. For the same reason it is best to avoid too many colors in an image in order not to overcharge the observer visually. This is especially obvious with title slides with a lot of colors, which quickly tire the viewer by making him or her focus on the various colors at various planes.

✓ The background color should not affect that of the object (Fig. 5.26). This is avoided by isolating the object and using a glass support which is about 10–15cm above the color background.

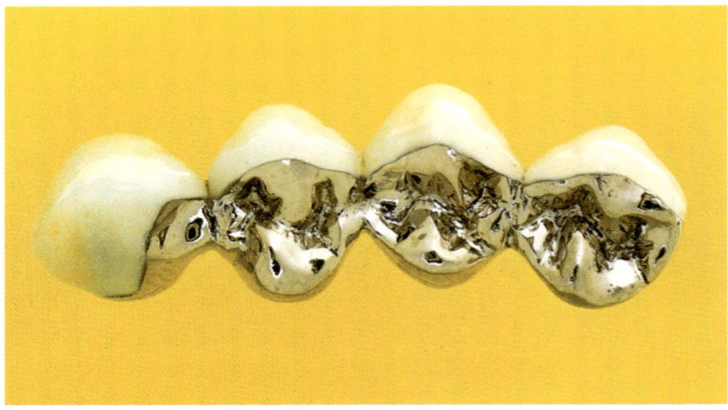

Fig. 5.23 Insufficient isolation of an object in front of a background with a similar color.

Other sensory physiological and psychological factors should also be considered. The phenomenon of simultaneous contrast makes an object on a brighter background appear darker than on a darker one (Fig. 5.27). In a slide series with varying background colors the successive contrast can lead to false color perception.

Another sensory physiological phenomenon makes brighter objects appear larger than darker ones. A woman's "small black number" makes her appear thinner than her other dresses (Fig. 5.28).

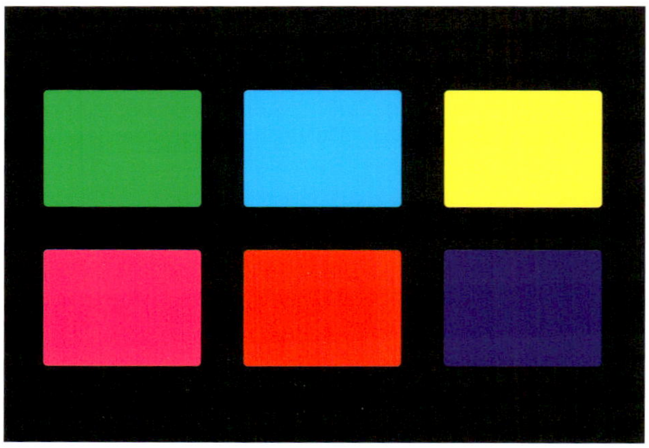

Fig. 5.24 Many color combinations appear harmonic, others are not harmonic and should be avoided. Generally the combination of blue and yellow is tolerable, but the complementary pairs of cyan-red and green-magenta are mostly felt not to be harmonic.

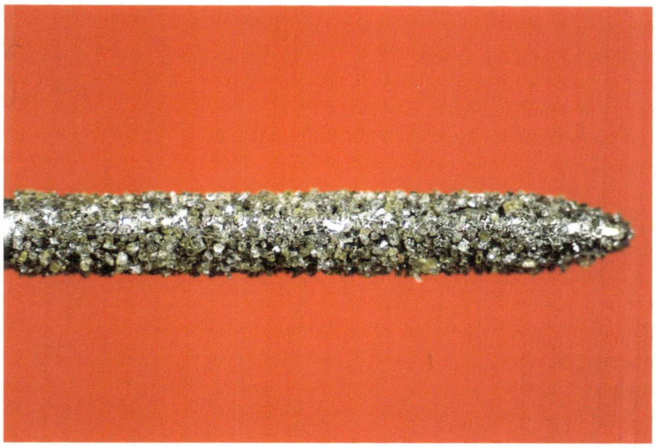

Fig. 5.25 Red is not a good background color, since visually it springs into the foreground.

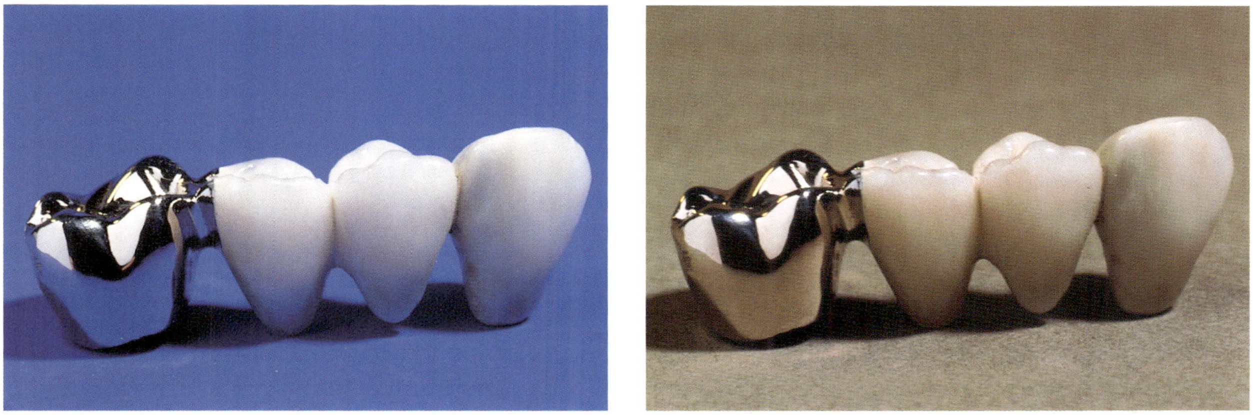

Fig. 5.26 If an object whose color is important is placed directly on a coloured background, its own color will be significantly changed (a,b).

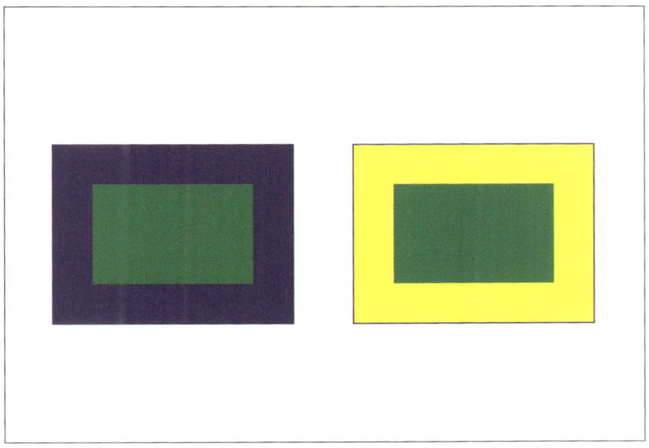

Fig. 5.27 Simultaneous contrast is a sensory physiological phenomenon which demonstrates that the color perception of an object is also influenced by the background color.

Fig. 5.28 Contrast in brightness: the band in the middle which is uniform gray not only appears to vary in brightness, but also in width.

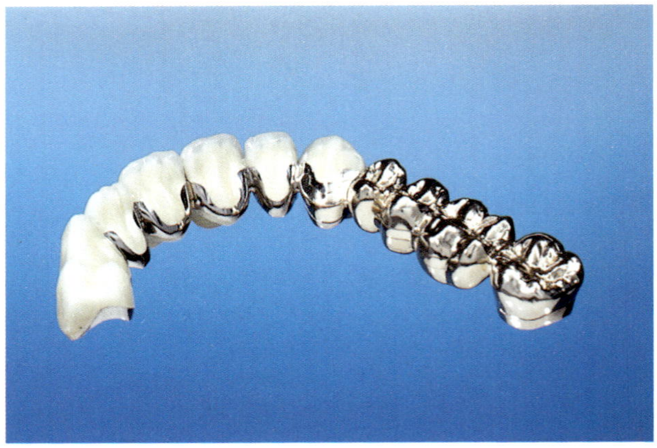

Fig. 5.29 Graduated backgrounds are pleasant to look at because they correspond to our everyday perceptions, for example, in the appearance of the sky.

If lighter and darker parts of an image are to have the same value optically, the brighter portion of the picture should take up one third of the image and the darker two thirds.

It is difficult to assess the emotional impact of an image since individual conditioning also plays a role. Red has strong impact and is attention getting (used for signals), blue is soothing, understated and sober.

Graduated backgrounds

Graduated backgrounds from one color to white or – less good – from one color to another avoid make objects appearing as if in a catalog. They give the image a certain depth. As a rule, the brighter part of the background is at the top and the darker at the bottom (Fig. 5.29).

Graduated backgrounds can be created through lighting, but it is easier to buy special graduated backgrounds from a photographic supplier. It is important to match the size of the card to that of the object. Photographing an individual crown against a 2 m long background does not make sense, since the blending occurs over the entire length and width of the card. In a small section of the image the blending is not at all evident.

5.3 Object Adequate Lighting

One of the most difficult tasks in dental photography is correctly lighting an object. The type of the light source and its direction must be carefully considered from various aspects. Light sources are divided into daylight and artificial light and the latter into flash and constant light sources.

Light can be either incident or back lighting. Incident lighting is either axial (e.g. by using a ringflash), oblique or texture lighting which clearly emphasizes the surface details of the object (Fig. 5.30). In general, lighting should be as simple as possible. As a rule, a single light source is sufficient. It should also be noted that the main light should come from above. Since in the course of our evolution we are accustomed to having light from above from the sun, the pattern of light and shadows give us an idea of the three dimensional quality of an object (Fig. 5.31). A rim of light on the upper part of the object and shadow underneath are perceived as a raised surface and the opposite as a depressed one. If this principle is ignored it can lead to irritating optical effects. An image of an impression if lit improperly can appear to be a dental cast and vice versa.

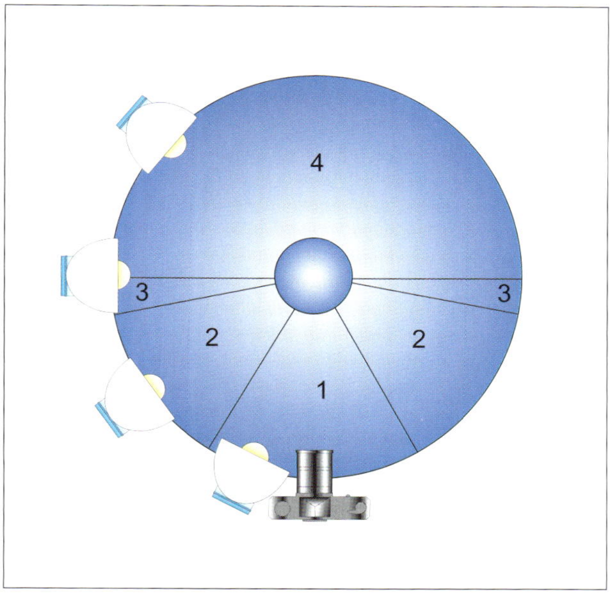

Fig. 5.30 Lighting is divided into axial front lighting (1), incident light (2), texture lighting (3) and back-lighting (4).

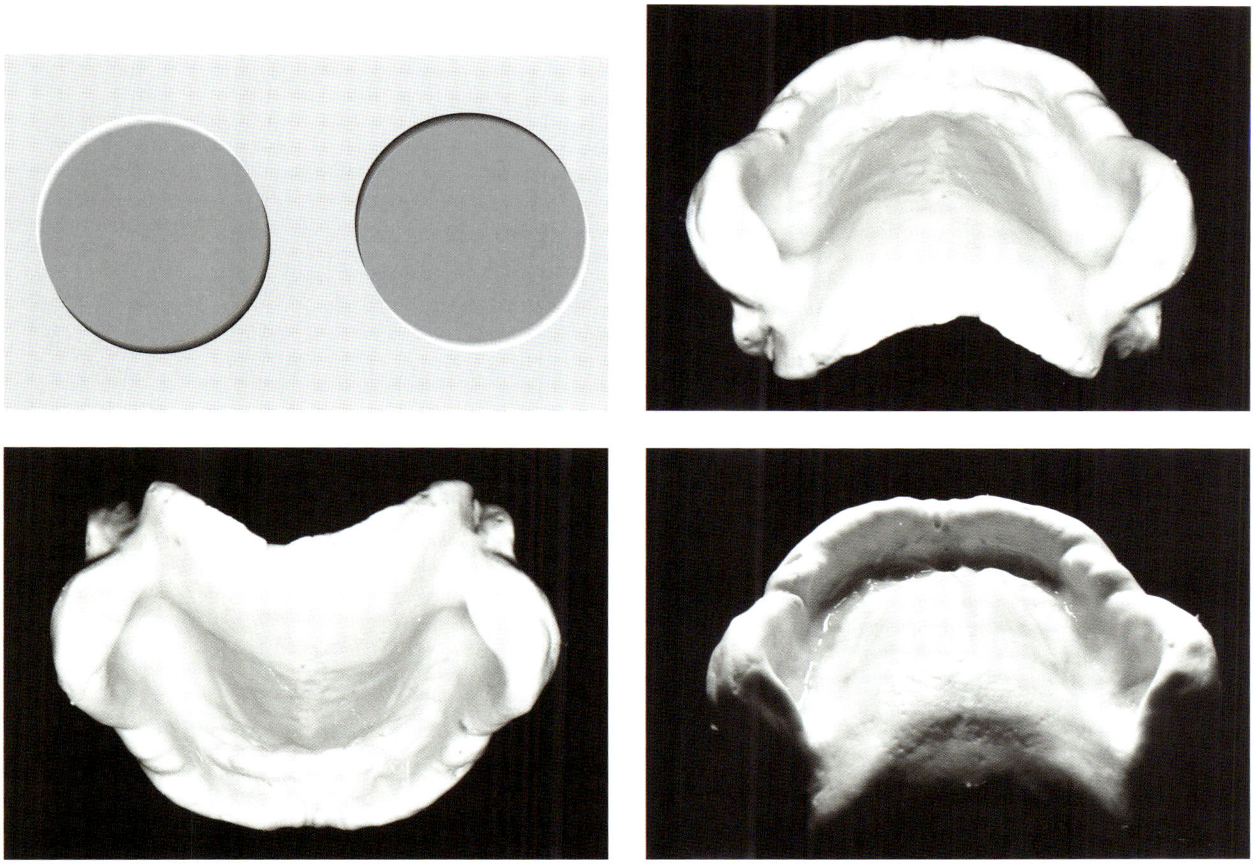

Fig. 5.31 The distribution of light and shadow edges influences our perception of depth. If the edge of the shadow is below and the light above, the object appears raised, otherwise as recessed (a). For this reason in photographs of impressions the recessed areas frequently appear as raised areas (b and c). Thus in object photography the light should always come from above (d) to create an image with correct rendering of the third dimension.

5.3.1 Types of lighting

Daylight-Northlight

Using daylight to light an object seems at first completely old-fashioned and insufficient. However, using daylight from a northern direction can achieve completely professional results without having to invest practically any money (Fig. 5.32). In the early days of photography many photographers had studios which had a series of north-facing windows and a window in the roof which faced north. The northerly direction avoided the sun shining in directly. For us, light from the north also has the most constant color temperature throughout the day and time of year and largely avoids color casts.

Photographing with light from the north is very simple. A work table is set up near a north-facing window. The light can be diffused by fixing drawing paper or a special diffusion foil to the window. The object is positioned, possibly isolated on a glass plate. The camera is placed on a tripod. The image is framed through the viewfinder and the aperture selected for the required depth of field (checked by using the depth of field preview button). Still checking through the viewfinder, the photographer illuminates the side of the object away from the light source using small reflectors (styrofoam from a hardware or home hobby store or reflectors from photographic suppliers). The shutter is tripped using a cable release to avoid camera vibrations. To begin with an exposure bracketing se-

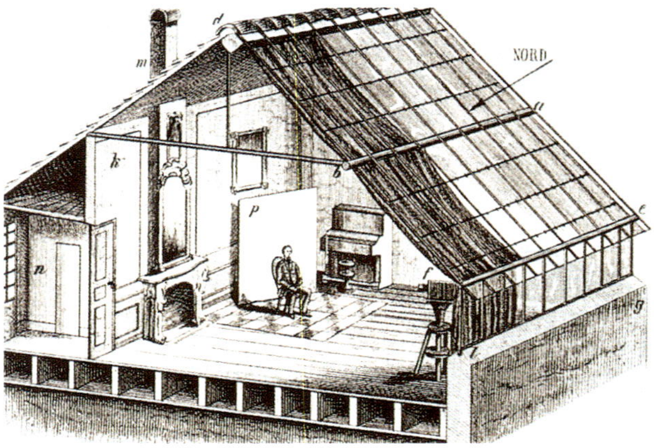

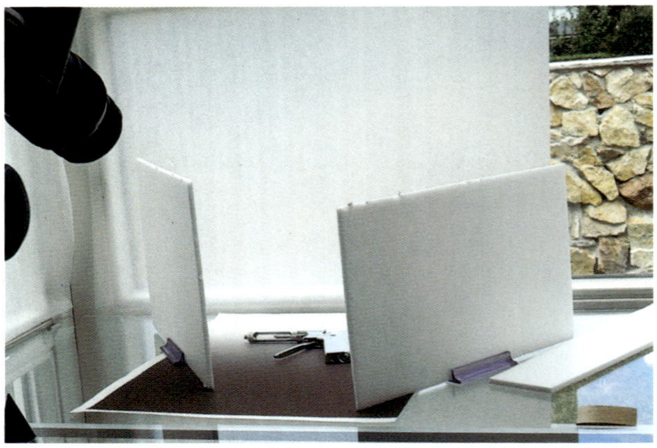

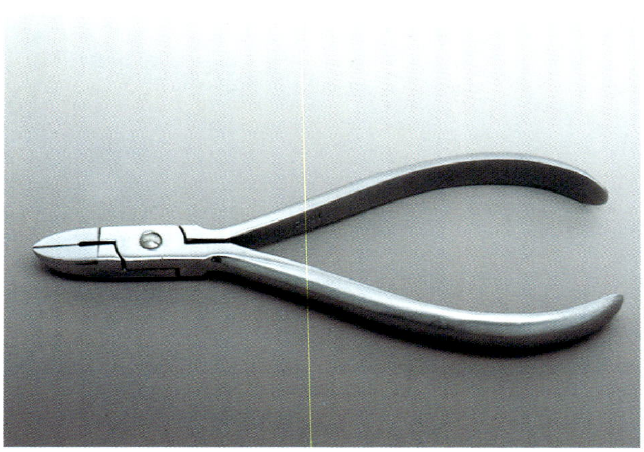

Fig. 5.32 Photography using north light. In the early history of photography photographers worked in north-facing studios (a). This prevented the sun shining in directly. A north-facing window is just as suitable for today's object photography (b). This ensures that the light has the most consistent color. With some experience the photographer can achieve fine results which do not reveal their simple set up (c).

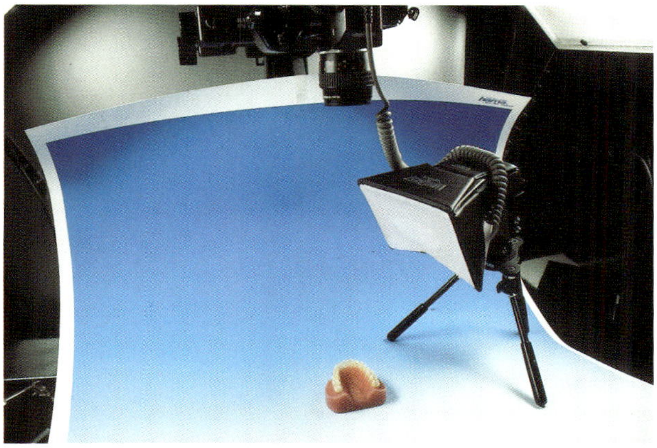

Fig. 5.33 If electronic flash is used for technical photography the beam of light should be spread by using a diffuser.

ries is useful, though later this is necessary only with objects which are difficult for exposure metering. With some practice this type of inexpensive lighting can achieve very good results.
This type of work can be improved by using a color temperature meter and corresponding filters.
A disadvantage of north lighting is dependency on daylight. In order to solve this problem artificial light must be used.

Artificial light

If a lot of object photography must be undertaken artificial light is more commonly used. This type of lighting is divided into flash lighting and constant light sources. Both can be used and have their advantages and disadvantages.

Electronic flash

Electronic flash is frequently used, as flashguns suitable for dental photography are available anyway (Fig. 5.33). Other advantages are the daylight character of the light (its color temperature is balanced for daylight film) and the short duration of the flash which eliminates the problem of camera shake. Electronic flashguns are compact, do not take up much room, and are available in a wide range of types.
A disadvantage of flashguns is that the effect of the light can not be assessed because of its short duration. The photographer must have a lot of experience to achieve the best possible distribution of light and shadow or make a lot of exposures to achieve a good image.

Studio flash

Professional flash units overcome this disadvantage of electronic flash by adding a constant light source to the flash tubes (Fig. 5.34). Using the viewfinder, the photographer can adjust the flash position until the desired light-shadow combination is created. The object is then photographed using flash. The flash output is ascertained in advance using a flash meter. Such studio flash units are available in a very wide range with many accessories which concentrate or diffuse the light. Purchase of such lighting units for dental photography is worthwhile only if they are frequently used.

Constant light

Constant light allows the photographer to assess the effect of the lighting and the distribution of light and shadow in the viewfinder before the exposure is made. The disadvantage of studio lights is their color temperature. Each source of light has a different color temperature. Daylight film, which is usually used in clinical photography, is balanced for daylight. Lights which have a color temperature of about 5500 degrees K to 6000 degrees K render color as we perceive it. Halogen light sources or electric light bulbs have a lower temperature and cause the image to have a red-yellow cast. Halogen tube lights create a definite green cast. To the human eye, these color changes are barely perceivable or not at all, since our brains make adjustments for color. If a person reads a book by a daylight balanced light and then switches on a lightbulb the paper appears yellowish only in the first few seconds. After a brief time the paper again looks as white as it did with the daylight balanced light.
If the color temperature of the light source is known a color conversion filter can be used in front of the

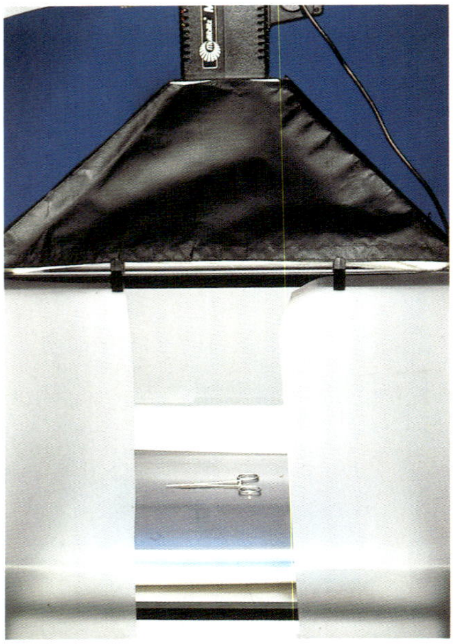

Fig. 5.34 Studio flash lights have a built-in constant light source which can be used as modeling lamp. This allows control of the distribution of light and shadow.

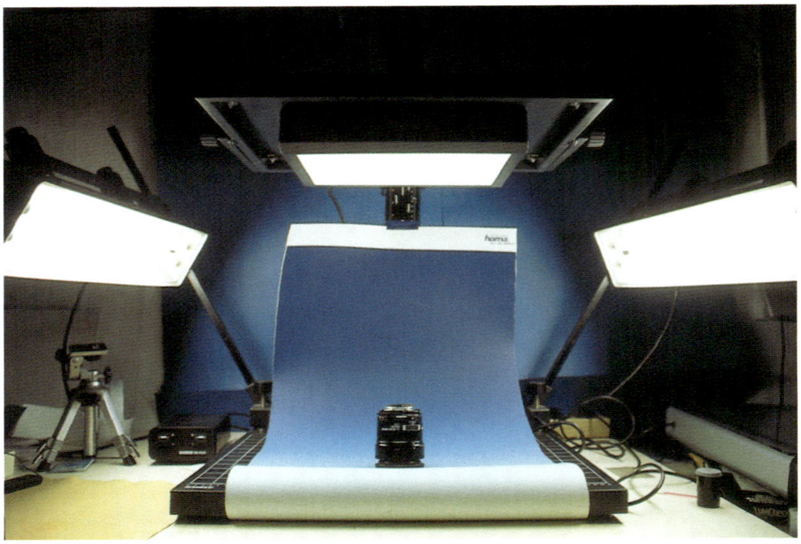

Fig. 5.35 Constant light sources such as the light banks and the light box mounted above allow the illumination to be checked in the viewfinder.

light source or the camera lens to change the color of the light. Another possibility is to use film balanced for artificial light which has an emulsion balanced for about 3200 degrees K.
If the color temperature of the light source is not known it can be determined using a color temperature meter.
For our purposes it is simpler to use a daylight balanced constant light source such as lights which are supplied for copy stands (Fig. 5.35). Light boxes which are used for examining slides can also be used for this purpose since they are generally daylight balanced.
Experience has shown that using daylight balanced light sources leads to more predictable results than using electronic flash, unless the photographer has had a great deal of practice.

5.3.2 Direction of light

The direction of light is also as important as the type of light source. Typical examples are given below which can be achieved with either constant light sources or electronic flash. The direction of the light is the main factor in the character of the image and the rendering of the object's surface.

Incident light

The most common practice is to light the object from above (Fig. 5.36). Generally this requires only one light source. Lighting an object symmetrically from the right and the left side leads to a flat appearance since the object is largely without shadows, giving very little information about the three dimensional nature of the object (Fig. 5.37).

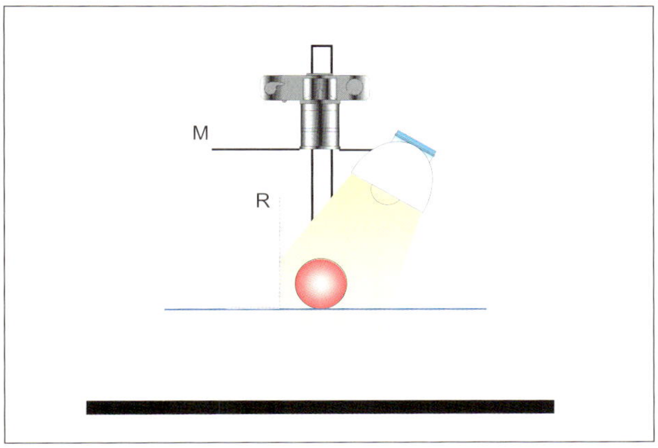

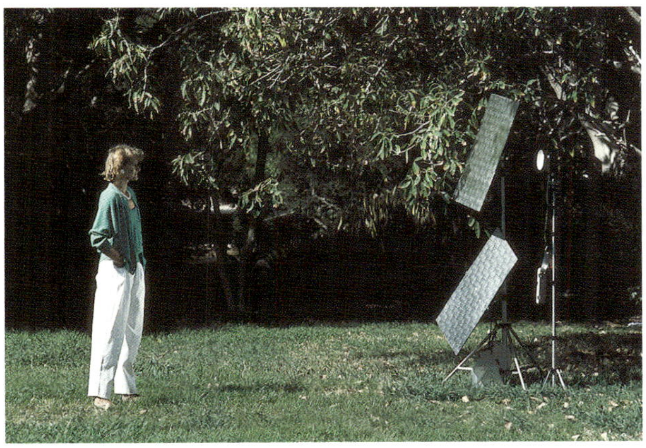

Fig. 5.36 Object photographs generally require only one light source. The unlighted side of the subject is illuminated by a reflector (R) (a). This principle is also used in professional photography (b).

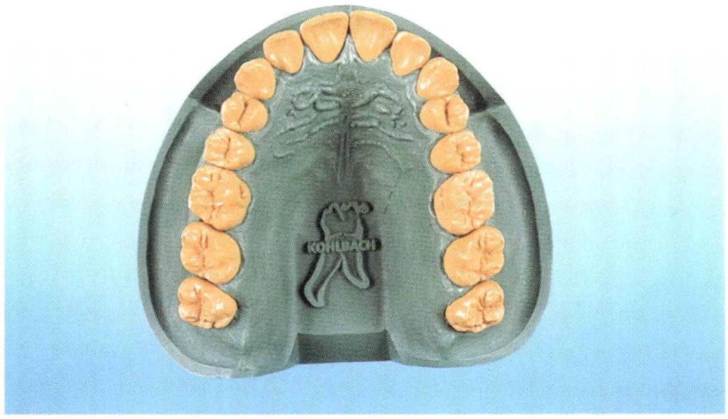

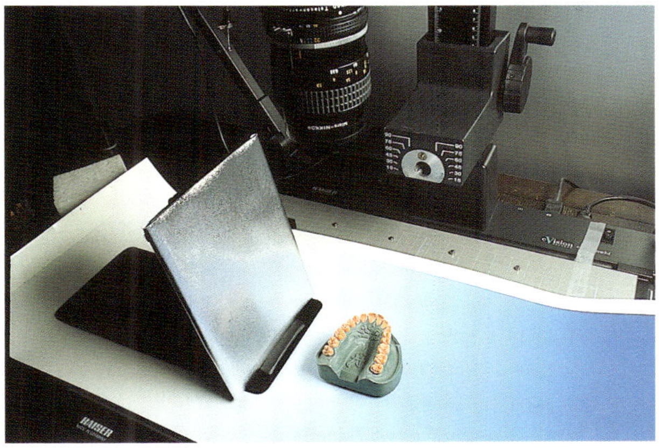

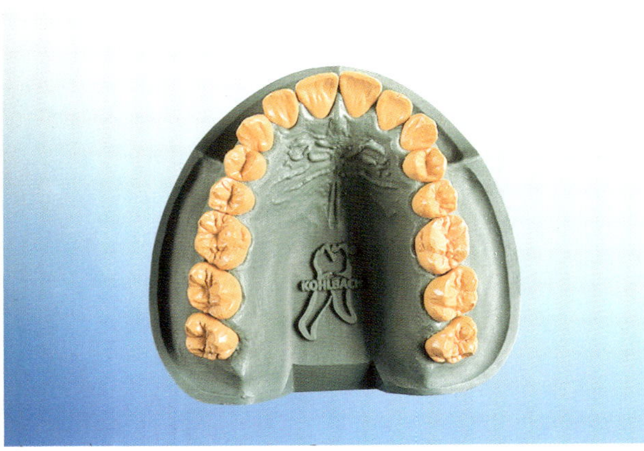

Fig. 5.37 Symmetrical lighting frequently results in images which are not sufficiently plastic (a). If a single light source and a reflector (b) are used the images appear more three dimensional (c).

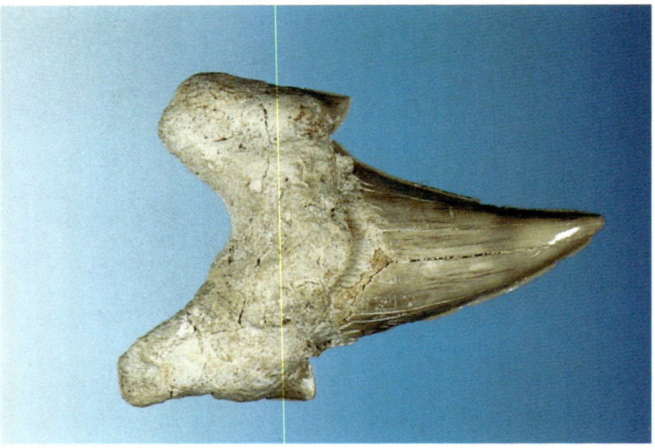

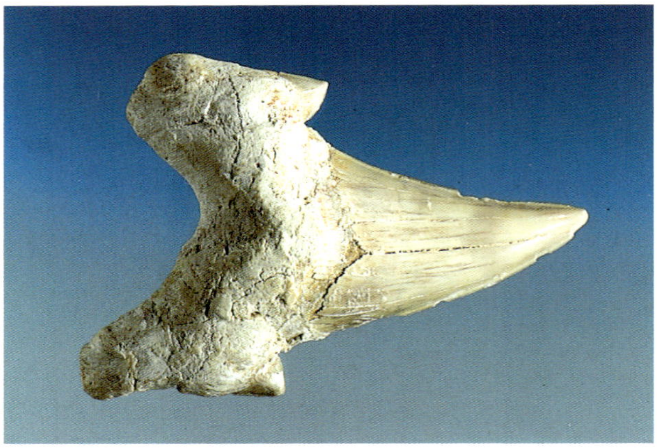

Fig. 5.38 Symmetrical lighting of a fossil using a copy stand (a). A better result is achieved using direct lighting with a reflector illuminating the shadow details (b).

Light falling from one side is supplemented by reflectors which illuminate the side of the object away from the light. Such reflectors can be obtained from photographic suppliers. Small styrofoam sheets are just as good for this purpose and less expensive; these can be positioned next to the object. If the sheets are moved closer to the object the light is intensified; if moved further away the image has more lighting contrast (Fig. 5.38).

Diffuser-reflector lighting

Using a point flash with a small reflector rarely achieves satisfactory results. To achieve pleasant lighting the size of the light emitting surface and the object should be in a good relation to each other (Fig. 5.39). A very small light source leads to harsh lighting with a lot of contrast and marked divisions between light and shadow. A typical example of this is illumination by the sun on a cloudless day which results in unflattering portraits for example. It is better when the emitting surface of the light source is increased, as is the case for example on an overcast day.

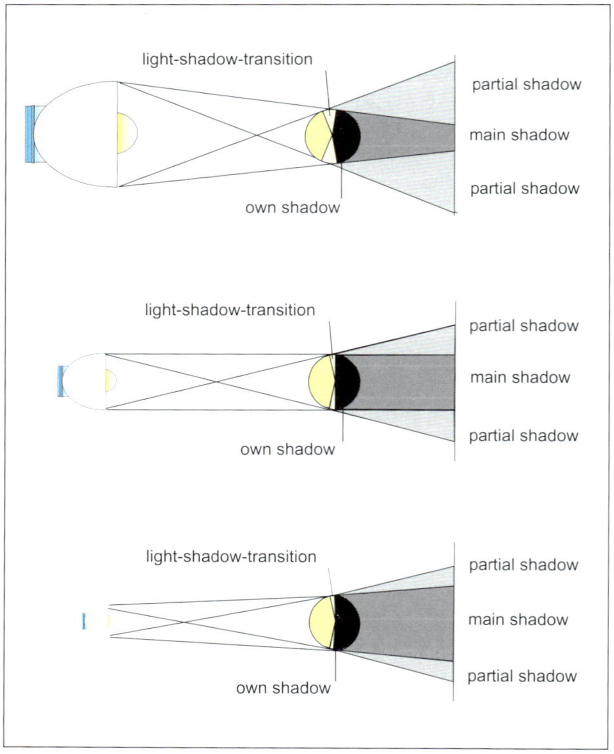

Fig. 5.39 The illuminating surface of a light source should be significantly greater than the object. Only in this way can soft transitions between light and shadow and pleasant lighting effects be created.

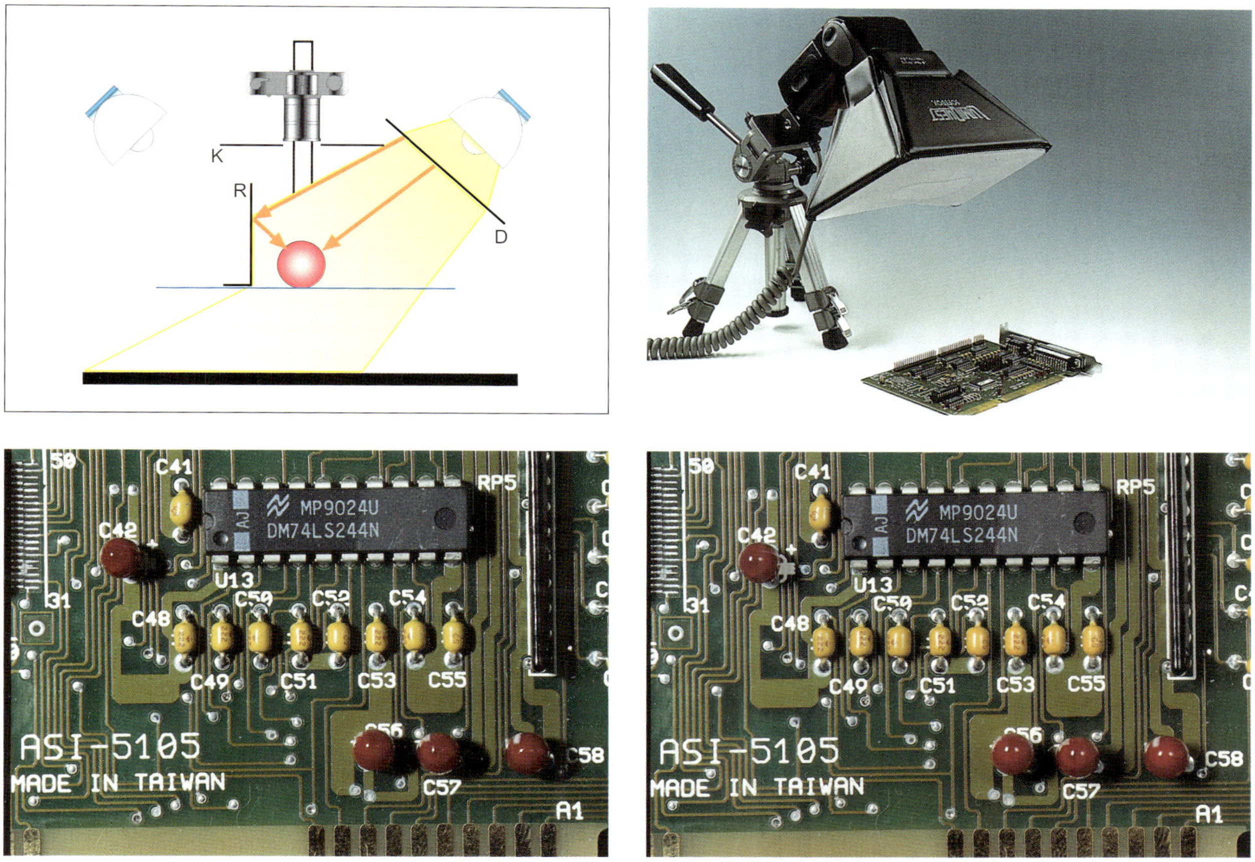

Fig. 5.40 Diagram of lighting using a diffuser and reflector which achieves the best results in technical photography (a). The light emitting surface of a flashgun can be increased using a soft box (b). This produces less harsh lighting (d), in contrast to the image made without using a soft box (c).

The emitting surface of the light can be increased by placing a diffuser, that is, a transparent medium which scatters light, in front of the light source (Fig. 5.40). Special diffuser gels and accessories for flash units (e.g. soft boxes) are designed for this.
Another way to increase the size of the illuminating surface is to use indirect flash or indirect lighting. The least expensive way of doing this is to fire the flash at a styrofoam sheet, but special umbrellas are also available.
Light banks and light boxes have very large illuminating surfaces; these generally have a "diffuser" in the form of an opal screen (Fig. 5.41).

If the size of the illuminating surface is increased and one or more reflectors are moved closer to the object it is possible to bathe the object in light and achieve the effect of a light tent.

Light tents

Objects made of highly polished metal and chrome instruments not only reflect the light source(s) but also their dark surroundings, as these are far removed. This creates very light highlights and practically black surfaces, making it difficult to assess the object's surface and its natural color. It is therefore advisable to photograph such highly reflective objects using a light tent (Fig. 5.42).

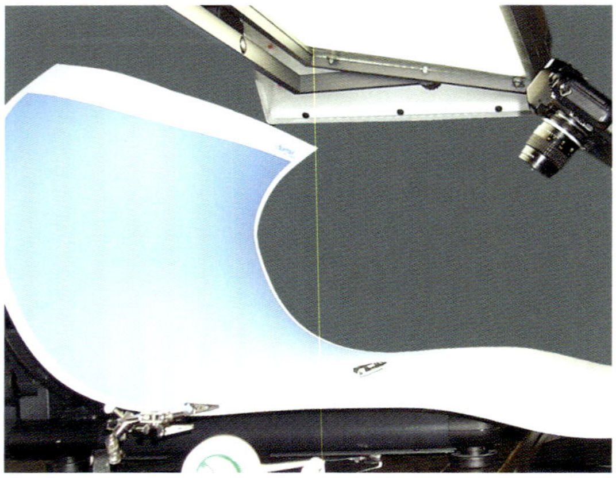

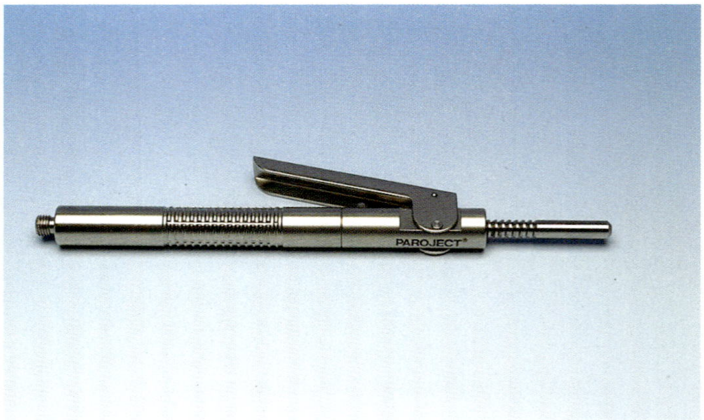

Fig. 5.41 A light box is ideal for incident lighting since it puts out a broad, soft light. Check to make sure it is daylight balanced (a). Images taken using this simple arrangement do not betray this simplicity (b).

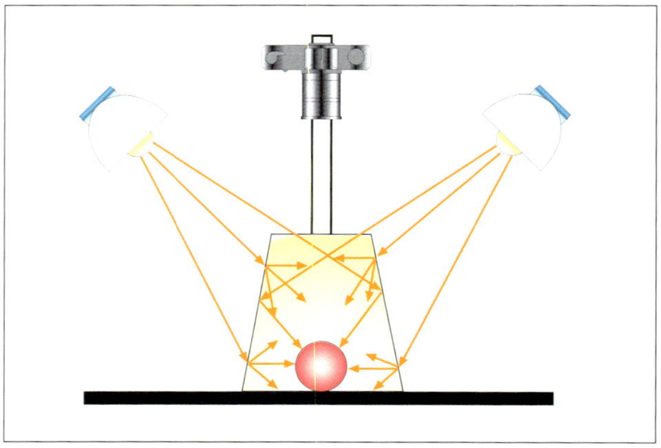

Fig. 5.42 A light tent surrounds the object from all sides and thus creates large, enclosed reflections.

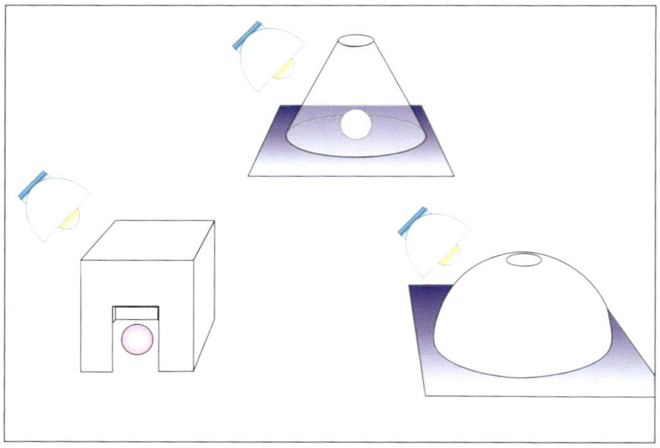

Fig. 5.43 Light tents can have many forms. In principle, they surround the object with a transparent medium and are generally lighted from outside.

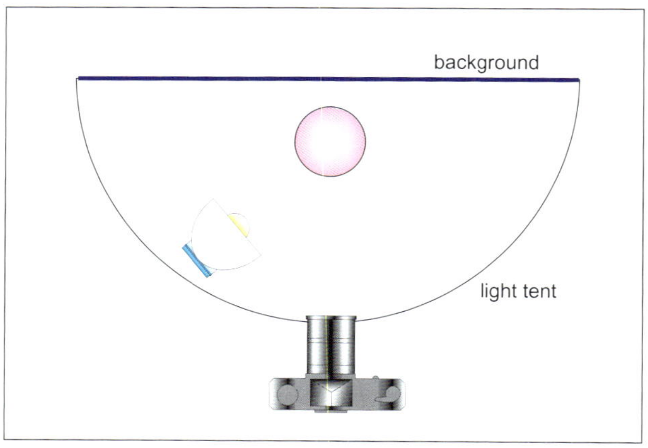

Fig. 5.44 A light source within the light tent provides more directional light.

Fig. 5.45 If direct light of a point flash is used to photograph an object the lighting is harsh (b). If the object is placed in a light tent and a flashgun is fired from outside (a), shiny objects are better lit and have much better color rendition (c)

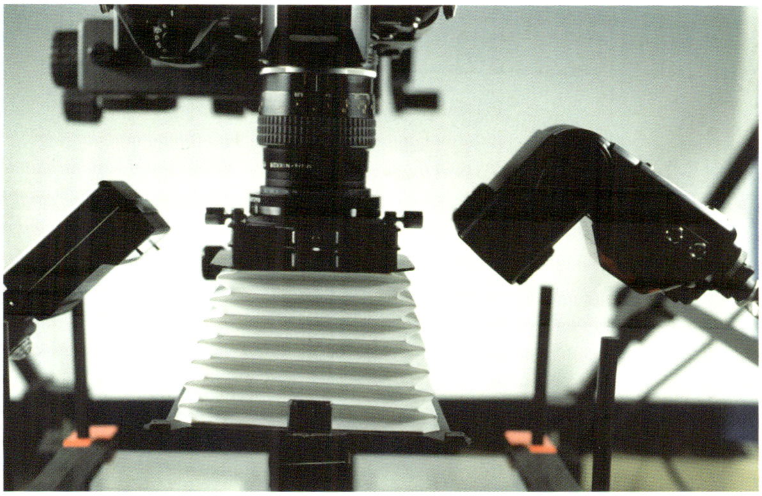

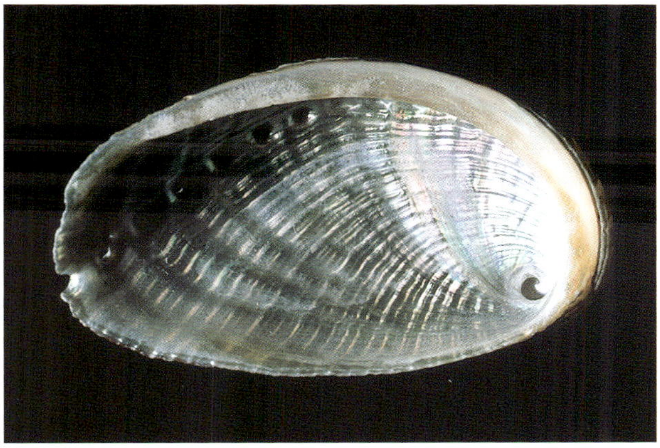

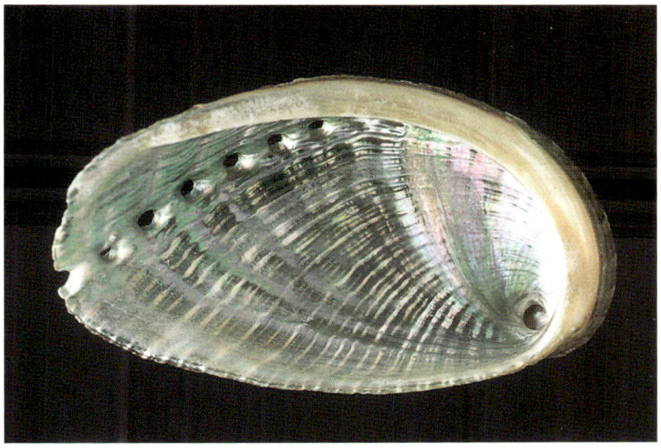

The combination of reflective and diffusing surfaces creates large reflections on the metal surface, leading to a better rendering of the object's surface.
Such light tents are sold by photographic suppliers in many types and sizes. With a little skill and talent for improvisation however, the photographer can build her or his own light tent from materials available from hardware stores. All light tents are principally cylindrical, conical, cubic or semi-round forms which can be made of transparent paper or other transparent materials. Plastic drinking cups with the bottom removed or white silk which is intended for silk screening can be used. The photographer is limited only by his or her imagination. Conical and cylindrical paper shapes have proven themselves; these can be made in different sizes for different reproduction ratios. Since light tents create not only large, enclosed reflective areas but also lighting which is practically without shadows, the objects can often be placed directly on a photo cardboard without creating irritating shadows.
If the object needs sharper contours a black piece of cardboard can be glued in the transparent cylinder; its reflection falls on the surface of the object as a shadow, or a light source can be positioned in the light tent (Fig. 5.44)
Using a dulling spray is another possibility to improve the appearance of highly polished metal surfaces.
Figures 5.45–5.52 show a step by step demonstration of how to photograph a highly reflective object. The prototype of the Kaiser TopTable system was used.

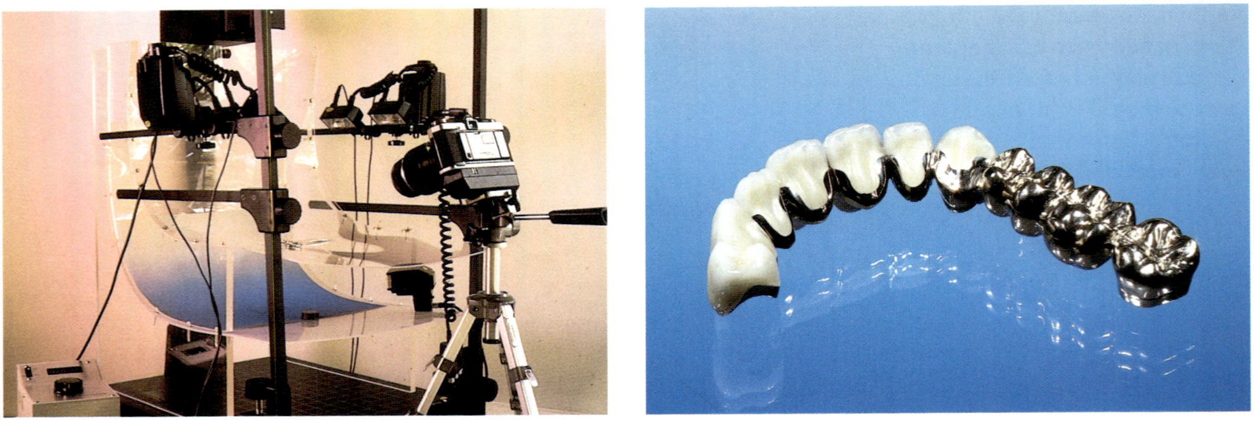

Fig. 5.46 Set up for photography using the prototype of the Kaiser TopTable system. The object is photographed using direct flash (a). Result: poor rendition of the metal surfaces due to black areas and highlights. Disturbing reflections from the object on the Plexiglas plate (b).

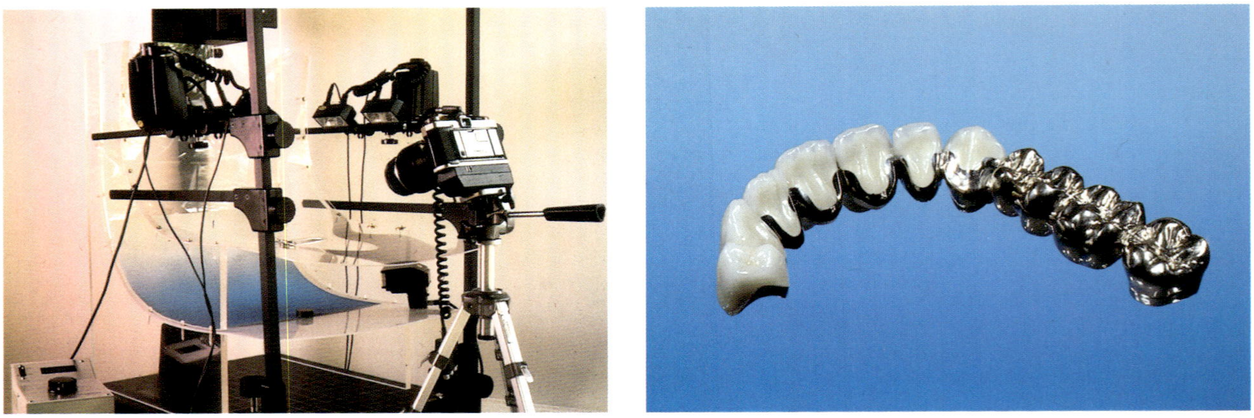

Fig. 5.47 A polarizing filter is placed in front of the lens (a), eliminating the reflections from the object (b).

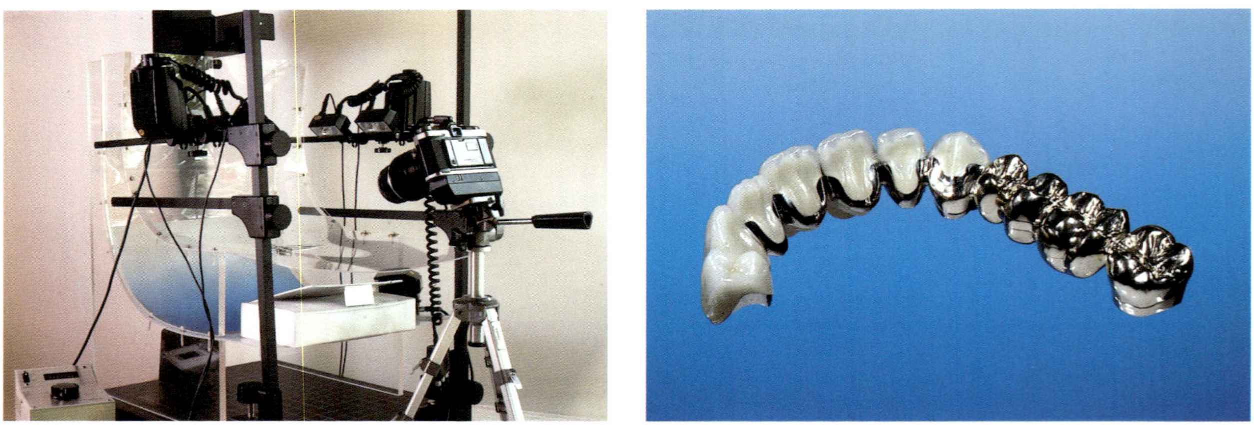

Fig. 5.48 A reflector is positioned below (a), lighting the lower part of the metal (b).

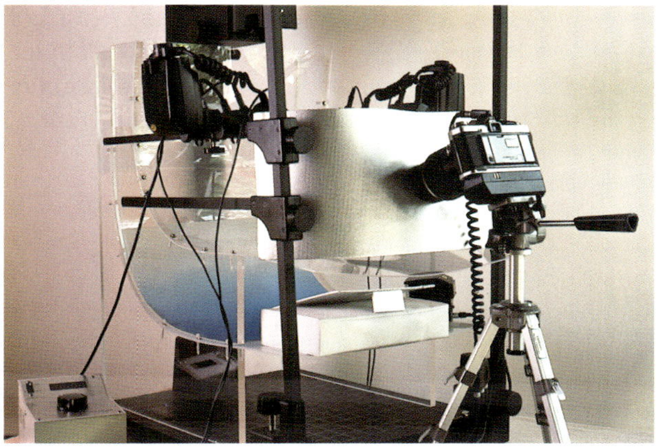

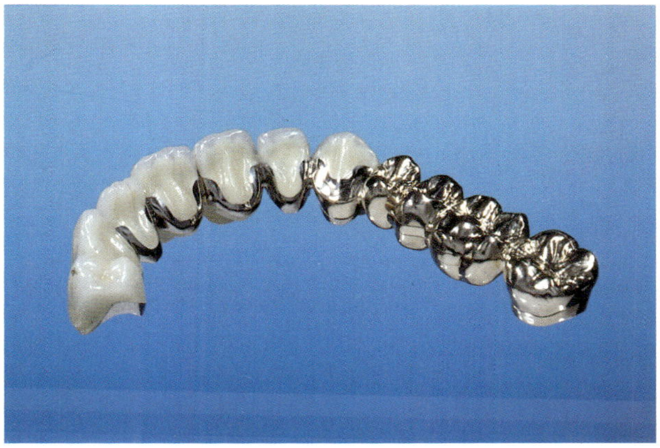

Fig. 5.49 A styrofoam reflector is placed in front of the camera with an opening for the lens (a). Metal surface now brighter (b).

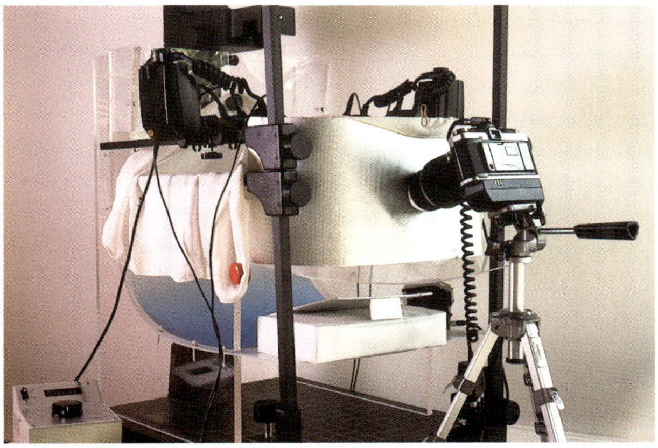

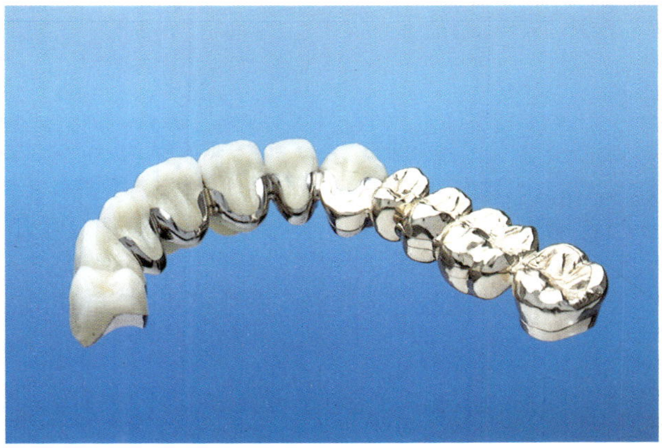

Fig. 5.50 Silk cloths also placed over the light sources (a) which achieves very soft lighting of the object (b).

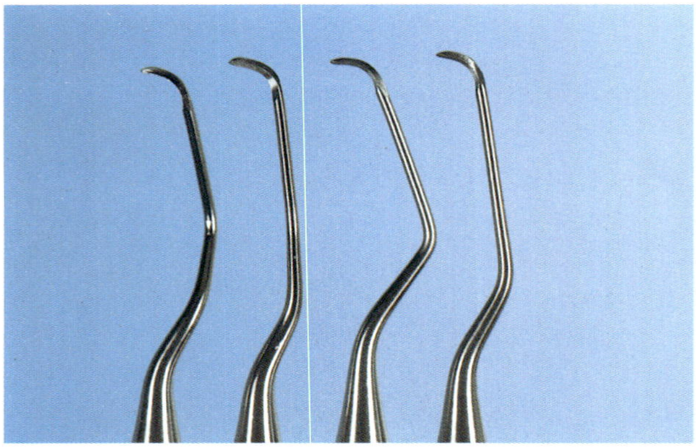

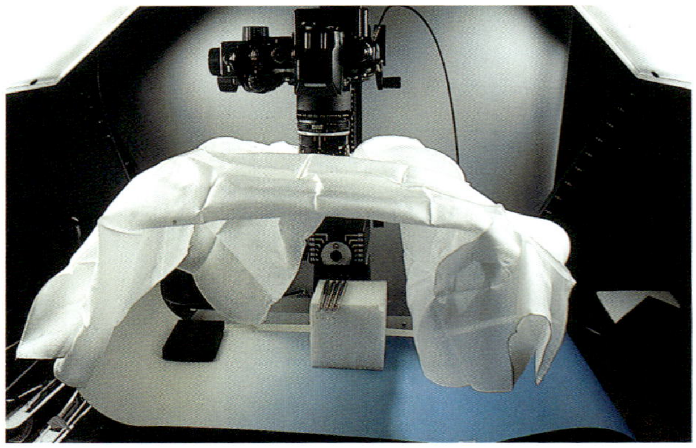

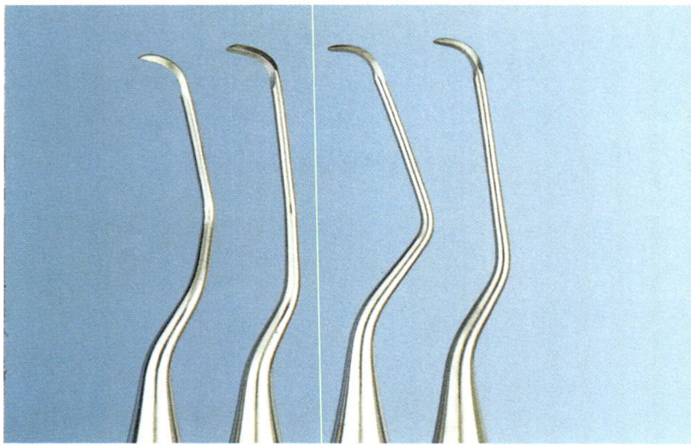

Fig. 5.51 Curettes lit by two light banks (a), set up of a simple light tent (b) and the result of photographing using the light tent (c).

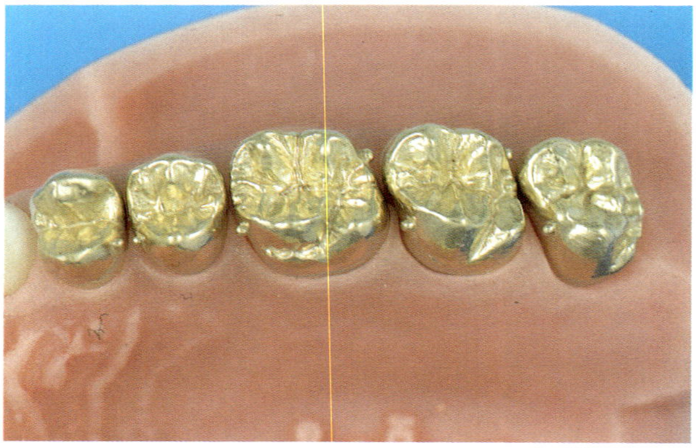

Fig. 5.52 Sometimes the illumination using a light tent is too "soft" (a). In these instances a simple reflector (b) can be used to improve results (c).

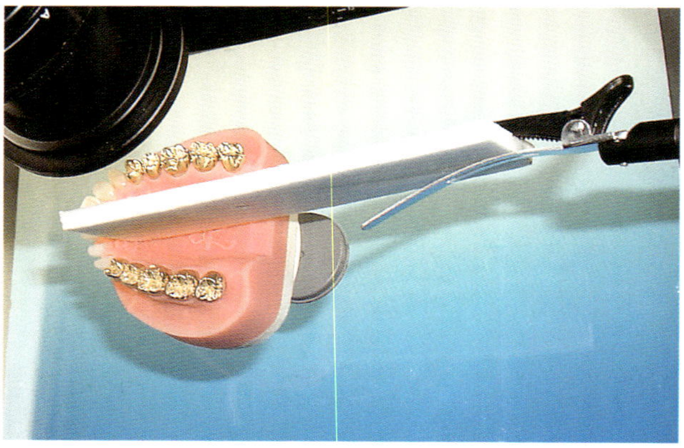

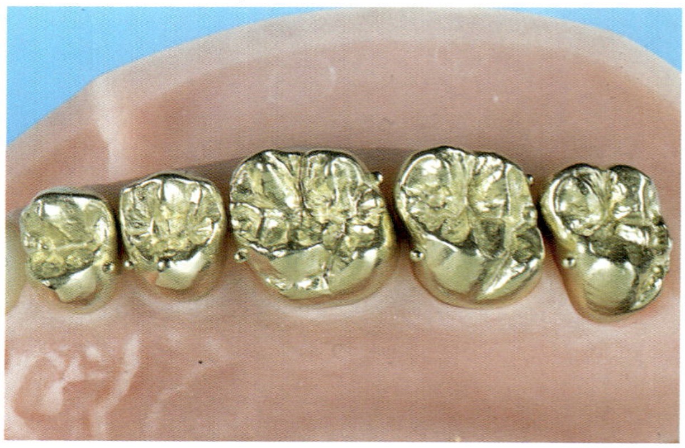

Especially for lighting coins it is recommended that a thin glass plate should be placed 45 degrees to the optical axis and photographed through. The glass plate is lit from the side and part of the light is directed vertically off its surface onto the coin.

Rendering surfaces of small objects

A photographer trying to recreate the morphology of a tooth's surface in a light tent soon discovers that this is possible only to a limited extent, since there is not much contrast on the predominantly white occlusal surface. To do this, a flat, directed light (texture lighting) is required in order to show the surface morphology by creating shadows. Various manufacturers produce fiber optic light sources for this purpose (Fig. 5.53 and 5.54). The most important qualities to look for in this type of equipment is the rigidity of the light conducting arms, the variety of accessories and the ability to change the color temperature of the integrated halogen light source permanently by using a blue filter in front of it. One recommended system is the fiber optic light source from Novoflex; its light arms are positioned on the top and thus their position is easily retained. This system not only has color and polarizing filters which are placed in front of the light emitting arms, but also a slot in which a conversion filter can be left long-term. An electronic flash system can be used in place of the halogen light source; its flash can be directed into the light pipes through a mirror system. This arrangement allows moving objects to be photographed.
Very creative solutions for lighting, especially of very small objects, can be achieved in this manner (Fig. 5.55–5.57).

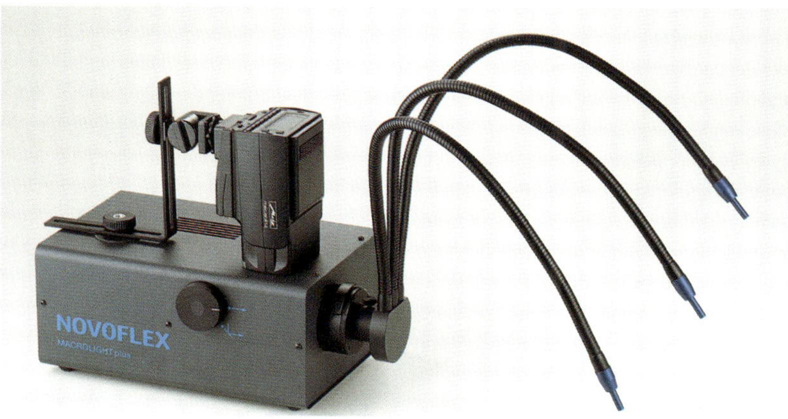

Fig. 5.53 Novoflex Cold Light Source Macrolight Plus (Photo: Novoflex).

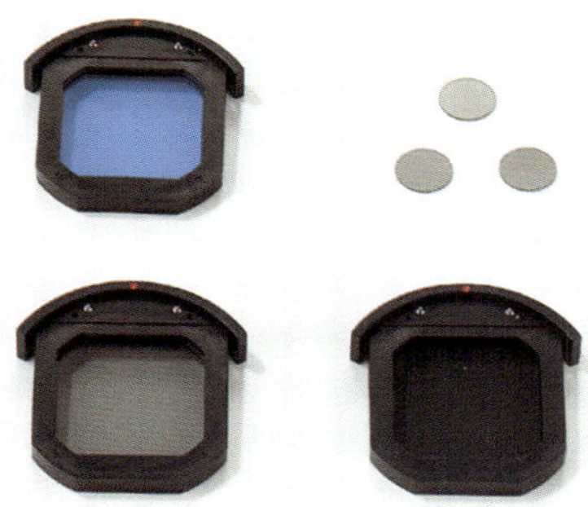

Fig. 5.54 A blue filter can be placed in front of the light source to provide daylight balanced light. Light output can be reduced if necessary by using a gray filter (Photo: Novoflex).

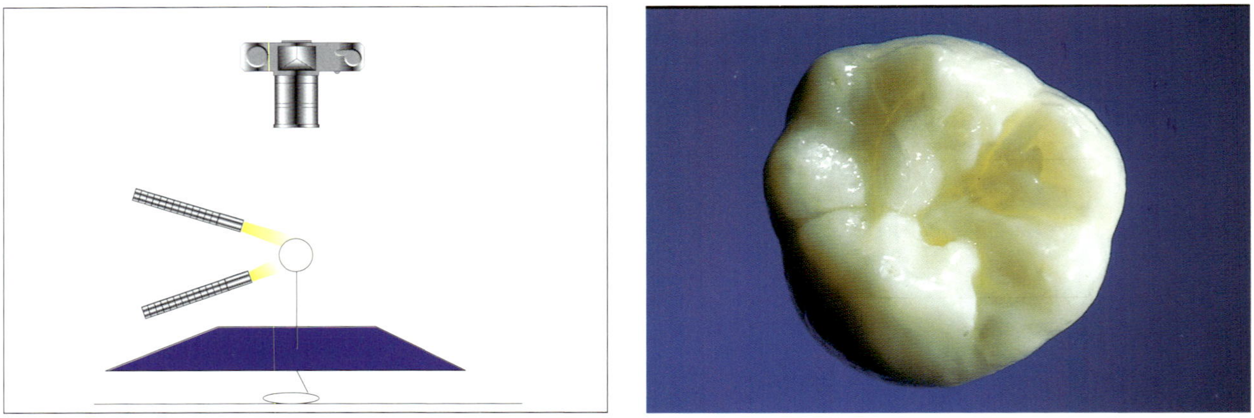

Fig. 5.55 Fiber optic light sources permit individual and creative lighting effects using only one piece of equipment. Arrangement of fiber optic light sources (a) and the result (b)

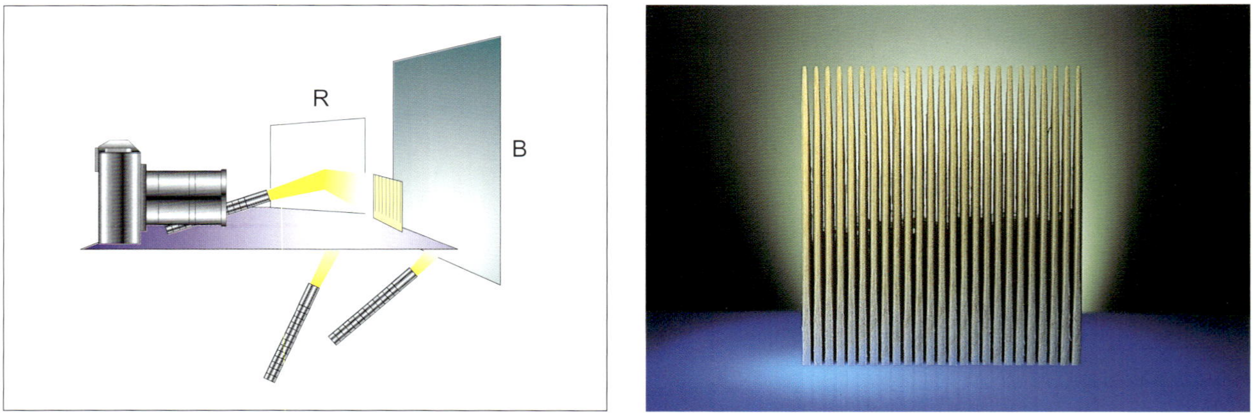

Fig. 5.56 This image too does not reveal the secret of its simple set up. Diagram of the fiber optic light sources (a) and result (b).

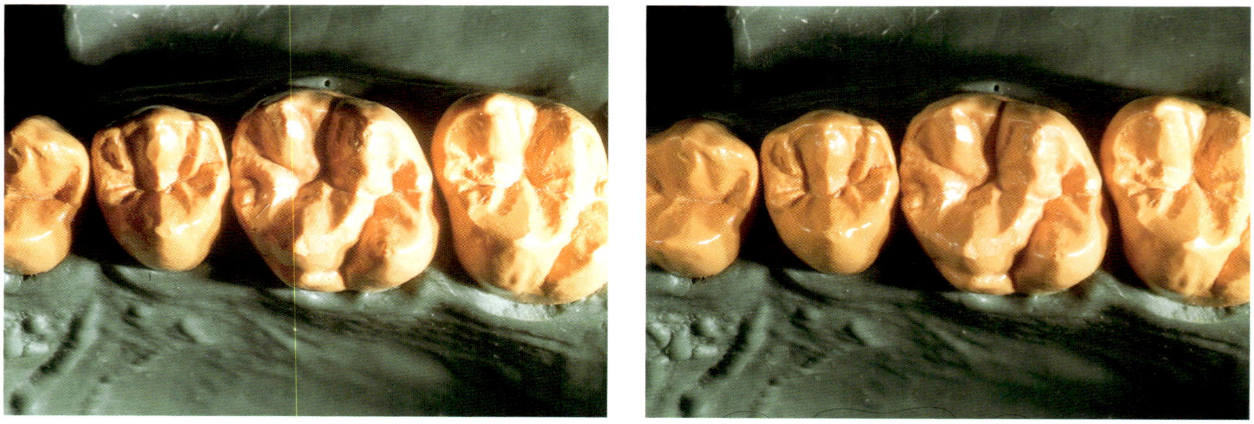

Fig. 5.57 Due to the small opening the light from a fiber optic light source is too harsh for larger objects (a). Better results can be obtained by adding a reflector (b).

Transmitted lighting

When the light source is positioned behind an object we call this transmitted lighting; this is naturally useful for (semi-)transparent objects.
As in microscopy we use the term bright field illumination when the object's surroundings appear bright. If they are dark or black, they are termed dark field illumination.

Bright field illumination

In this instance the light source is in back of or below the object within the camera's field of view. This light, coming from behind or below, passes through the object and the light which passes the object to the side creates the brightness around the object (Fig. 5.58). This allows transparent or partially transparent objects to be photographed.
To avoid flare and unnecessary loss of brilliance due to the dispersed light falling on the lens the area surrounding the camera's field of view should be covered with black cardboard (masking).
A plus exposure correction should be used when photographing an object with a white background in order to achieve correct exposure (Fig. 5.59).

Dark field illumination

In this case the light source, for example, a light box, is behind or under the object, however, its surface, about the size of the camera's field of view, is covered with black cardboard so that it is opaque (Fig. 5.60). The object itself is about 10cm in front of or above the light source. This allows the light rays from the light source to strike and illuminate the object (Fig. 5.61). This type of illumination achieves striking effects. Objects with partially transparent surface structures are particularly suitable for this and show up very clearly against a black background. Minus corrections of exposure must be made to avoid overexposure, depending on the size of the object's surface in relation to the frame.
Glass supports must be free of dust and dirt when used to photograph objects in isolation, since dust particles also light up in the dark field and make the image unusable (Fig. 5.62).

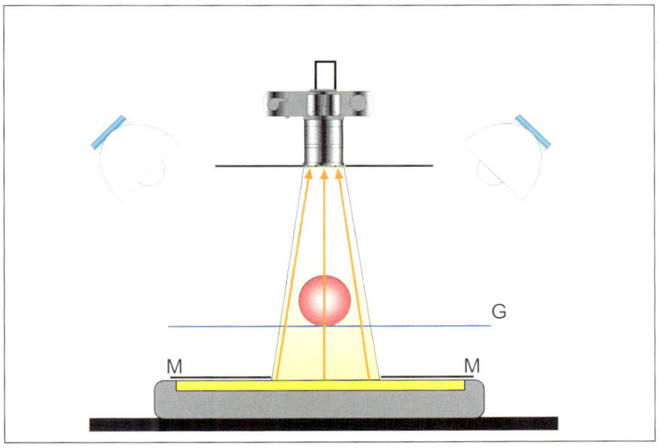

Fig. 5.58 Diagram of a transmitted light arrangement (bright field illumination). The object is placed on a glass support (G) and is illuminated from beneath. The light box outside of the camera's view is masked off with black cardboard (M) to prevent stray light from entering the lens.

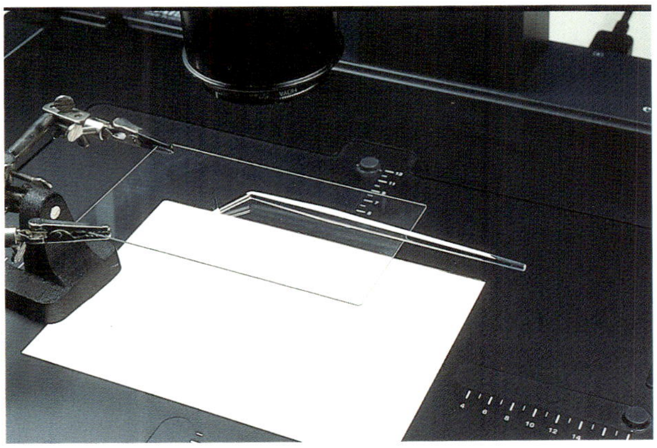

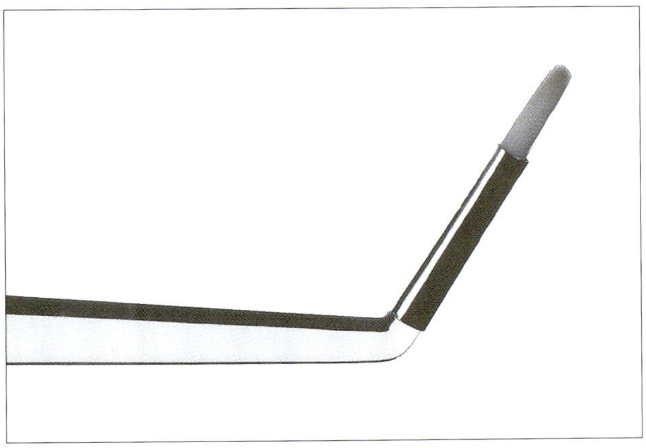

Fig. 5.59 A simple arrangement for a bright field illumination photo (a) and the result (b).

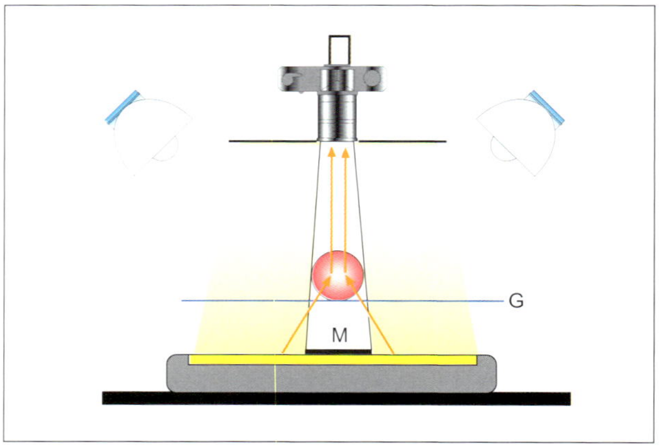

Fig. 5.60 Schematic of a dark field illumination. The background of the object is covered using an opaque mask (M). The object is lighted by the light surrounding the mask.

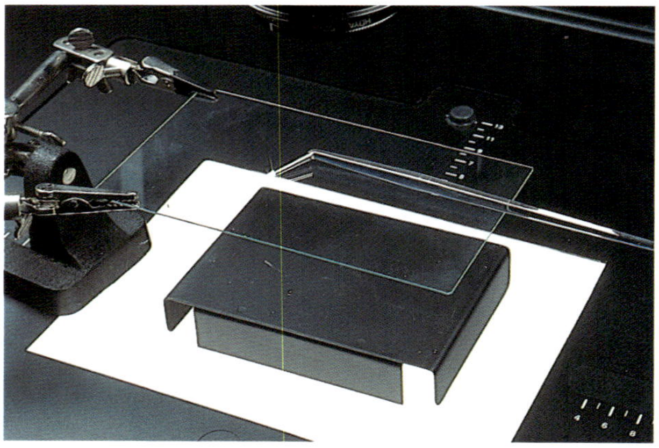

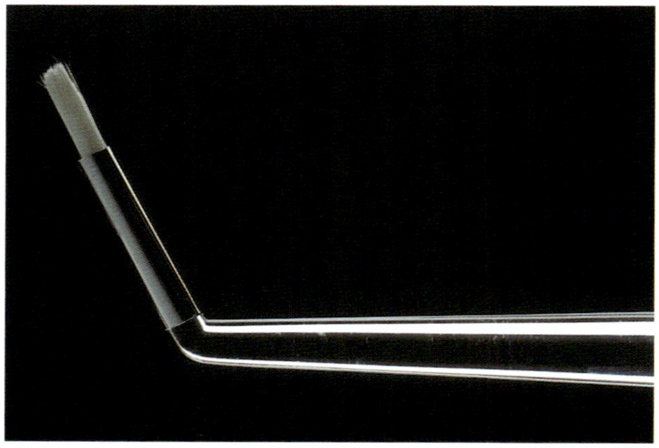

Fig. 5.61 Set-up for a dark field illumination photo (a) and the result (b).

The room should be darkened to improve the visability of the dust particles to be removed. Once the photographer's eyes have become adjusted to the dark, he or she can use the depth of field preview button to check for dust and remove it with a small brush or cotton tip. A minus correction is required for dark field illumination to achieve a truly black background (Fig. 5.63–5.65).

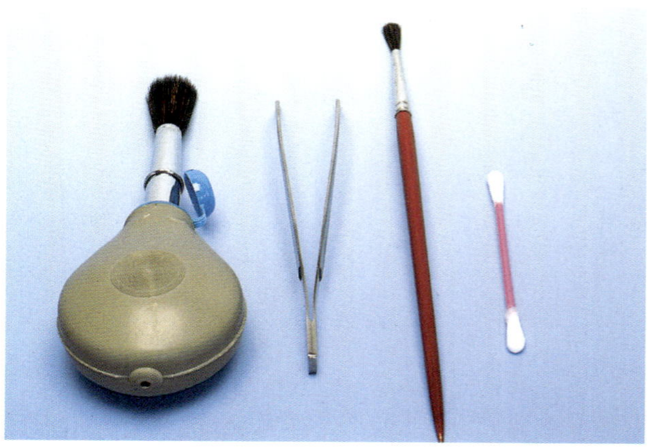

Fig. 5.62 Small tools helpful in cleaning off dust particles for dark field illumination photos.

Photographing with polarized transmitted light

This type of lighting, which is very easy to achieve, results not only in very impressive images, but also allows the background brightness to be infinitely varied. A polarizing filter sheet is placed in front of the light source and the second polarizing filter on the camera lens (Fig. 5.66 from 5.67). The light

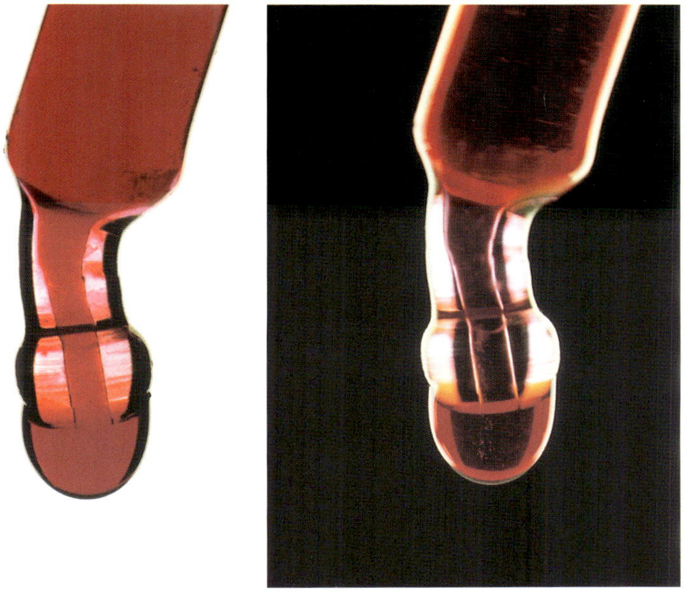

Fig. 5.63 Transparent objects appear differently in bright-field illumination photos (a) and dark field illumination photos (b).

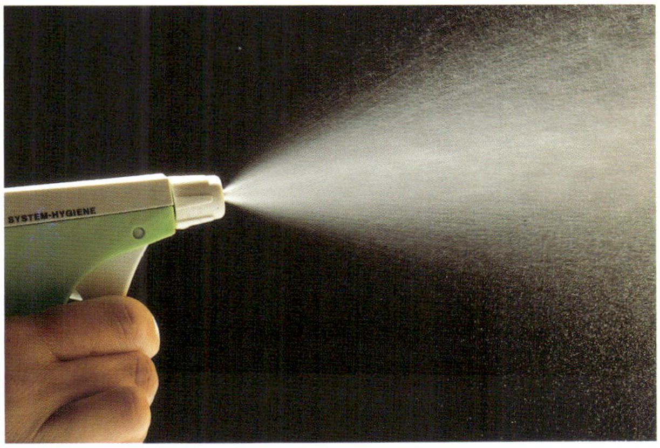

Fig. 5.64 Very fine structures such as these spray droplets are illuminated in dark field technique. The spray would not be visible in a bright field illumination photograph.

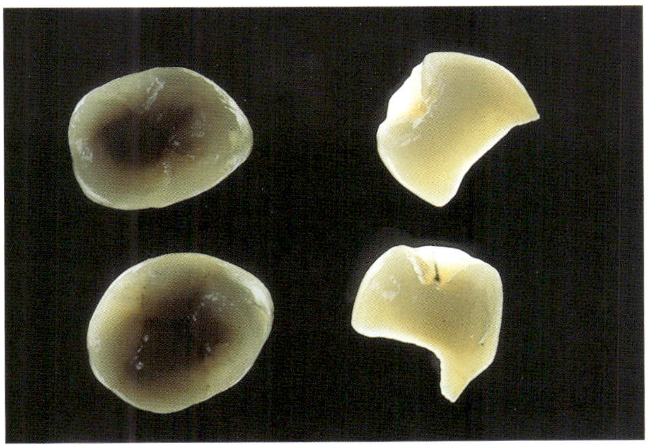

Fig. 5.65 Dark field illumination photo to illustrate the varying transparency of metal ceramic crowns (left) and Procera crowns (right in photo).

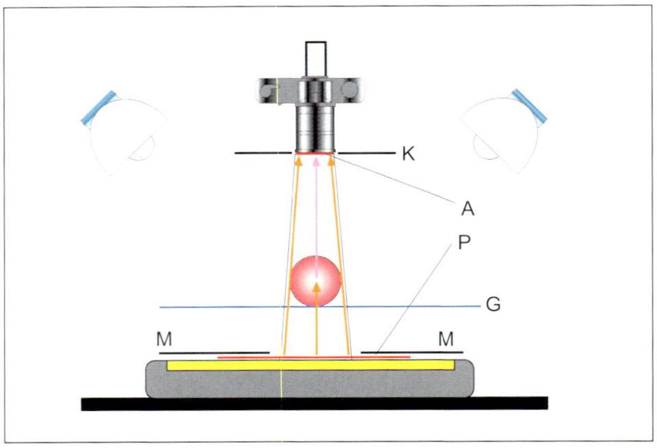

Fig. 5.66 Polarized transmitted light creates interesting effects. A polarizing filter (called a polarisator = P) is placed on the light box; the second one, the analyser is fitted on the lens (A).

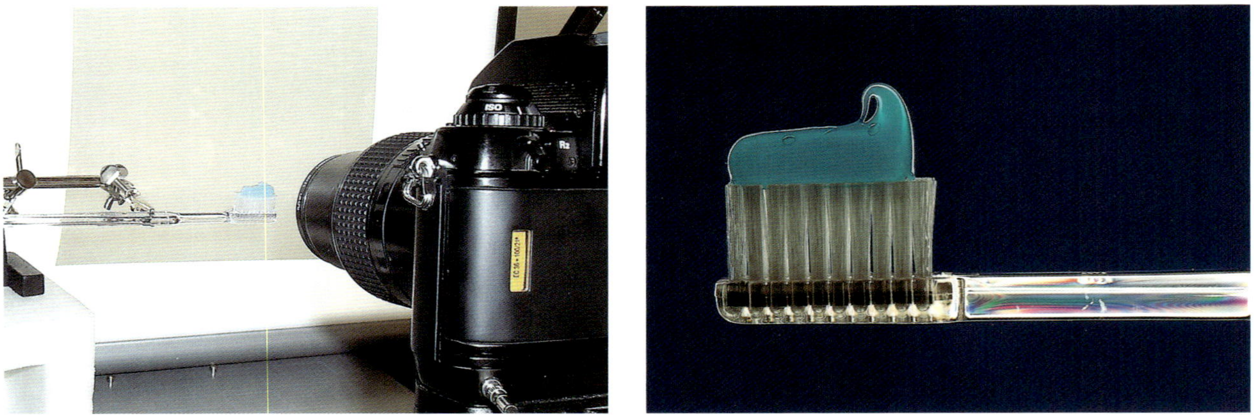

Fig. 5.67 Photographing horizontally using polarized transmitted light (a). A polarizing sheet has been fixed to a light box stood vertically. A second polarizing filter is fitted to the lens. If both polarizing filters are adjusted nearly completely perpendicular the background appears dark blue (b).

falling in the direction of the camera is polarized by the polarizing filter. The photographer rotates the second polarizing filter on the camera lens while checking in the viewfinder. If the polarizing axes of the two filters are perpendicular to each other all the light is cut off. However, the direction of the vibrations of the light passing through the object are altered and are thus not blocked completely by the polarizing filter on the camera lens. The result is that the object appears in its natural colors in front of a background which appears to be bright, gray, blue or black, depending how the filter is rotated (Fig. 5.68).
Materials which are double refractive appear in all colors of the rainbow in polarized transmitted light. Sections of teeth, for instance, can be photographed very impressive in this manner (Fig. 5.69). Inner stresses of plastic objects can also be shown when they are photographed using two crossed polarizing filters, which are known in photoelastic strain analysis as the polarizer and analyser. The molecular formations occurring under mechanical stress cause varying degrees of shifts in the main vibration direction of the polarized light and the analyser thus blocks the light to varying degrees. The result is a rainbow of colors within the object; their arrangement gives some information about the stress peaks (Fig. 5.70). In this way, for example, implant forms were studied in order to investigate the load of bone.

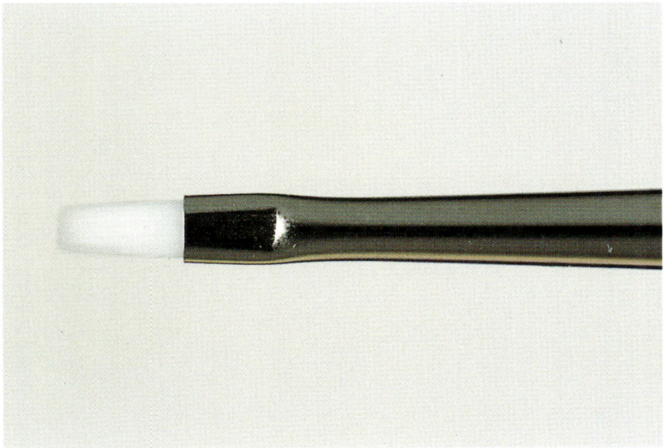

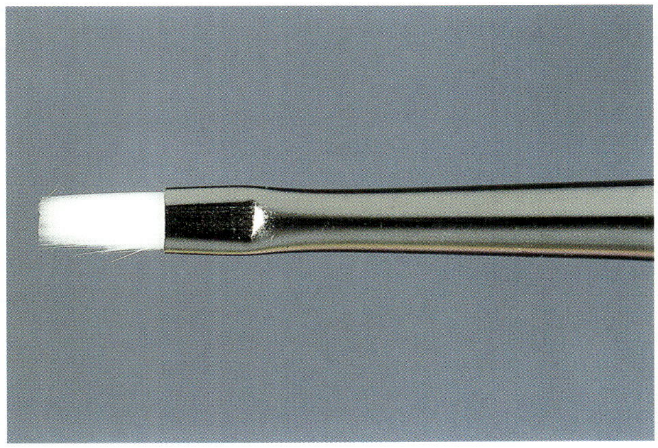

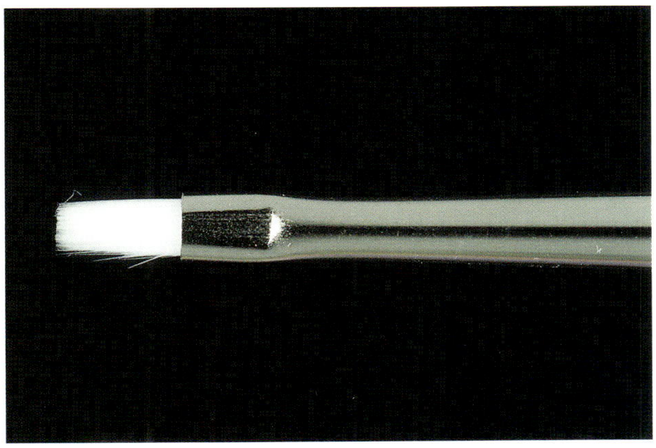

Fig. 5.68 The brightness of a background can be infinitely adjusted by using polarized transmitted lighting. The brightness varies in accordance with the adjustment of the filter on the camera (a-c). The surface of the object was additionally lit from the top.

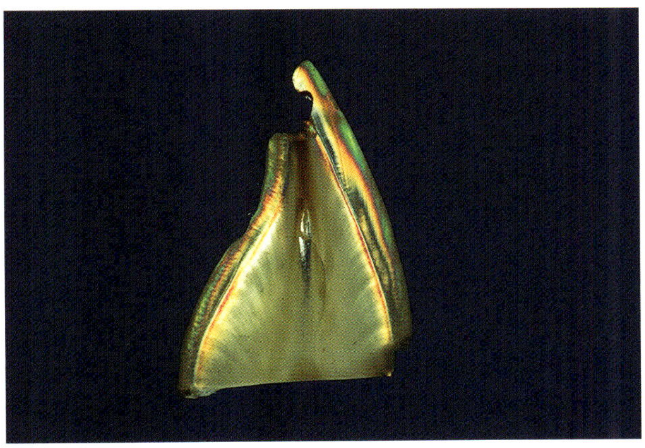

Fig. 5.69 Many materials are double refractive, such as this tooth, which is shown as a section in all the colors of the rainbow.

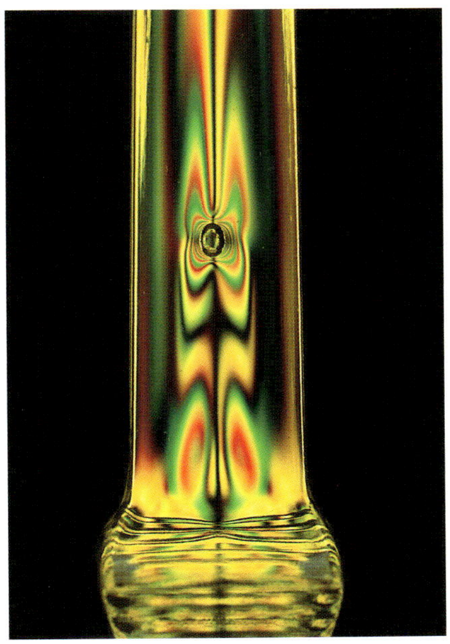

Fig. 5.70 Polarized transmitted lighting is also used for showing mechanical stresses. Internal mechanical stresses are rendered as color bands. The image shows this type of mechanical stress surrounding a small air bubble in the handle of a toothbrush.

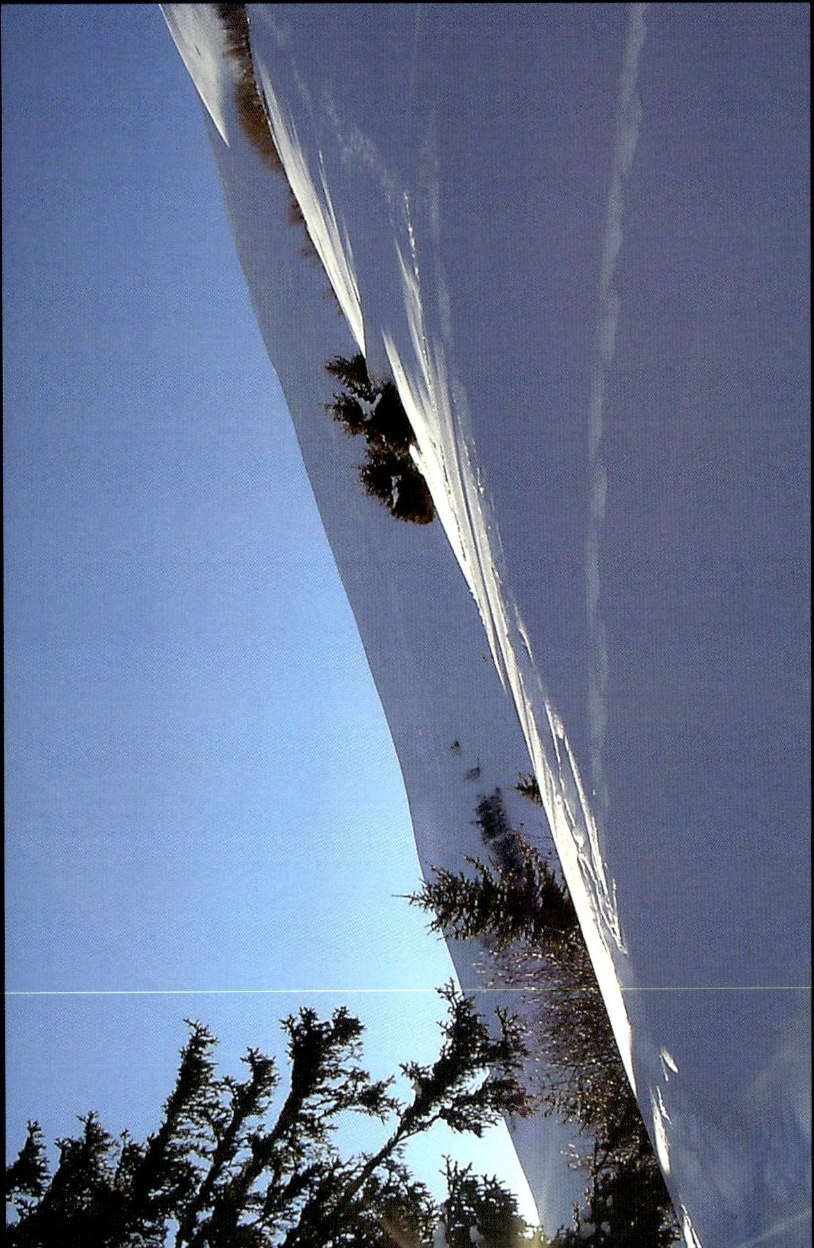

6 Photography of Dental Casts

The assessment of casts is one of the important bases of diagnosis and treatment planning not only in orthodontics, but also in prosthetic dentistry and periodontal therapy.
For the purposes of organization and improvement of documentation it makes sense in many instances to take photographs of the models. Due to its intrinsic problems, photography of casts is dealt with in a chapter on its own.

Special problems in photographing casts
Models not only provide information about the three dimensional arrangement of the teeth in relation to each other, but also about their size and the size of the dental arch. Thus it is recommended that a millimeter scale be photographed along with the model which should be placed about the level of the occlusal plane. This permits copies to be made subsequently at the correct scale.

In shadow areas where the direct rays from the sun are blocked, only the blue light from the sky is seen. The side of this hill away from the sun is not only darker, but the shadows appear bluish. We do not see this, any more than we do the color of artificial light. This is evident to us only in photographs. For this reason, photos which are taken in shadow often show an ugly bluish color (Photograph taken with Kodak DC260).

Casts are generally of uniform color and often white, with very low level of contrast.
Pretreatment of the models with soap, talcum powder or special polish, which is done as a normal practice to protect them from dirt, gives these models a shiny surface; this in turn improves the three dimensional nature of the image due to the resulting highlights. Close attention should be paid to lighting in order to increase the three dimensional appearance of the model.

6.1 Technical Considerations

6.1.1 Camera

There are no specific requirements for the camera other than those for clinical photography. It is important to use a lens with a focal length of about 100mm in order to avoid distorted perspective (Fig. 6.1). A focusing screen with a grid aids in achieving good results.

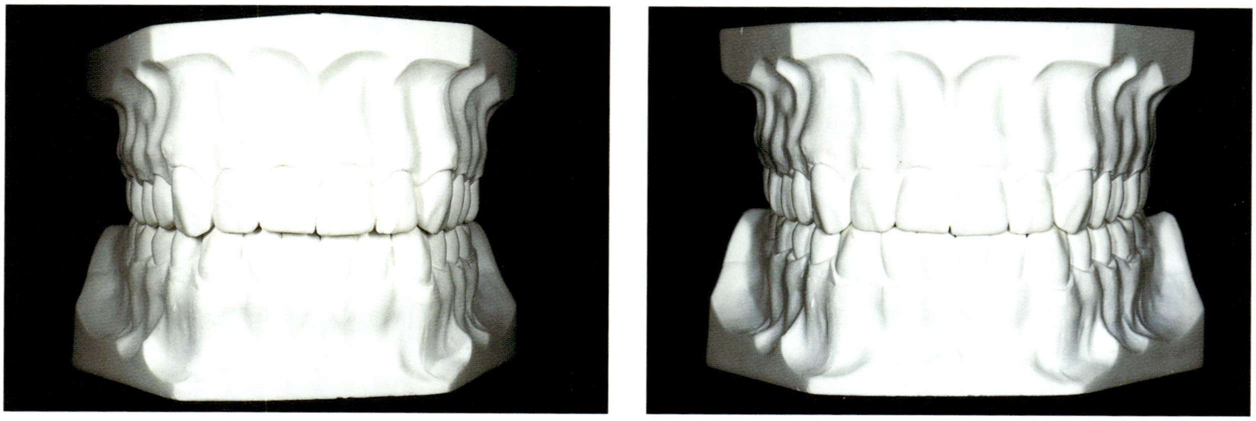

Fig. 6.1 Too short a lens – here a 50mm lens – distorts the perspective of the cast (a). A 105mm lens reproduces the cast as it would normally appear to us, when viewed from a normal distance (b).

6.1.2 Stabilization of camera and model

It should be the goal to produce images which are taken under defined and therefore reproducible conditions.

If models are photographed frequently a copy stand should be purchased (Fig. 6.2). A prerequisite for speedy work is a correct trimming of the casts which should always remain in the correct position without having to be supported.

A copy stand can be fairly easily modified for photographing models. Two screw clamps can be used to attach a plate perpendicular to the baseboard. By rotating the entire copy stand almost 90 degrees, which brings the vertical column almost into a horizontal position, the models can be placed onto the plate so that they do not fall off (Fig. 6.3).

The Novoflex macro/reprostand is also suitable; this allows the camera to be attached in a similar manner to it as on an optical bench (Fig. 6.4). However, the camera guide rail length must be increased.

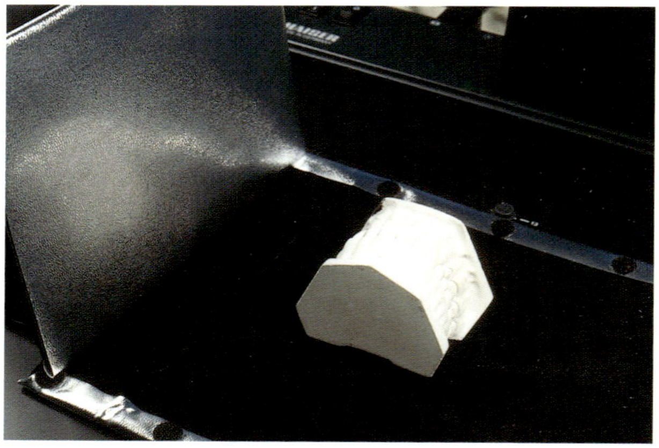

Fig. 6.2 Model on a copy stand. In this case too only one light source is needed. The side away from the light is illuminated by using a reflector.

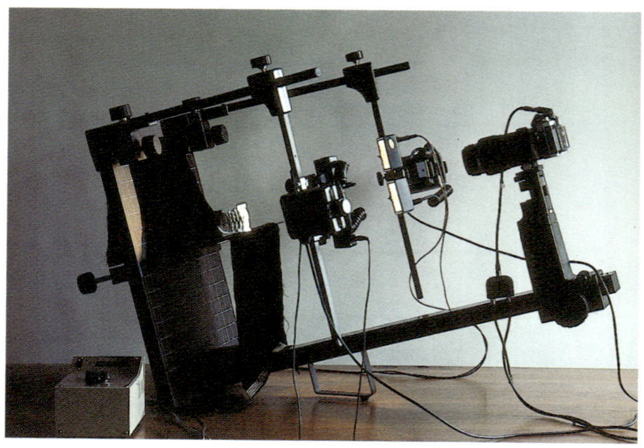

Fig. 6.3 A copy stand modified with a perpendicular plate fixed to the ground board.

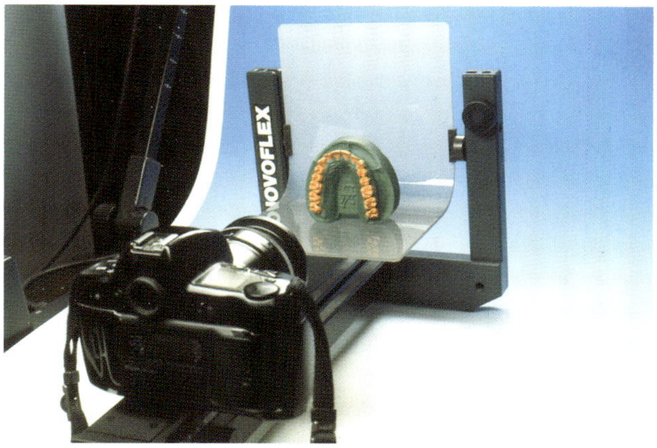

Fig. 6.4 Macro/Reprostand from Novoflex.

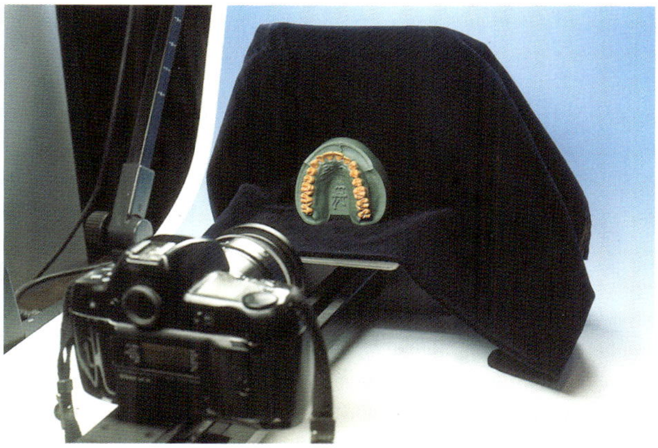

Fig. 6.5 A black silk cloth is used to isolate the model in front of a black background.

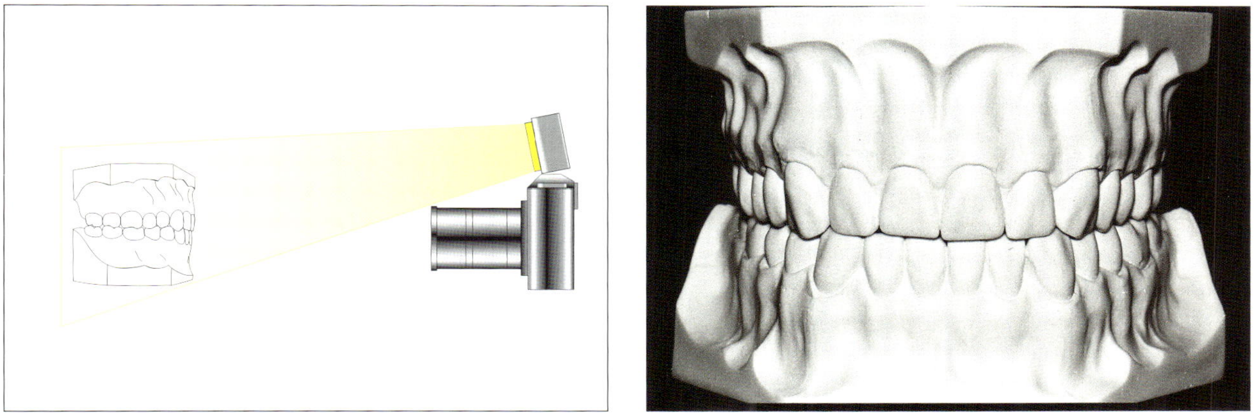

Fig. 6.6 Frontal view of the model with flash in 12:00 position. Diagram (a) and result (b).

6.1.3 Background

The most common background is black velvet or black cardboard or a corresponding black plastic sheet (Fig. 6.5). The normally light colored casts show up well against these backgrounds and the shadows they produce are not visible, as they are "swallowed".

If color backgrounds are desired, these can be selected and arranged in accordance with the principles covered in the chapter on object photography.

6.1.4 Lighting

In this instance also the principle applies that a single light source, whether electronic flash or a constant light source, is sufficient.

A side flash which can be rotated and is attached to the camera, or a side flash with cable release separate from the camera are suitable.

If a copy stand is used, its lights can of course be used. Figures 6.6 to 6.12 show typical lighting arrangements and their results.

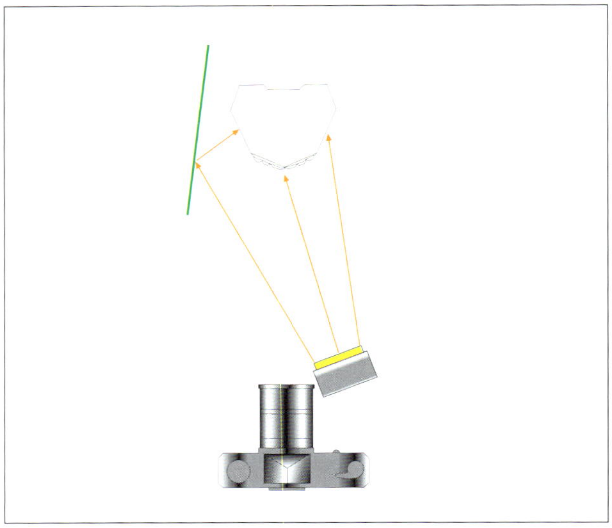

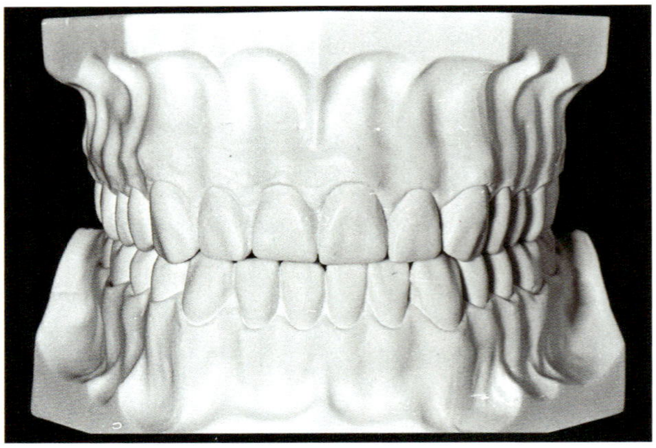

Fig. 6.7 Frontal view with directional side lighting. The side away from the light is illuminated with a reflector. Diagram (a) and result (b).

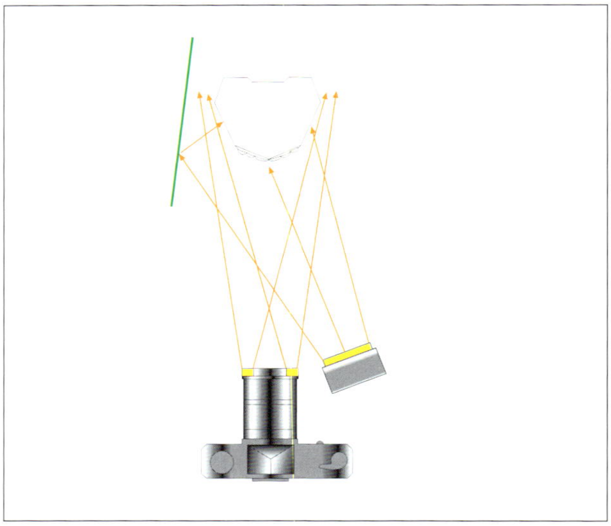

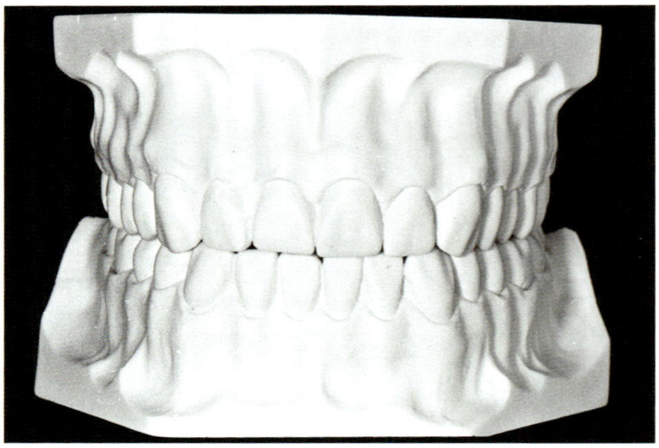

Fig. 6.8 Frontal view with ring flash/point flash combination. Diagram (a) and result (b).

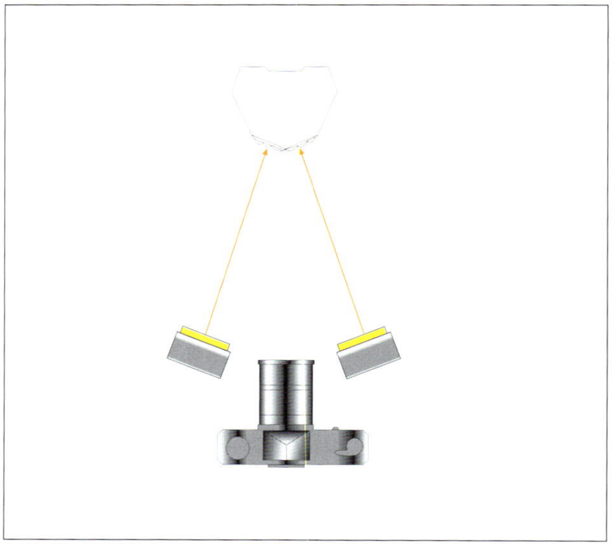

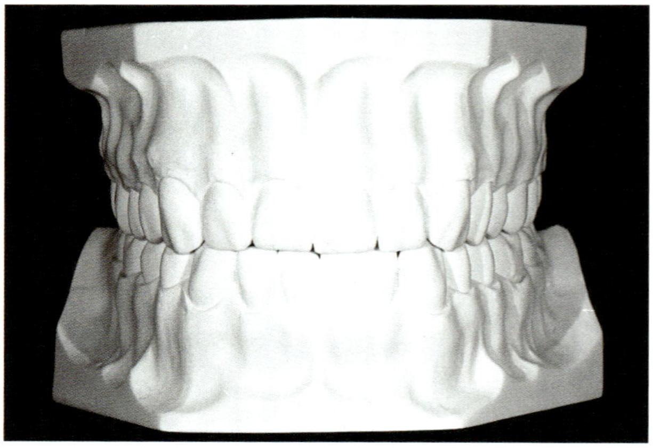

Fig. 6.9 Photograph of a cast with a twin flash system. Diagram (a) and result (b).

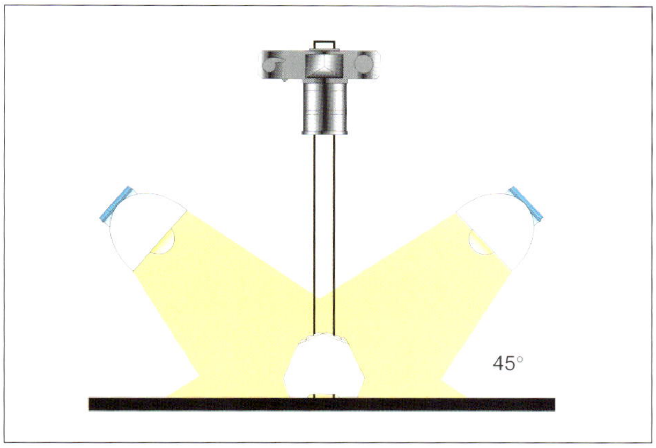

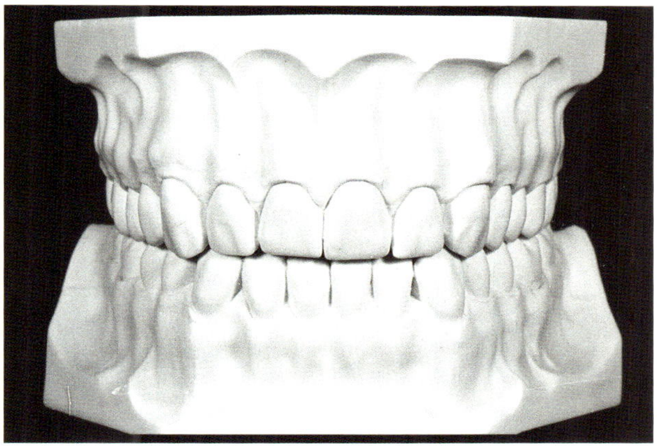

Fig. 6.10 Frontal view of a cast taken using a copy stand. Diagram (a) and result (b). If the top lamps only are switched on, the light forms a shadow line below the upper incisors which clearly separate the upper and lower jaw.

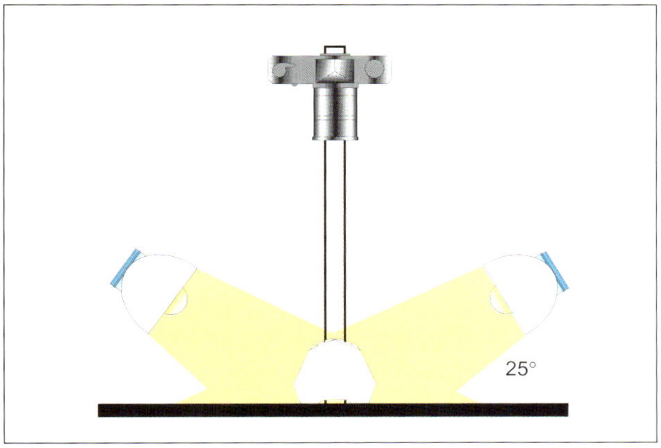

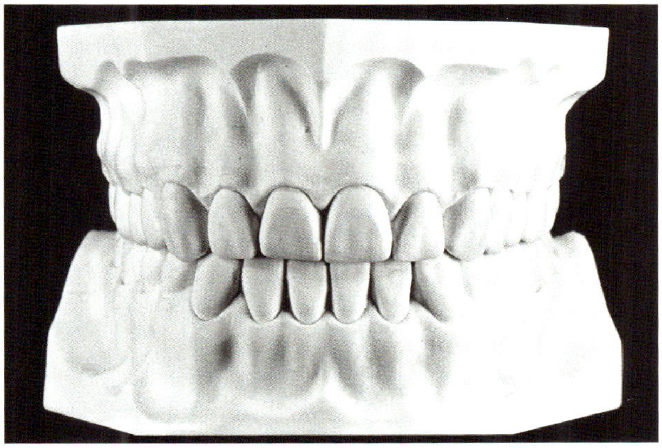

Fig. 6.11 Light angled on a copy stand at a shallow angle increases the plasticity of the front teeth. Diagram (a) and result (b).

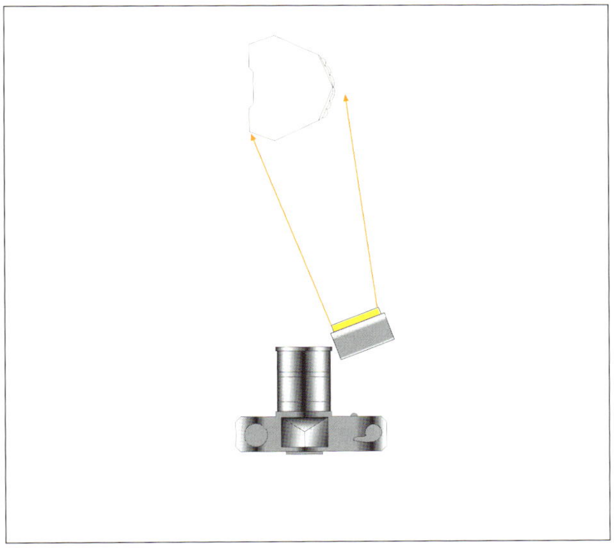
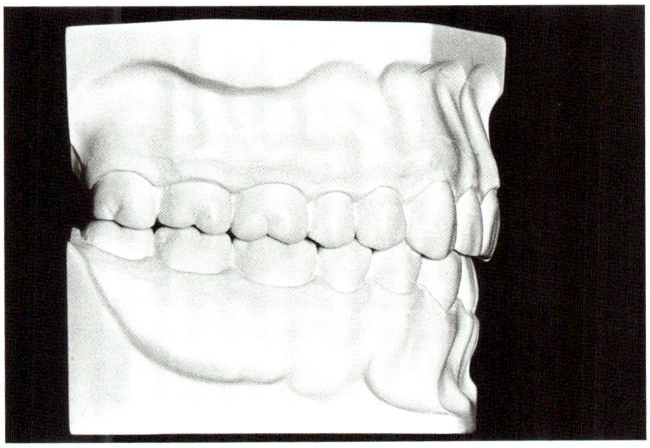

Fig. 6.12 When photographing a lateral view of a cast, the side flash should always be positioned on the side with the front teeth. Diagram (a) and result (b).

6.2 Standard Images – Model Status

The standard views correspond in general to those of intraoral photography: frontal view, two lateral views, two occlusal views. Thus there are five standard views.
All images are made in horizontal format. If white models are photographed an exposure compensation of about 1 – 1 1/3 stops is required so that the surface is reproduced bright enough.

6.2.1 Frontal view

The center of the photograph is at the contact point of the upper incisors. Focus on the canines (Fig. 6.13). The occlusion plane is horizontal. The model is illuminated with a flash fitted to the camera at the 12:00 o'clock position or a light source from the side plus illumination of the opposite side using a reflector. If the photographer has a copy stand with two lights on the right and the left, the lights on the lower jaw side should be switched off. This achieves a fine shadow contour below the upper incisors.

6.2.2 Lateral views

The center of the photo and the focus point are both around the second premolars or first molars (Fig. 6.14). Lighting should be from the side of the front teeth. The lighting should be angled so that the side teeth are separated by fine interdental shadow lines. This angle also shows up the jugae alveolariae and the inserted ligaments well.

6.2.3 Occlusal views

In this view the centre of the picture is at the cross-section of the line joining the premolars and the sagittal plane (Fig. 6.15 – 17). Focus on the fissures. Illumination is either with camera flash at the 12:00 o'clock position used with a reflector or with a side light plus reflector. If symmetrical lighting is provided by lights on a copy stand, it should be flat enough to clearly show the contours of the fissure.

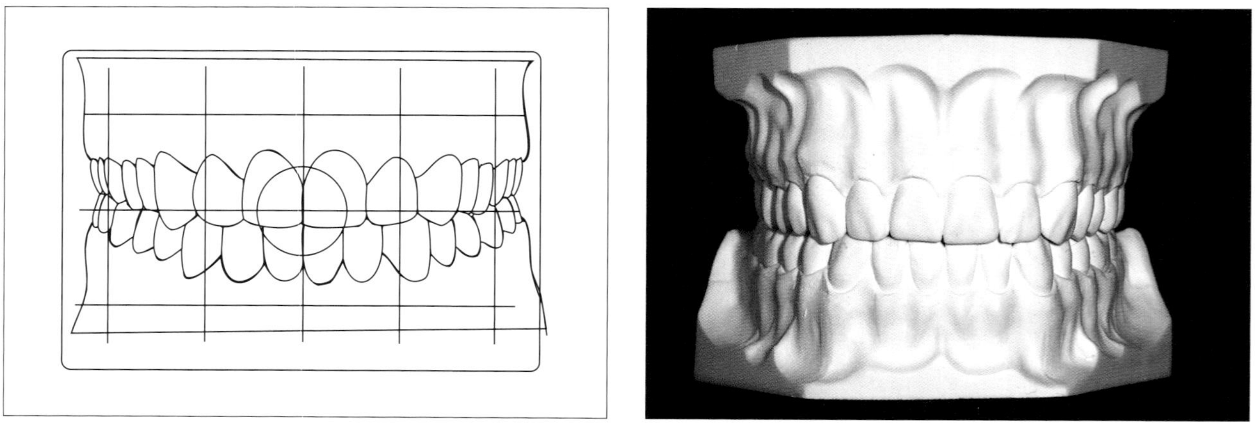

Fig. 6.13 The composition in photographing the frontal view of a model should correspond to the conventions of intraoral photography. Diagram (a) and result (b).

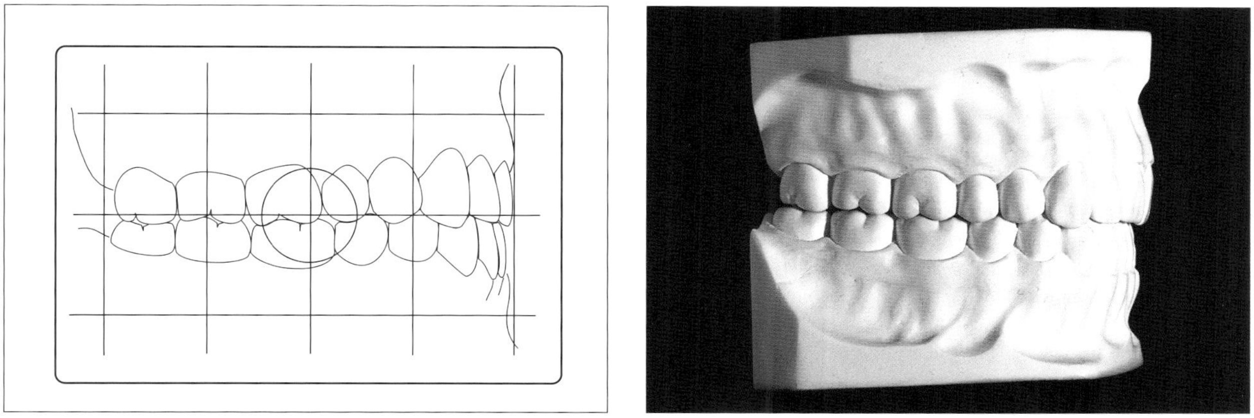

Fig. 6.14 Lateral view of a cast. Diagram (a) and result (b).

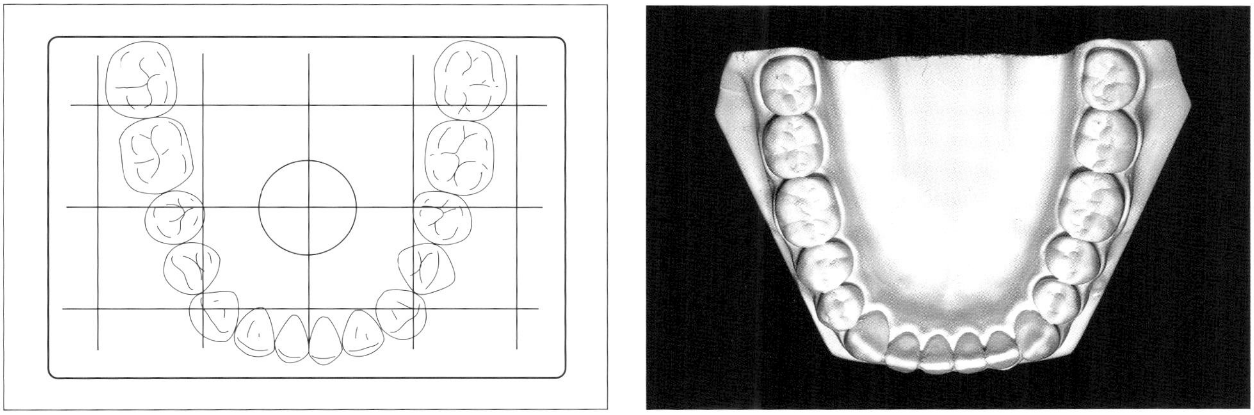

Fig. 6.15 Lower jaw – occlusal view. Composition (a) and result (b).

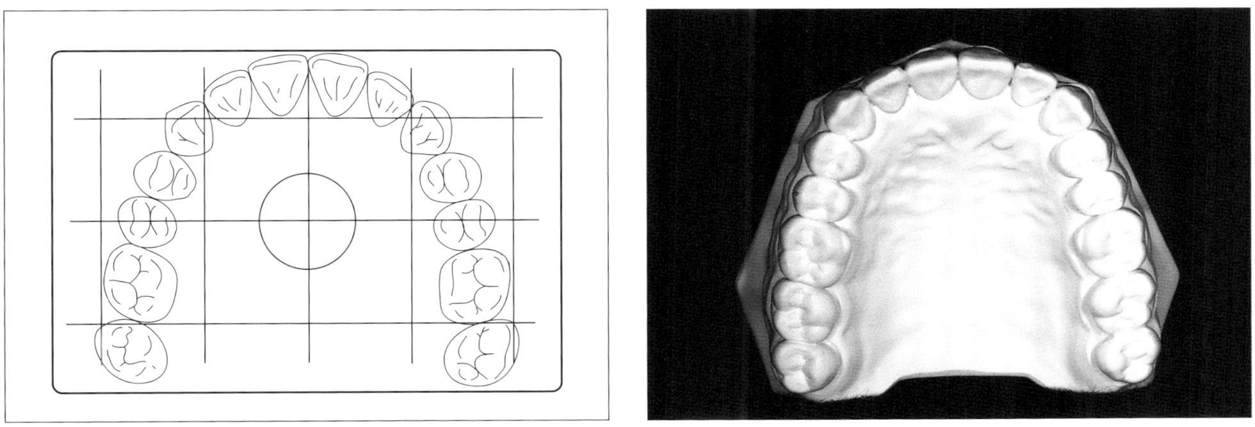

Fig. 6.16 Upper jaw – occlusal view. Compositon (a) and result (b).

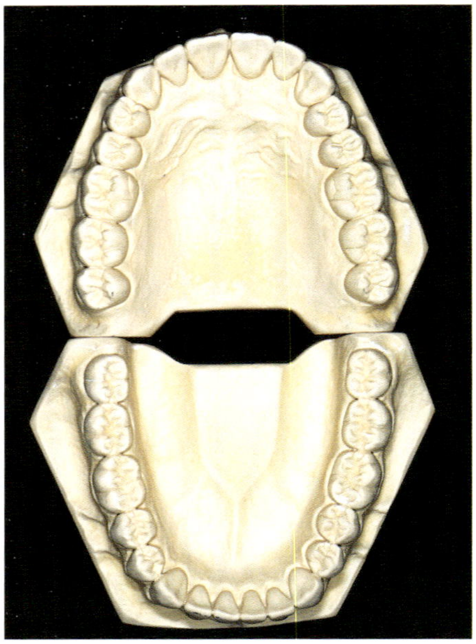

Fig. 6.17 Both occlusal views can be photographed in a single image.

6.3 Special Equipment

Only a few systems recommended in the literature and by commercial firms have proven of practical use.
One of these is the Keil 3D model photo stand; this is an angled mirror which allows simultaneous photography of frontal and lateral views. Another system is the model photostat from Voss and the photo stand from Hinz which permits photography of the entire photostat in one image by the use of multiple exposures (Fig. 6.18).

Checklist for photography of models

- ✓ Camera with 100mm macro lens
- ✓ Exposure correction +1 - 1 1/3 stops for white models
- ✓ Positioning of the model using grid focusing screen

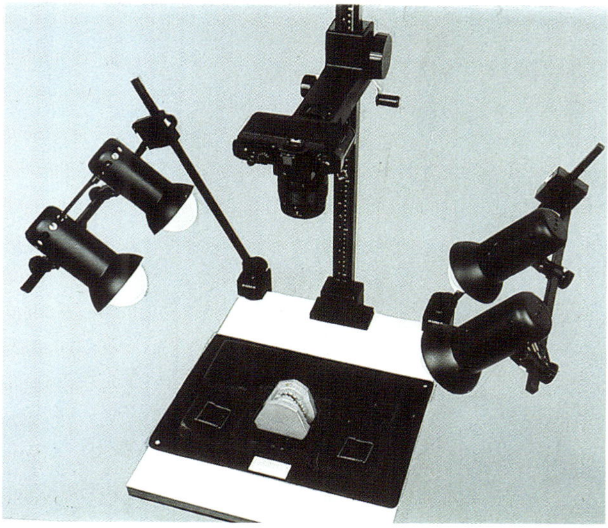

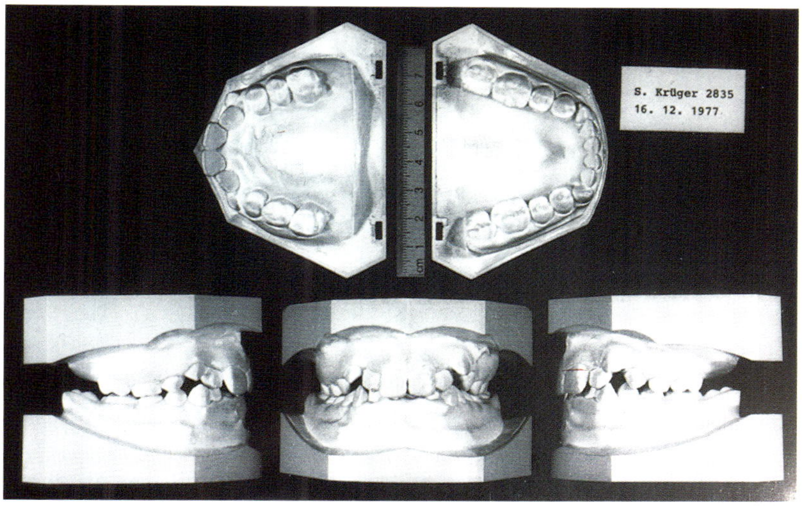

Fig. 6.18 Hinz photo stand (a) and the resulting image with the standard arrangement in one photograph (b) (Photos: ZFV-Verlag).

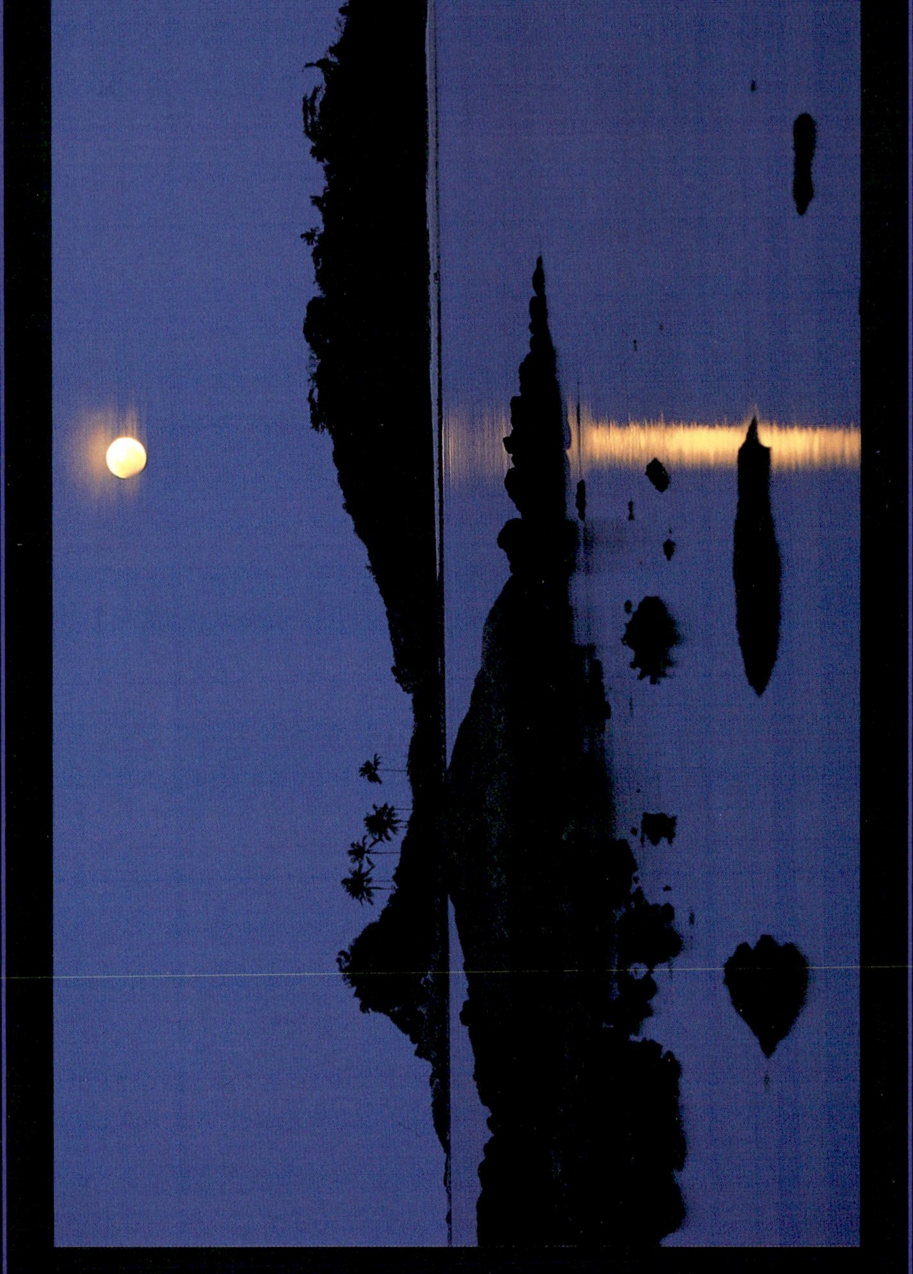

7 Copy Work

The term "copy work" means the reproduction of images, text or objects for which the third dimension is not important (i.e. coins). In dental photography copies are used for instance for:

✓ Reproducing originals (text or images) for lectures or publications
✓ Reproducing patient records relating to treatment in order to save space
✓ Reproducing patients' photos for the dental technician.

Slide copying and copying X-ray images are treated in separate chapters due to their specific requirements.

◄ As the light falls its color becomes darker and darker blue ("blue hour"). We however hardly notice that the late light is dark blue, since our color perception lessens with decreasing brightness ("At night all cats are gray"). Here too the color adaptation of the brain is responsible for the fact that this scene in Thailand looked different to the observer than on film.

7.1 Technical Considerations

7.1.1 Camera

A camera suitable for clinical photography also can be used without problems for copying. A 100 mm macro lens is not necessarily required. Since there are no major perspective problems to be expected with flat documents a 50mm macro lens can be used too.

7.1.2 Film

Color reversal film as used in clinical photography is generally suitable for most purposes. Otherwise film selection is determined by the purpose of the copy and the type of document being copied.

High-contrast line copy

Line drawings require only the reproduction of pure white or black tones with none in between. The most suitable film for reproduction in black and white is the orthochromatic high contrast black and white film. Recommended negative films for example are Agfa Ortho 25 Professional, Kodak Ektagraphic HC Slide , and the panchromatic High-Contrast Copy Film 5069.

Copying halftones

Originals with halftones have tones between black and white. Black and white negative film is best for reproduction in black and white.

Medium		Original	
	Line art	Halftone	Color
Black and white negative	Document film	Panchromatic film	Panchromatic film
Black and white slide	Reversal development	Copy from negative film	–
	Black and white slide film	Black and white slide film	Black and white slide film
Color slide			Color reversal film

Color originals
Originals which have color in them and are to be reproduced in color are photographed on color slide film.

Black and white slides
It sometimes is desirable to include black and white slides in a presentation with color slides. This can be to attract attention or to emphasize the form of an object independent of its color.
For our purposes a black and white slide film (Agfa Scala) is most suitable. However, it is also possible to copy a black and white negative onto documentary film or reverse development based on Agfaortho 25 material.

7.1.3 Camera stabilization – copy stands

In principle it is possible to stabilize the camera using a tripod, but if a lot of copy work is required it is better to purchase a copy stand, which – as has already been demonstrated – can also be used for other photographic purposes (Fig. 7.1).
The following criteria should be considered in the purchase of a copy stand:

- ✓ Good overall stability
- ✓ Modular design
- ✓ Large enough baseboard
- ✓ Tall enough vertical column
- ✓ Uniform illumination with daylight balanced lamps

Many types of copy stands are available from photographic suppliers for the dedicated amateur or professional photographer.
If daylight balanced lamps are not available attention should be paid to the color temperature of the light sources or the film sensitivity for reproducing color originals (Fig. 7.2). Opal lamps have a color temperature of about 2400 degrees K to 2800 degrees K. Nitraphot lamps have a color temperature of 3200 degrees K. In both cases either a film balanced for artificial light should be used or the color of the light needs to be changed by using a blue filter on the camera lens. Conver-

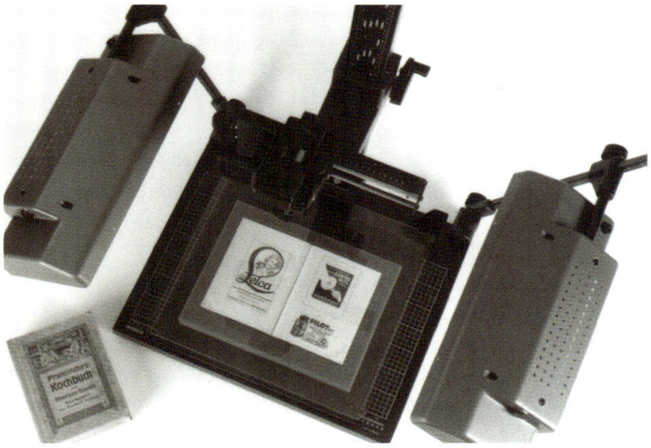

Fig. 7.1 For those who photograph frequently a copy stand is a sensible acquisition – and not only for copying (Photo: Kaiser).

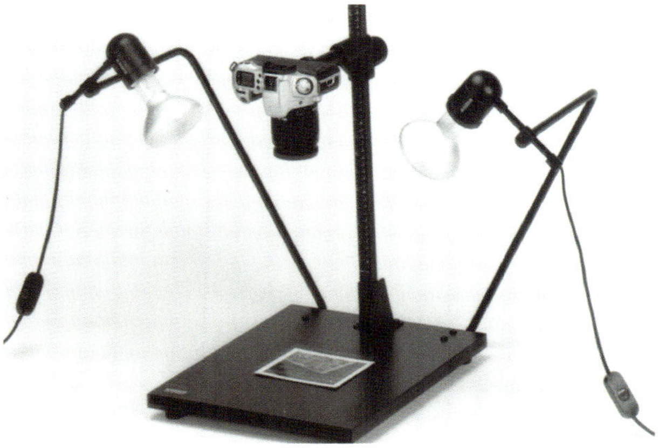

Fig. 7.2 When using artificial light, care must be taken that the color temperature of the light sources and the film balance are the same (Photo: Kaiser).

sion tables list the exact type of filter to be used. In any case, it is far simpler to use daylight balanced slide film with daylight balanced lamps.
Just as constant light sources can be used, so too can electronic flash. If only one flash is available this should be placed as far away from the document as possible to achieve uniform lighting. As a rule of thumb, the distance between the flash and the document should be about six times the width of the document (Fig. 7.3).

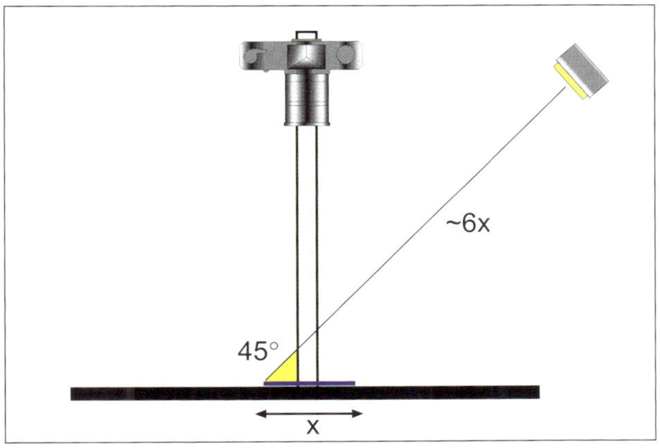

Fig. 7.3 If only one flashgun is available it should be positioned at a distance six times the width of the original. Only in this way can an evenly lit copy be made.

7.2 Practical Considerations

The original is placed on the baseboard and the camera fixed on the copy stand. Its exact vertical placement can be checked with a spirit level, but it is even simpler to use a mirror placed on the base plate. By looking through the viewfinder the camera position can be altered until the lens opening is directly in the mirror.
The lamps should be positioned symmetrically. The axis of the light should be about 40 degrees to the baseboard to prevent reflections from the document's surface entering the lens (Fig. 7.4). The symmetry of the illumination can be checked by noting the shadow of a pencil placed in the middle of the original (Fig. 7.5).
The copy is framed by moving the camera vertically on the column and then adjusting the focus. The shutter is released using a cable release or the camera's self timer with the setting for aperture priority ("A" marking) and the aperture set at f/8 or f/11.
If the originals are particularly light or dark it is recommended that a gray card be used (see below).

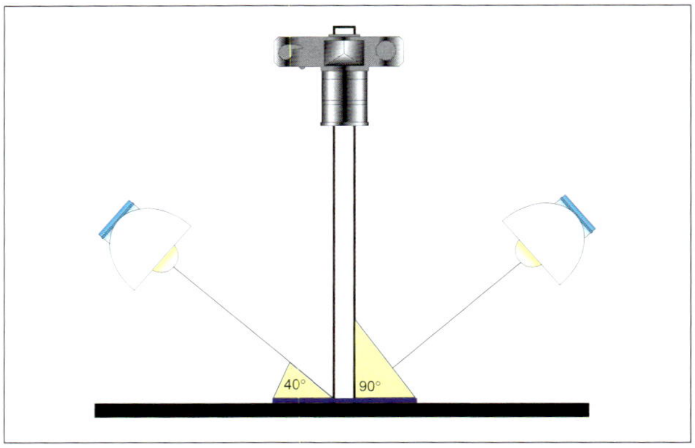

Fig. 7.4 The lighting should be set up so that reflections do not strike the camera. A lighting angle of 40 degrees to the baseboard can achieve this.

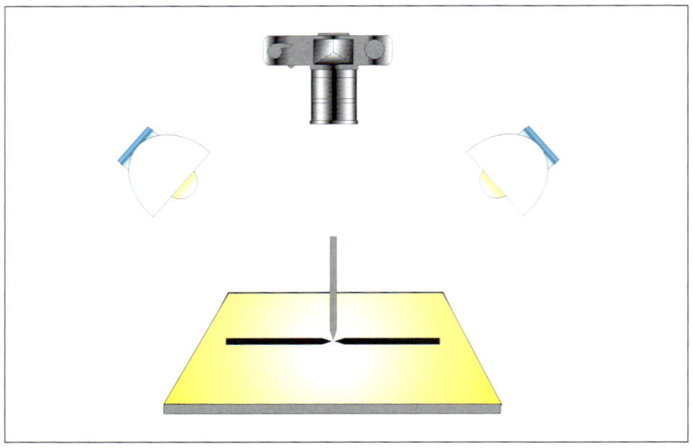

Fig. 7.5 If the shadows of a pencil placed in the middle of the orginal are symmetrical it can be assumed that the lighting is also symmetrical.

Measuring exposure with a gray card – substitute readings

Light meters, either handheld or those built in to the camera, are calibrated to give settings that will produce an average tone. This means this is for an object which reflects just under 18 % of the light falling on it. The exposure is set so that the object is rendered as a mid-gray. If the object is brighter than average the resulting image is too dark. Using a gray card is helpful in such cases; this is a sheet of cardboard or plastic which reflects light at approximately 18 %. Instead of the object, the exposure is measured with the gray card (substitute reading).

To do this the camera and the original are placed in position and the image framed (Fig. 7.6). The gray card is then placed on the original. The camera is set for manual exposure ("M" symbol) and the aperture set to the "copying" apertures of f/8 or f/11. Using the viewfinder, the shutter speed is adjusted to achieve the proper exposure. The gray card is then removed from the original and the copy is made.

The result is that the original is reproduced at its correct brightness and the camera light meter is not fooled into trying to achieve an "average" exposure for the image. The shutter speed can be used for copying originals of a similar size as long as the other parameters (aperture and placement

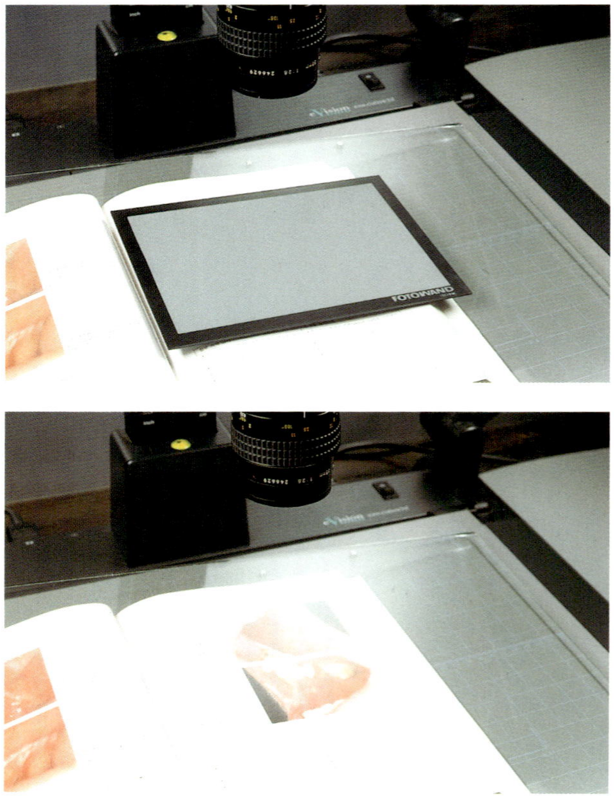

Fig. 7.6 A gray card is helpful in copy work in achieving correct exposure. The image is framed and with manual exposure, the aperture set at the "copying apertures" of f/8 or f/11 and the shutter speed adjusted to create the correct exposure (a). The gray card is then removed and the image is made (b).

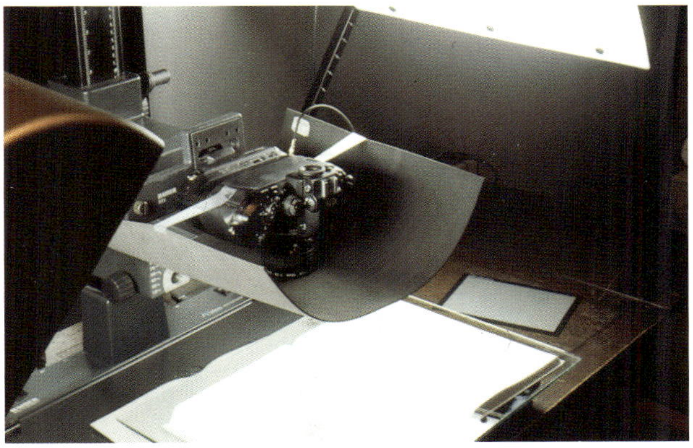

Fig. 7.7 Uneven originals can be flattened using a glass plate. The black cardboard in front of the camera prevents reflections on the surface of the glass.

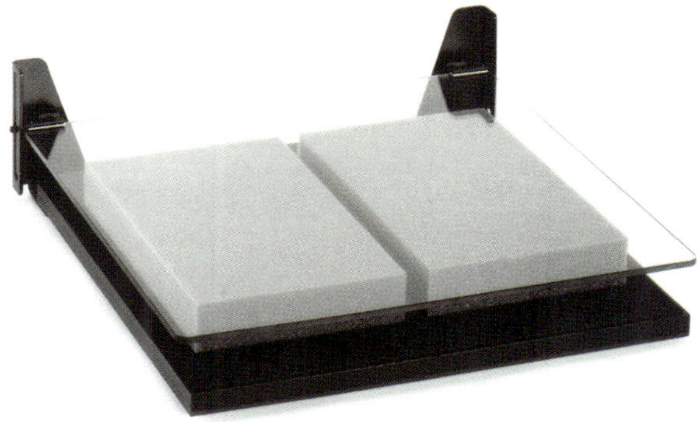

Fig. 7.8 If copies are frequently made from books a book holder is a good investment (Photo: Kaiser).

of the lamps) remain the same. Setting exposure with a gray card is to be preferred to using the camera's own light meter as it achieves better results.

If flash is used, a flash meter is necessary. Generally, plus or minus corrections are made based on experience.

7.3 Tips for Problematic Originals

- ✓ Uneven originals should be flattened under a glass plate (Fig. 7.7). However, care should be taken to avoid unwanted reflections. Reflections of the camera itself can be avoided by using black cardboard shield with an opening for the lens, placed in front of the camera.
- ✓ If there is print-through from the reverse of thin originals, this can be remedied by using a sheet of black cardboard underneath.
- ✓ Transparent paper originals can be copied by laying a white sheet of paper underneath to improve the contrast of the print.
- ✓ Damaged originals can be copied by using a sheet of paper with the same color as that of the original.
- ✓ A book holder is useful if books are frequently copied; this also flattens thick books (Fig. 7.8)

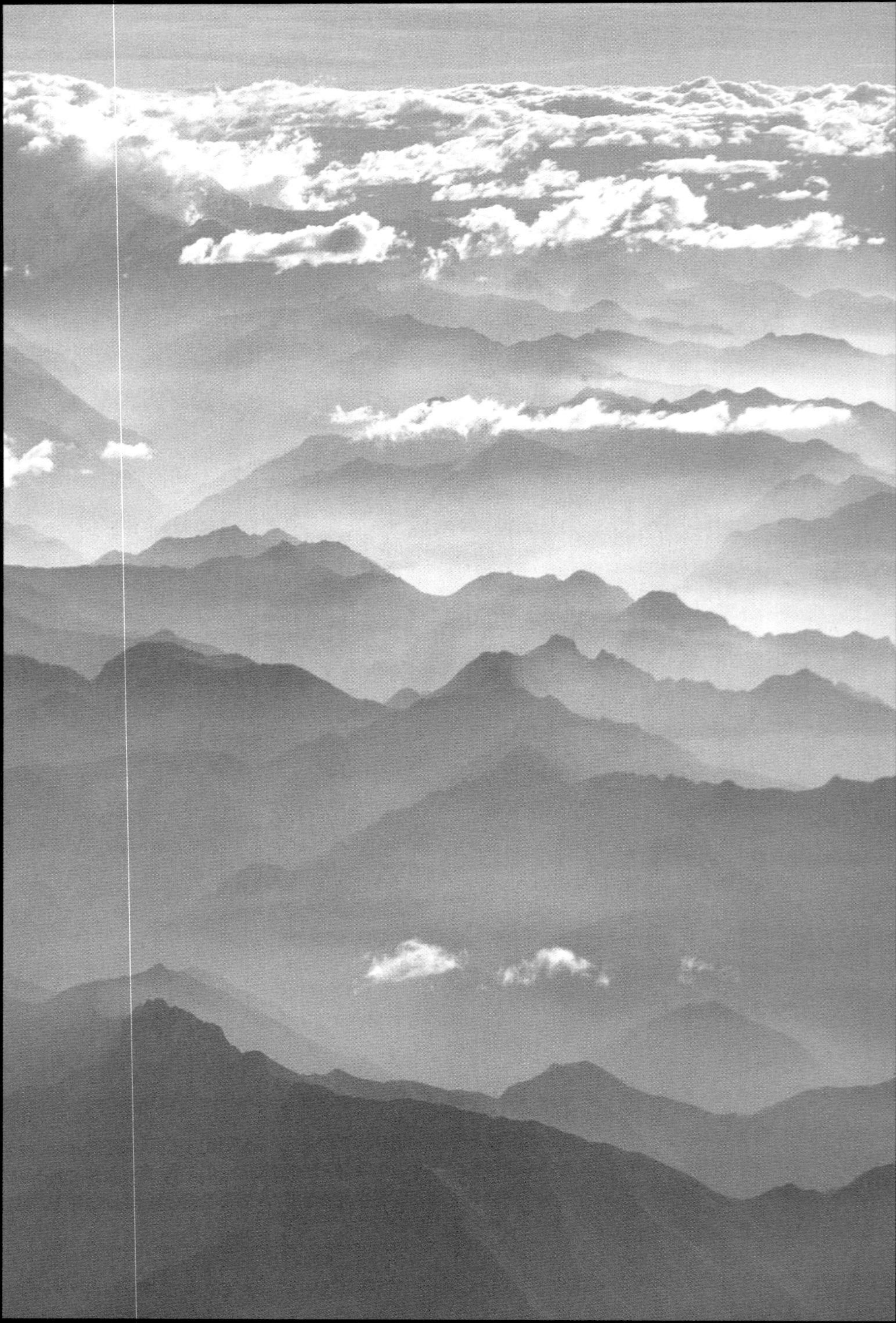

8 Copying X-ray Images

An X-ray image is one of the most important sources of information in dental diagnostics. It can be necessary to copy them to illustrate publications and lectures, but also to copy important documents for treatment given to colleagues for the dentist's own records.
Special films and processes are available to produce contact copies. This section deals with photographic techniques of copying using 35mm film. In principle, copying X-ray images is the same as copying originals with transmitted light. Thus a light source which shines through the X-ray image is needed in addition to the equipment for copying.

8.1 Camera Stabilization

X-ray images are by nature unsharp (two layer films, fluorescent dispersed illumination, patient movement). To avoid intensifying this unsharpness, handheld copying is out of the question due to its relatively long shutter speeds. The camera must be stabilized.
A copy stand is of course the most suitable for this, optimally one with a daylight balanced light source integrated in the base board (Fig. 8.1). Naturally a tripod which allows the camera to be mounted for a vertical shot can also be used.

8.2 Accessories for Transmitted Light

Any light box which provides even lighting is suitable for copying X-ray images. This includes those used for viewing X-ray images, which are normally found in the practice anyway, and slide viewers (Fig. 8.2).
Slide viewers generally have daylight balanced light sources. X-ray image viewers for the most part have halogen tubes; using them with daylight balanced slide film results in a greenish-blue color cast.

◄ So-called aerial perspective, which makes these mountains gradually become bluer as they recede in the image, is also due to diffusion of light. The light is not only scattered by the air molecules in the atmosphere but also by haze particles. It can be seen in this image taken from an aircraft that there is more moisture in the valleys. The larger haze particles generally cause whiter or brighter blue colors. The "aerial perspective" not only gives us an idea of the scattering of light but is also a clear indication of depth, that is, perception of the third dimension.

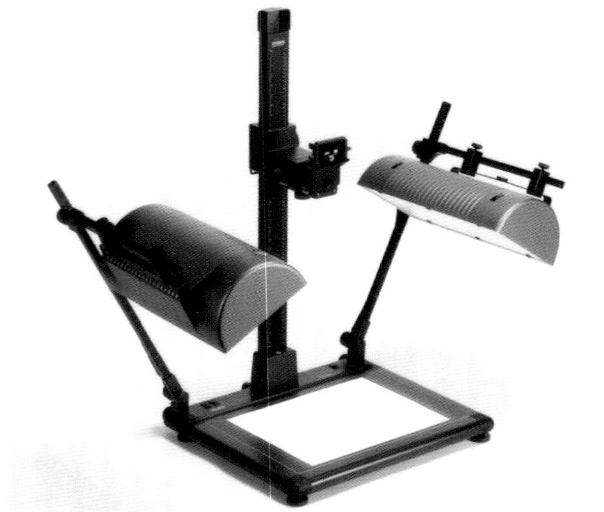

Fig. 8.1 The Copylizer is a modern copy stand with an integrated light box in the base board (Photo: Kaiser).

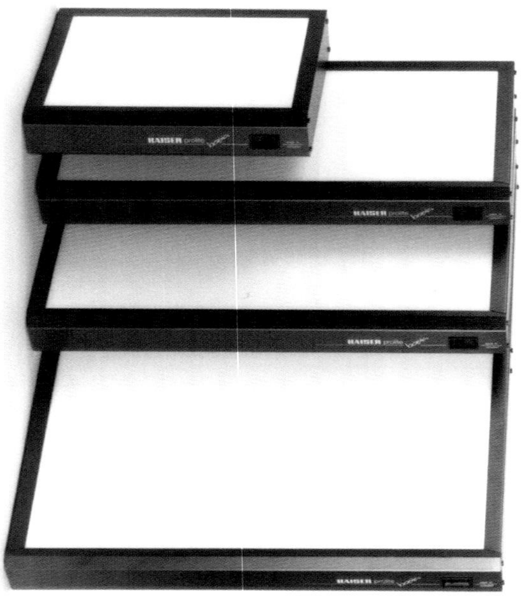

Fig. 8.2 Light boxes are available in various sizes. If possible, one with daylight balanced light should be selected (Photo: Kaiser).

It is important that the area around the X-ray image be masked off with black cardboard (Fig. 8.3). This prevents stray light from entering the lens and reducing the brilliance of the image. Masks with various size openings are also available for this purpose from photographic suppliers (Fig. 8.4)
An electronic flash can also be used if necessary. The X-ray image is placed on a glass plate about 15cm above a styrofoam sheet which is illuminated by two flashguns.
Dental x-ray films can also be copied with a slide copier holder, since they are about the same format as 35mm slides.
If copies need to be made only occasionally X-ray film can be copied by using a window (optimally north-facing). The X-ray film is fixed to the window with transparent tape and the camera attached to a tripod.

8.3 Positioning

The aim of the copy is to fill the frame as much as possible. For a dental radiograph a reproduction ratio of 1:1 is necessary.
Series of X-ray images are best copied by attaching the individual images one by one to a transparent sheet. Overlapping areas of the images can be cut away and the edges covered with black tape. Using the conventional X-ray image holders allows a lot of light between the individual images and leads to exposure problems. In order to avoid this X-ray image archive holders with opaque individual frames are available (Trollhätteplast, Sweden) (Fig. 8.5).
When copying a series of dental X-ray films with 14 individual frames an approximately 45% increase over the individual films can be achieved by arranging the individual frames in a sequence other than the normal one (Fig. 8.6).

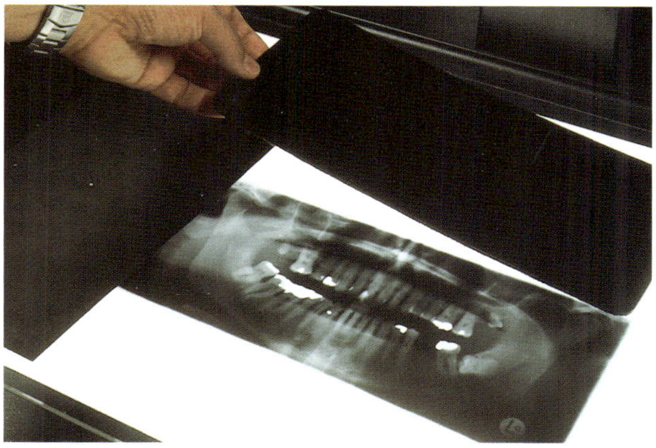

Fig. 8.3 To prevent stray light from entering the lens, which reduces the brilliance of the image, the area surrounding the X-ray image is masked off with black cardboard.

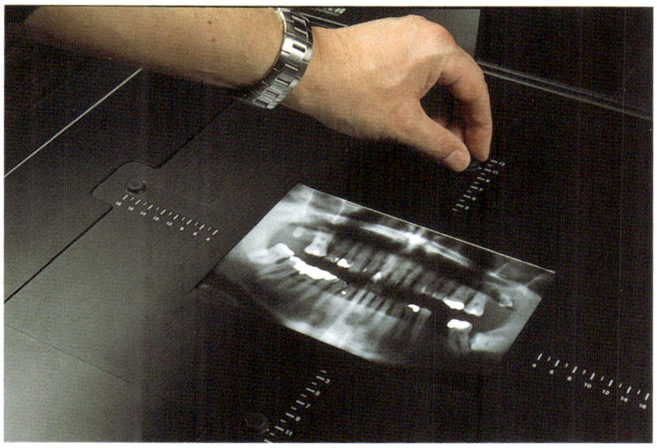

Fig. 8.4 If X-ray images are frequently copied, then the mask frame from Kaiser is worth considering (Photo: Kaiser).

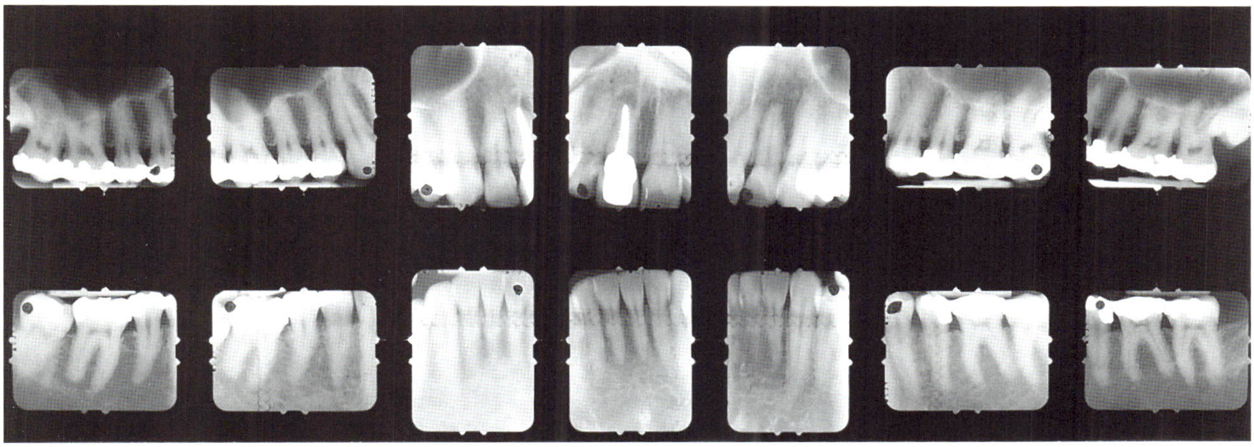

Fig. 8.9 X-ray holders with opaque frames between the individual images are very well suited for copying as they help avoid incorrect exposures.

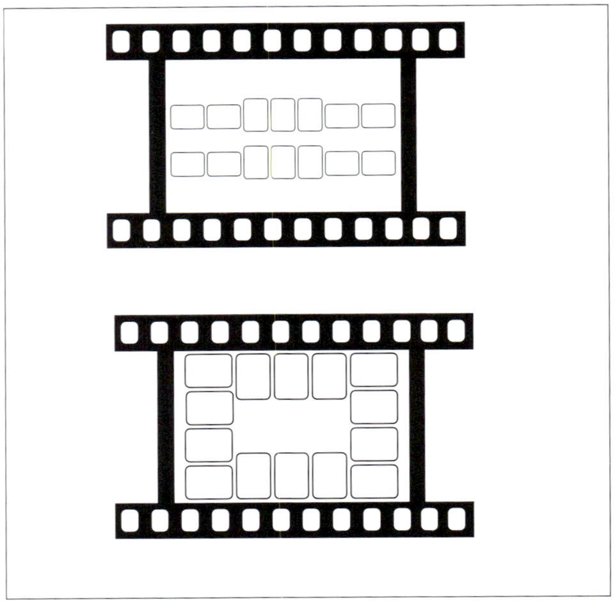

Fig. 8.6 There are various ways of arranging X-ray films, which results in different sizes of these individual images.

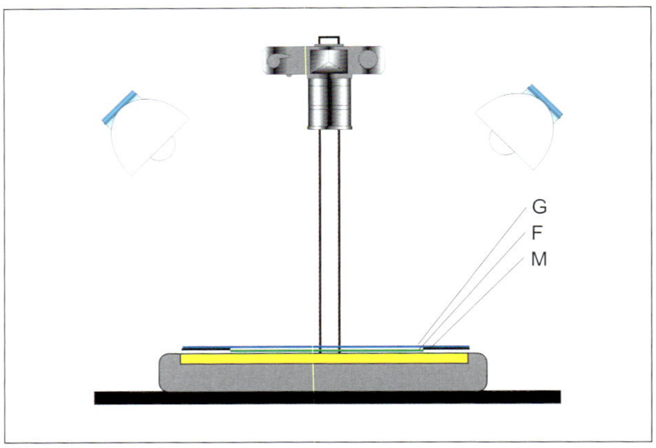

Fig. 8.7 Diagram of arrangement for copying X-ray images. Flatness of the film (F) is achieved by laying a glass plate (G) on it. Areas of the light box around the film are masked off with black cardboard (M).

When making a panorama copy consideration should be given as to whether it is necessary to reproduce the entire image, or whether, by leaving out the side portions, a better side ratio and thus to a more format-filling copy can be obtained. The unexposed middle section of panorex images can be cut out. This not only improves the side ratio but also reduces the chances of incorrect exposures. If the original needs to be flattened a glass plate can be used (Fig. 8.7).

8.4 Film

Daylight balanced slide film, as used in clinical photography, is generally also suitable for our purposes. Copies have different color casts depending on the type of lighting used (Fig. 8.8).
If X-ray image viewers are used as a light source the resulting color cast is greenish-blue, which is not necessarily a disadvantage. Many authors are even of the opinion that the subjective perception of the image's contrast is improved.
If a daylight balanced light source is used the resulting copies have the same color as that of the original.
Black and white slide film (Agfa Scala film) can also be used, but does not achieve any better results than color slide film.
If maximum rendering of gray scale nuances is important, which does not apply in dentistry, panchromatic black and white negative film can be used (for use in print). High contrast slides can be achieved by copying the negative onto orthochromatic film (Agraortho 25). This process is not viable for a dental practice simply due to the high cost of the laboratory work.

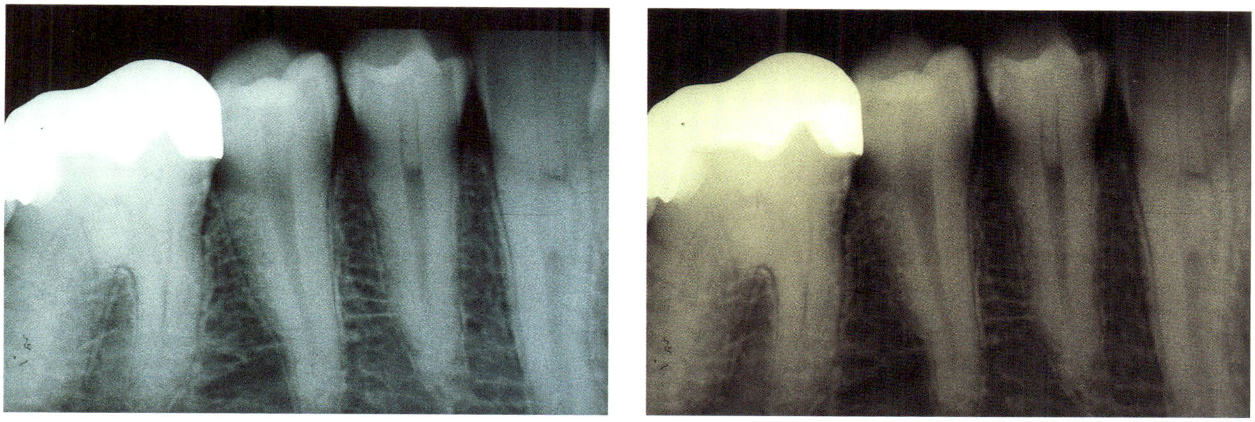

Fig. 8.8 Different light sources create different color rendition with color slide film. (a) shows the image taken with electronic flash, (b) the use of artificial light.

8.5 Step-by-Step Procedures

- Place the X-ray image to be copied on the light source (light box) and cover the surrounding area with black cardboard.
- Determine the framing of the copy by changing the reproduction ratio.
- Set the camera to aperture priority ("A" symbol) and aperture to f/8 or f/11.
- Turn off ambient lights.
- Trip the shutter with a cable release.
- Use bracketing with apertures in increments of 1/3 for originals which pose difficulties (very dark or bright, high contrast). In general, this is not necessary however.

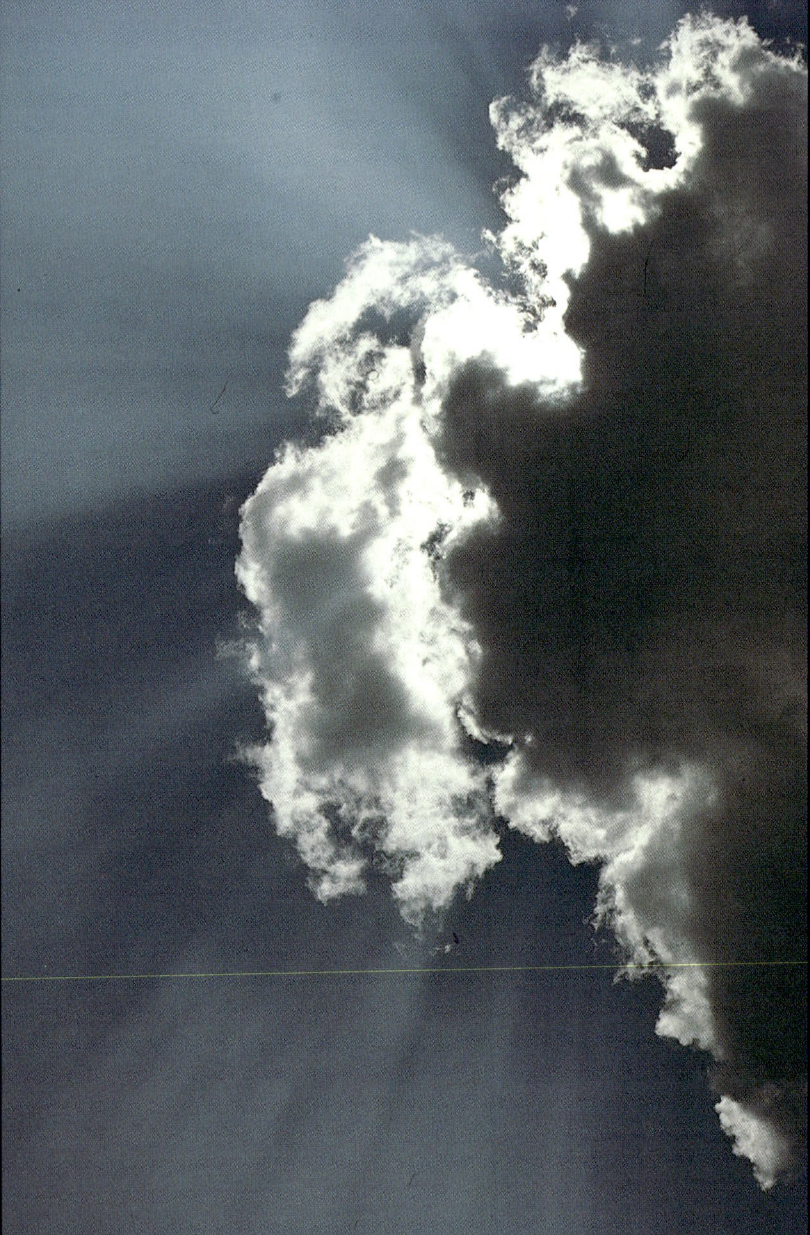

9 Copying Slides

Slide copies are reproductions of slides with transmitted light. For the most part this is to create duplicate slides to avoid having to use originals. This is necessary in order not to give away the precious originals In general it is sensible to use only duplicates for lectures, publications, etc in order to preserve the originals and keep the archive complete.
Duplicate slides also allow the content of the originals to be altered. Framing can be improved, multiple exposures allow text to be added (today mostly now done by computer) and color casts can be removed or deliberately added by the use of filters.

◄ Scattering of the light from the sun behind a cloud into a hazy atmosphere has created these rays. Part of the light is blocked by the edges of the cloud and the cloud's shadow creates the dark areas of the fan. Even the brightly lit edge of the cloud is due to scattering, although in this instance it results from the droplets in the cloud. The interior of the cloud appears dark because the sunlight is more scattered here; only a bit of the sunlight can penetrate the cloud in the original direction of the rays.

9.1 Basic Considerations

Color slide film is designed to achieve the brightest possible image with high brilliance. Among other things, contrast is increased. If a slide film is copied using a normal slide film there is a marked and irritating increase in contrast and mid-tone values are lost.
Moreover, every color slide film has its own color characteristics and if a slide is copied on the same slide film this color characteristic is increased, creating a sort of "photochemical incest" which is generally evident by a marked color cast (Fig. 9.1).
There are two main ways to avoid these basic problems:

- ✓ Using normal slide film and deliberately reducing contrast with carefully measured diffused light.
- ✓ Using special slide duplicating film

In both cases it is generally necessary to avoid color casts by using filters.

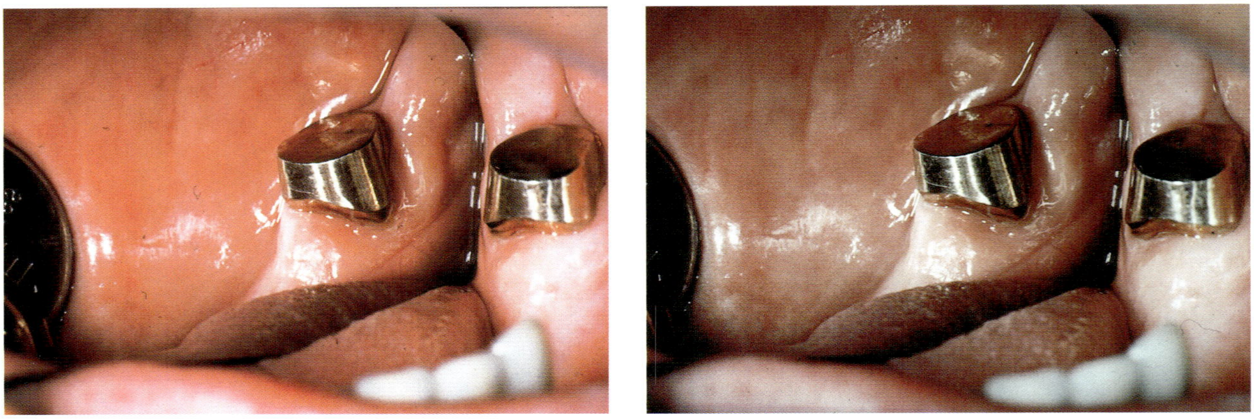

Fig. 9.1 If copies are repeatedly made on the same film the color characteristics are intensified and the contrast increased. (a) shows a copy of an Ektachrome image, (b) shows the second copy, which already clearly evinces the results of this "photochemical incest".

9.2 Duplicating Systems

If slides need to be copied frequently the purchase of a slide duplicating system is to be recommended. Various makes and models of these are available through photographic suppliers. Some of these systems allow measured dispersed light to fall into the camera lens to reduce the increase of contrast.

9.2.1 Slide copying mounts

A slide copying mount consists of a second bellows unit or a tube system which connects the slide mount into which the slide to be copied is inserted to the camera lens with no light leaks. The front of the slide mount has a translucent screen to disperse the light as evenly as possible onto the film (Fig. 9.2). Electronic flash units are most commonly used although a constant light source is another possibility. The light source determines whether daylight or artificial light duplicating film is used. It is not possible to add any further dispersed light to reduce contrast when using a slide copying attachment and thus special slide duplicating film should be used. Generally these attachments allow a color correction filter to be inserted.

9.2.2 Color head for slide duplicating

Prints from color slides or color negatives are produced on a color enlarger. The heart of such a system is the color head – in principle a halogen light source whose light can be seamlessly converted into the primary colors (individually or in combination). If this color head is rotated 180 degrees it is a perfect light source for copying slides (Fig. 9.3). Kaiser offers a holder which allows this to be done very easily. However, in this case too it is not possible to add any additional dispersed light and thus special slide duplicating film should be used.

9.2.3 Special equipment

There are other systems available for professional use, though these are generally not recommended for use in the dental practice.
One of these is the Bowens Illumitran (Fig. 9.4). This system has a built-in electronic flash with an intensity control which illuminates the slide to be duplicated. The optional Contrast Control Unit changes the contrast of the film by making a very small "fogging" exposure via a 45 degree clear glass "mirror". Color correction is possible, and indeed necessary, and is done by inserting filters into a holder.

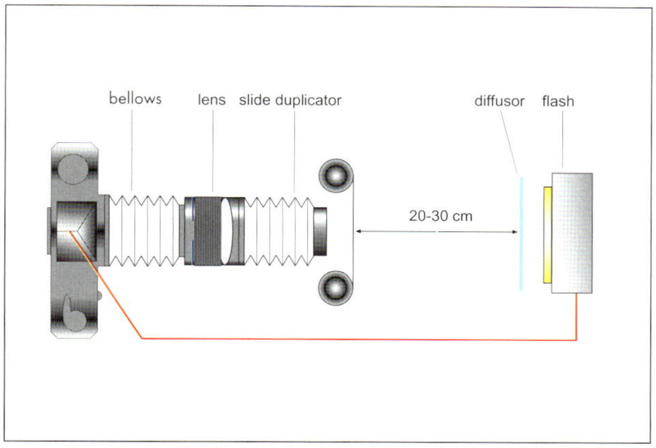

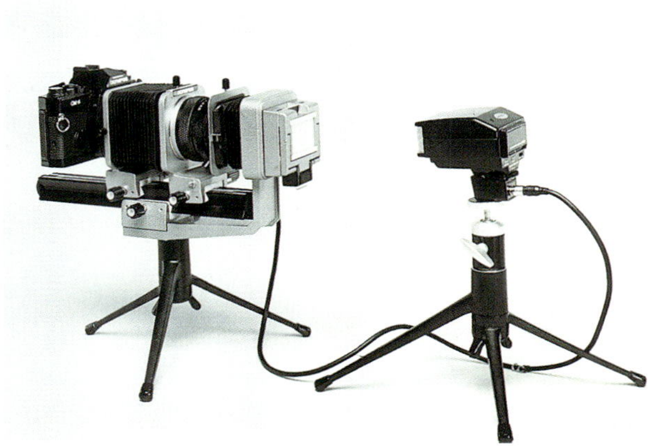

Fig. 9.2 Slide copying attachments consist of a second small bellows unit which forms a light-tight connection between the image holder and the camera lens. (a) diagram of arrangement, (b) photo of such a slide copying system (Photo: Olympus).

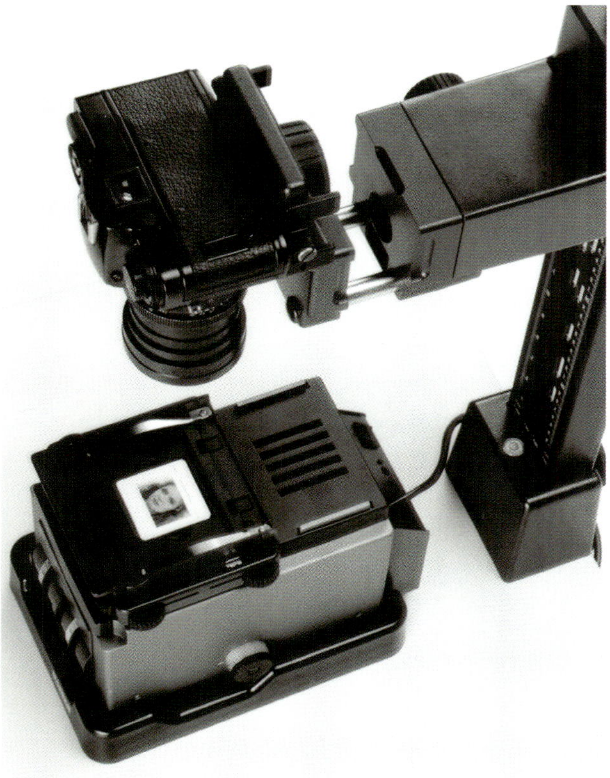

Fig. 9.3 The color head of a color enlarger is amply suited to slide copying since the color of its light can be changed as desired (Photo: Kaiser).

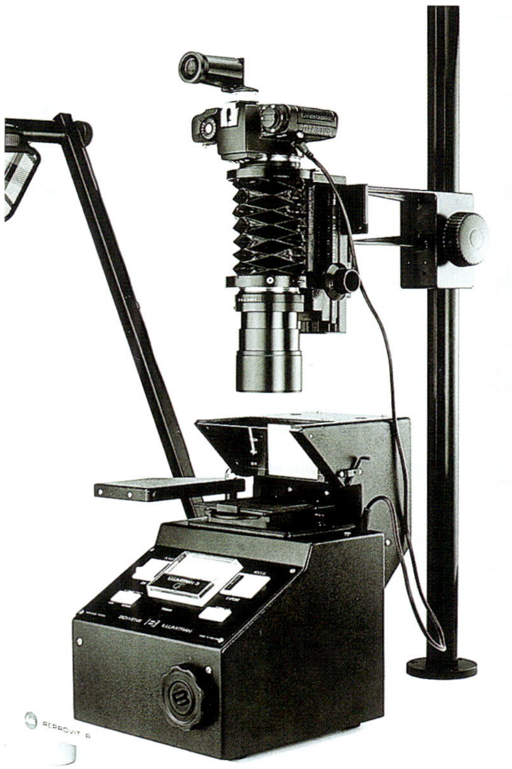

Fig. 9.4 The Illumitran collects stray light in the camera via a glass plate and thus prevents an increase in contrast (Photo: Bowens)

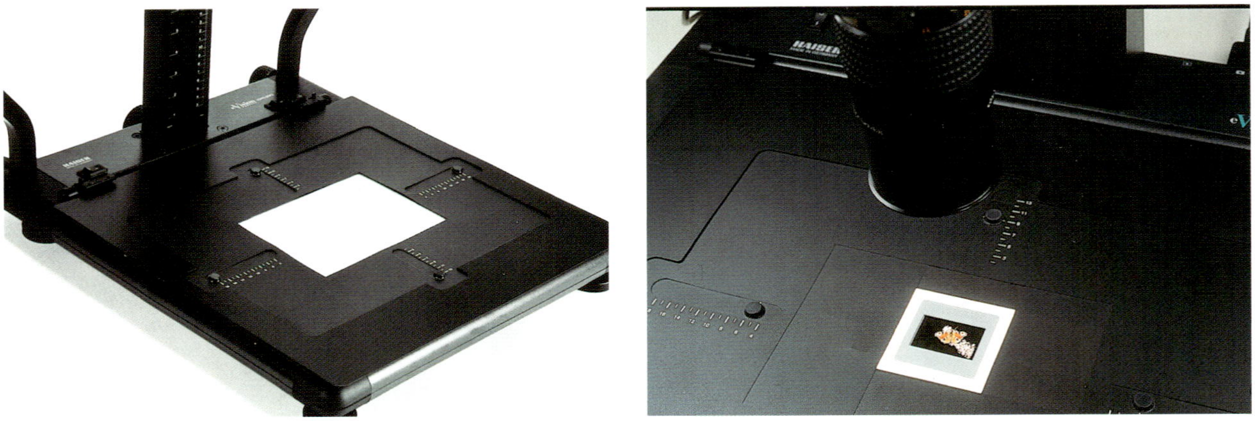

Fig. 9.5 A mask frame on a lightbox is also very good for copying slides (a). If the area around the slide being copied is left free to some extent this also reduces contrast (b).

9.2.4 A simple solution: the lightbox

If slides need to be copied only occasionally try the following procedure, which, with some practice, achieves satisfactory results.

Place the slide to be copied on a lightbox and fix the camera on a copy stand. Set the reproduction ratio on the camera lens to 1:1 and the aperture to f/8 or f/11. To avoid an increase in contrast the area surrounding the slide is not fully masked off with black cardboard and an area a few centimeters wide is left around the slide. This uncovered strip allows additional light into the lens when the copy is made and prevents the undesired increase in contrast (Fig. 9.5). At first, the width of the unmasked area should be varied to determine the correct amount of dispersed light to prevent the copy from showing too much flare but also to avoid an unwanted increase of contrast.

Additional color filtering is possible by placing color filter sheets on the lightbox.

9.3 Choosing Duplicating Film

Conventional slide film or special slide duplicating film can be used depending on the number of copies and the desired quality.

9.3.1 Normal slide film

In principle, a slide should not be copied on the same type of film for the above reasons. Increasing the film's color characteristics can be avoided only by using a different type of film. An increase in contrast can be prevented to some extent by using a faster film, but it is better to use calibrated dispersed light unless the slides to be copied show very low contrast.

Example: A Kodachrome transparency should be copied using Agfachrome or Ektachrome film. If the original slide has normal contrast, a faster Ektrachrome film (e.g. Ektachrome 200) should be used.

9.3.2 Special duplicating films

All the major film manufacturers produce special duplicating films for their own materials. However, their use is only sensible if duplicates are produced frequently, which is not usually the case in a dental practice. These duplicating films are "softer" than the original films and their color rendition is geared toward that of the original film. Nevertheless, to achieve optimum results in this case too, color filters should be used.
It should be noted that duplicating films can be balanced for either daylight (flash) or artificial light. Some of these are available in 36 exposures, while others are produced in meter lengths and must be cut into appropriate lengths.

Examples of duplicating films:

Kodak Ektachrome SE Duplicating Film SO-366
The SO-366 is designed to produce color duplicate slides of Ektachrome originals. It is available only as 135-36 exposures and allows the amateur to copy slides with a 35mm camera.

Kodak Ektachrome Slide Duplicating Film 5071
Designed for duplicating Ektrachrome originals, though available only in meter lengths.

Kodak Vericolor Slide Film SO-279
Designed for producing color slides from color negatives. Also can be used for title slides for presentations (see below).

Fujichrome Duplicating Film CDU Type II
Suitable for Fuji films.

9.4 Filters

Color correction filters should be used if optimum color rendition is important. Various manufacturers produce filters of varying densities in the primary colors of yellow, magenta and cyan.
Thus for example CC30 C 2/3 signifies a color compensating filter (Kodak), cyan filter, density 30, filter factor 2/3.
A data sheet is supplied by the manufacturer with every film which gives data about filters for the original film and the light source. The film box also contains additional information about filters, since every emulsion requires a different type of filter to compensate for color differences of the various emulsion numbers.
For filtration, first run a check using data from the film sheet and the film box.

Example: Copying Ektachrome slides with electronic flash using Kodak Ektachrome SE Duplicating film SO-366.

Data sheet values	+110y + 20c	
Plus values on film box	- 40y + 10c	-1 stop
Initial values for testing	+ 70y + 30c	-1 stop

If the color rendition is not optimal, the color values can be compensated for by adding a complementary color filter or eliminating filter of the same color.
It should be evident from the above that color slide copying requires a certain amount of effort. For this purpose, the procedure as described in 9.2.4 is recommended.
Nevertheless, the best results can be achieved by making a number of exposures of important images, thus producing a "second original" as a duplicate.

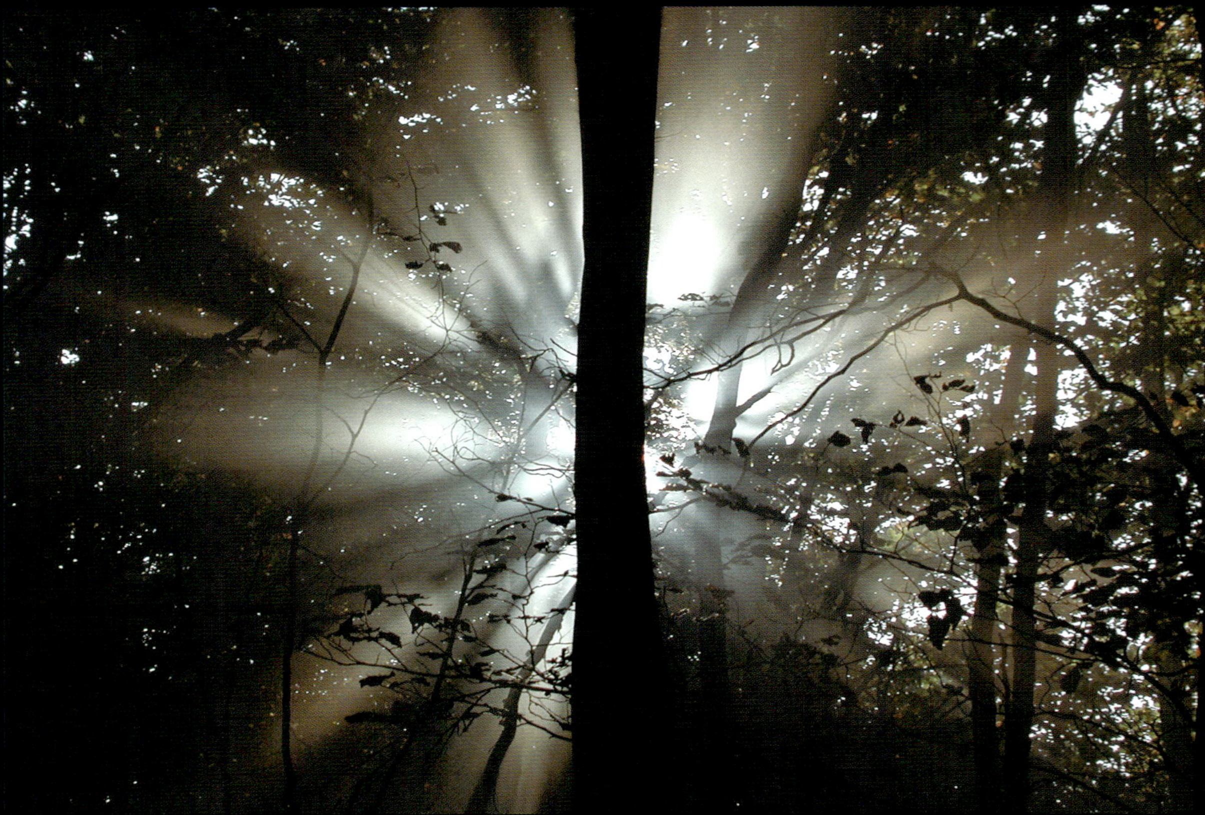

10 Making Presentation Slides

Computers have made no greater inroads in medical photography than in the production of slides for presentations. In the past, many medical photographers spent most of their time in producing originals for the production of presentation slides, but today most of this work is done on computer – and frequently by the lecturer him or herself. Many easily used programs are available for this. Often the medical photographer's work now frequently consists only of transforming computer generated files into transparencies by using a color film recorder.
Methods of presentation have progressed rapidly and today slide presentations are replaced more and more by computer presentations where the contents of computer screens are being projected by a beamer.
Even though the technology for producing title and presentation slides has undergone a revolution, the basic rules of graphic slide production have not changed, in keeping with the unaltered human perception.
The basic tenets of creating a graphic have remained unaltered, be it for a slide or a computer presentation.

Fan-shaped rays of light can also occur in forests and on their edges when sunlight shines in from a low angle and the air is hazy (Photographed with Nikon Coolpix 990)

The only transformation may be in our visual expectations. It can be assumed that people of the "video clip generation", who are constantly being bombarded by overpowering visual images, will need to have their attention held by different visual means than for their parents. Consumer surveys of US television audiences have shown that 35% of viewers are "flippers," that is, they keep changing from one channel to another. Even short periods of boredom are not tolerated, but are relieved by a quick click of the TV control. This of course has an effect on an audience's expectations of the visual content of a scientific presentation.
This chapter gives a brief introduction to the basic reasons for using slides in presentations, shows how to produce the materials for the slides and then the slides themselves.

10.1 Purpose of the Slides

"I listen and forget, I see and remember, I do and comprehend." (Oriental proverb)

The very ambitious goal of presenting a lecture is that the audience should retain as much as possible of that which we relate and show (Fig. 10.1). That which we perceive and have understood should remain as much as possible in our memory.

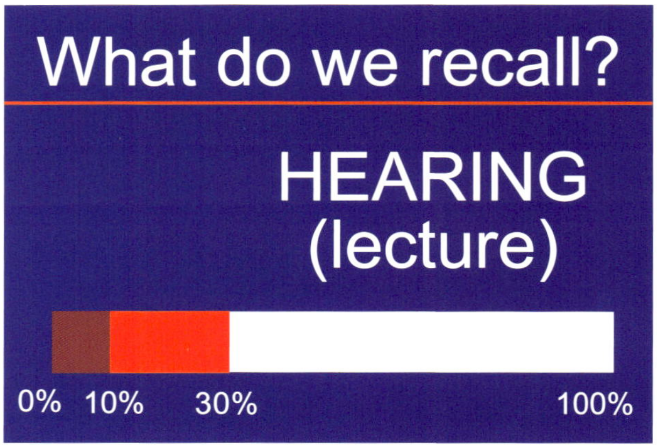

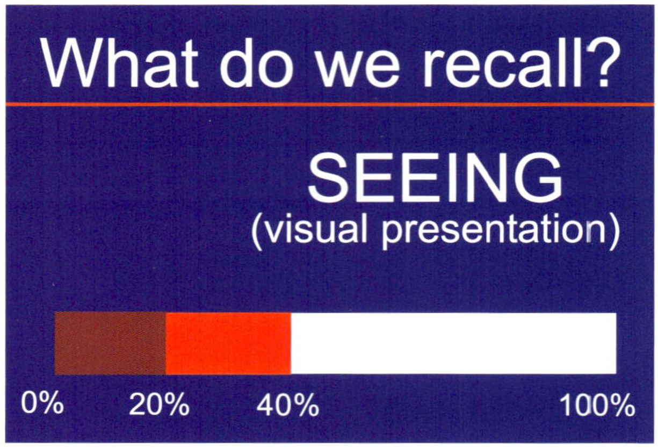

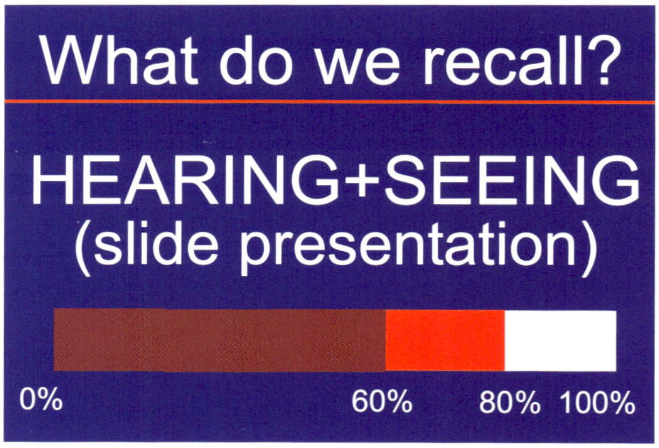

Fig. 10.1 We recall less of what we hear (a) than what we see (b). Both are significantly increased when we hear something which is illustrated at the same time, as is the case for example in a slide presentation.

Images and graphics are an aid to presenting complex concepts in a simpler manner. They improve understanding and reduce the amount of explanation needed: "One picture is worth a thousand words."
Presenting information in a visual form aids in remembering the spoken word, since a second "information channel" is being used. We remember more of what we have seen than what we have heard or read. The old boxer's maxim holds true here: "A punch on the eye is worth three on the ear." Combining oral and visual information increases the amount of information recalled. This is aided by images, which are the anchor for memory.
Real images intensify the impact of the information, since they appear authentic. Images are also able to sway an audience's emotions and intensify the message.
Text and graphic slides in particular are helpful in structuring the lecture. This not only helps the listener to better understand the ideas in context, but also forces the lecturer to better structure his or her presentation, with the slides being the main thread.

Types of slides

Various types of slides are used in presentations. Text slides are covered predominantly here, but other types of slides will also be discussed.
Real images always appear more authentic: "I've seen it with my own eyes." However, they can also manipulate the audience. Text slides emphasize certain points and structure a lecture. Graphic

slides and diagrams clarify contexts and show developments. Real image-text-graphic combinations can provide the greatest amount of information, but can also be overloaded and lose their effectiveness.

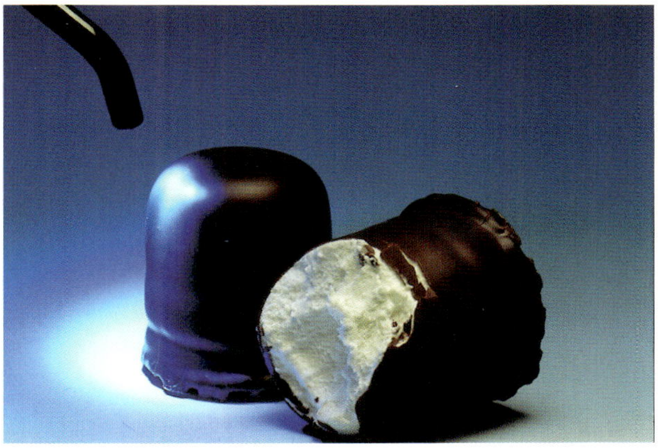

Fig. 10.2 Real images can jog the memory. This picture of a marshmallow cake which is illuminated by a polymerization lamp was used to clearly illustrate the problems of insufficient polymerization in composite fillings to an audience.

10.2 Producing the Slides

10.2.1 Real images

Slides are produced for different reasons. Their later use imposes various requirements on the images. Since the ultimate use of an image is not always known at the time it is created, it is generally advisable to take the images so that they can be viewed under difficult conditions.

Documentary images should be made under reproducible conditions. Images for print can be made with more detail than images for lectures, since the reader has better conditions under which to take in these images than a person looking at slides at a lecture. In the latter case, the length of time the slide is on the screen determines the time in which she or he can comprehend the content. With book illustrations the reader alone determines how long he or she wishes to examine an image. The viewer of a presentation does not have the ability to turn back the page, nor can she or he get closer to the image to see the details more closely as in looking at a book illustration. Real images are frequently used to implant the information in the listener's memory, in keeping with the motto: "Memory can not be forced, but it can be cajoled" (Fig. 10.2).

Requirements for a real image used in a lecture are thus:

- High technical quality
- Fill the frame; if possible, uniform horizontal format
- Reduced content
- Optimum perceptibility

Content can be reduced by:

- Using the whole format ("Get close to the subject!")
- Selective depth of field
- Selective illumination
- Isolating the subject
- Dividing complex content into several slides

Aside from its technical details, the perceptibility of an image is influenced by:

- correct orientation
- angle from which photo is taken permits three-dimensional perception of image content
- geared toward observer's experience (observer not overwhelmed; introduced to the subject)
- sufficient contrast with background
- correct illumination, main light from above
- correct arrangement of centre points of perception; with text slides, observing the direction the way in which the observer would read.

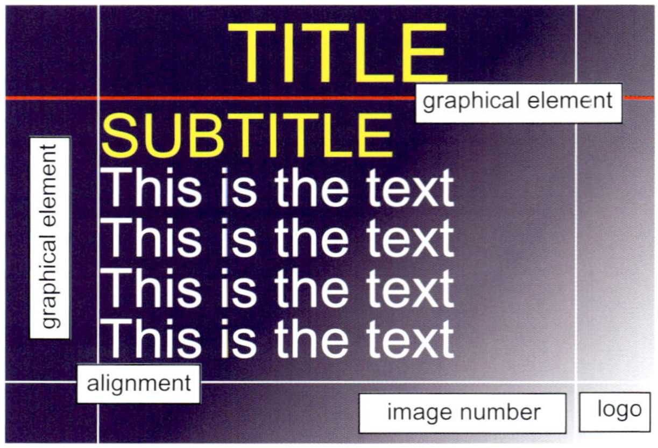

Fig. 10.3 Principal design of a text slide for lectures.

10.2.2 Text slides

The following relates to text slides, whether produced by photographic means or computer-generated, which is now more commonly the case. Thus these hints apply also to creating computer presentations.

The parts of a text slide are listed in Fig. 10.3:

- Background, possibly including graphics
- Text (including title and possibly sub-title)
- Possible logo
- Possible image number

Background

Producing the background for originals for optical slides is simple enough, the assumption being that black text will be used on a white background. The color of the background is not changed until the photographic process is introduced. However, today this is an exception.

For computer-generated slides the background is most important and its color should be chosen according to the following criteria:

- Select a medium tone: slides which are too bright tend to dazzle the audience and those which are too dark can make people feel sleepy, since the ambient light is reduced too much. Changing brightness in a series is to be avoided if possible.
- Good contrast with the text: light text on a dark background is more legible than vice versa.
- Background color should remain in the background in visual terms, that is, do not use red, since this color is focused at a different plane to those of other colors. Red is perceived in the foreground (Fig. 10.4).
- Reducing the number of background colors allows images from other series to be used.
- Uniform color for a series
- In case of doubt, blue should be selected as a background color. Since the human eye is relatively insensitive to blue, it provides good contrast and does not tire the audience if they have to look at a blue background for a long time.

Slides with a black background are easy to produce and also have the advantage of not showing dirty marks such as fingerprints or dust particles when projected. Black backgrounds should not be used with too many text colors. Blended backgrounds are pleasant on the eye and lively; they also correspond to our "normal" color perception and images thus tend to appear less like they are in a catalog. Blends from color to white

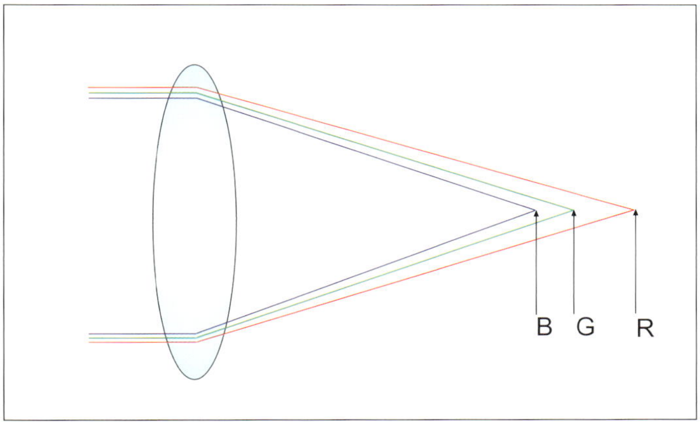

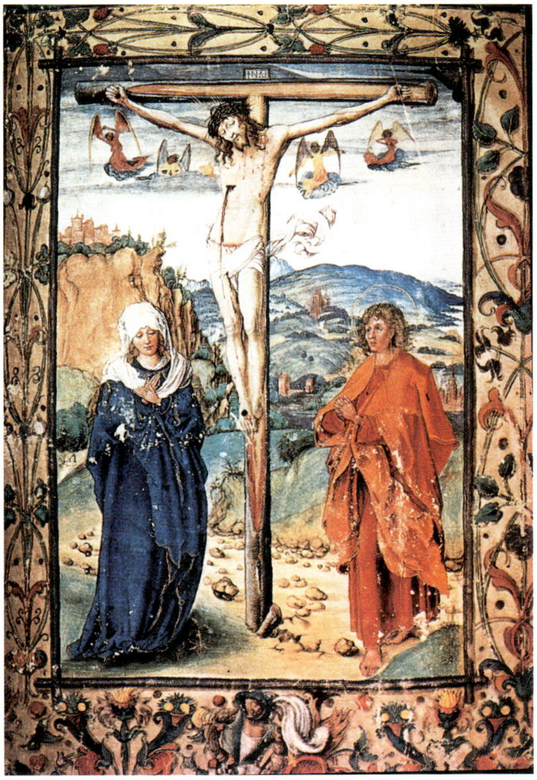

Fig. 10.4 Too many different colors overload the eye, as every color focuses at a different plane, since the eye, like many lenses, has the weakness of chromatic aberration (a). Red should not be used as a background color. The painters of the Renaissance were aware of this, since they clothed the saints who were "closer" to us in red, but Mary, who is "more removed" from us in blue (b).

are to be preferred. Color-to-color blends generally are too overpowering. Preferable colors (monochrome or blended) are gray and blue.

Graphic elements such as lines to divide up title text, bars along the side in contrasting colors and similar break up the image, but should be used sparingly.
Backgrounds with real images, as sometimes used by British or North American lecturers, should be avoided or used only seldom (title slide). Generally this reduces legibility since background structures obliterate the information.

The general rule of thumb: keep it simple. The listener/observer has attended the lecture to learn new information in his or her field and not what the latest computer graphics program can do.

Text
Text which provides information is characterized by:

✓ Font category
✓ Font style
✓ Font size
✓ Arrangement of text
✓ Color of type

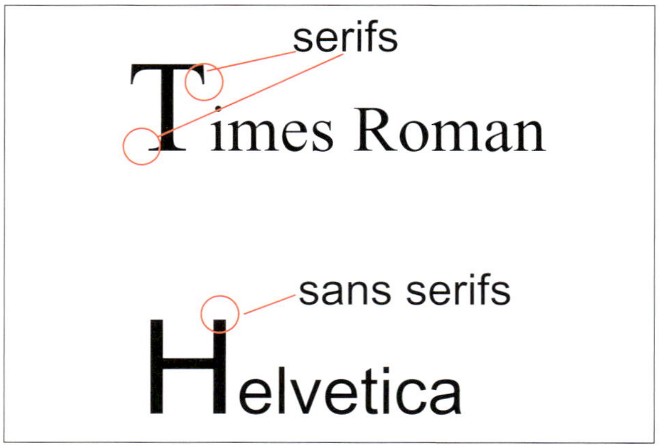

10.5a Serif typefaces are suitable for continuous blocks of text, since they guide the eye. However, sans serif typefaces are more suitable for lecture slides.

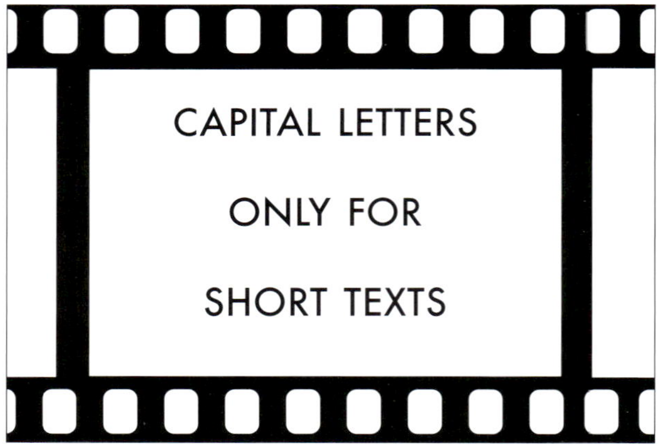

Fig. 10.5b Capital letters are suitable for short texts. Longer texts are better structured and more leg ble if upper and lower case are used.

Typeface
Clear, legible typefaces are to be preferred. Serif typefaces such as "Times" are to be avoided or used sparingly. Serifs are the thin lines on the top or bottom of letters. They are used to give a line of text more hold and replace lines such as those found in school notebooks. Serif fonts are very suitable for printed pages since they are legible because the eye is led and the reader does not lose the line (Fig. 10.5a). However, they are less appropriate for text slides since the thin cross lines create problems during projection and especially when shown on a computer screen.
Classical sans serif typefaces are for example Helvetica and its derivatives such as Avantgarde, Arial etc.
If at all possible typefaces should not be mixed. It is better to stick with one family of typefaces which are created by varying the basic typeface (e.g. Swiss, Swiss bold, Swiss light ...). "Bold" refers to a typeface with thick lines; "extra bold" is thicker still. "Light" typefaces have thinner lines, and "italic" cursive ones. "Condensed" refers to letters which are narrower than normal. All these should be used sparingly! Bold or very bold type improves legibility and italic type generally degrades it. Underlining also degrades legibility, particularly of letters with descenders (q, g, p).
Capital letters should be used for short texts only; longer texts are better structured, and thus more legible, by using the normal pattern of upper and lower case (Fig. 10.5b).

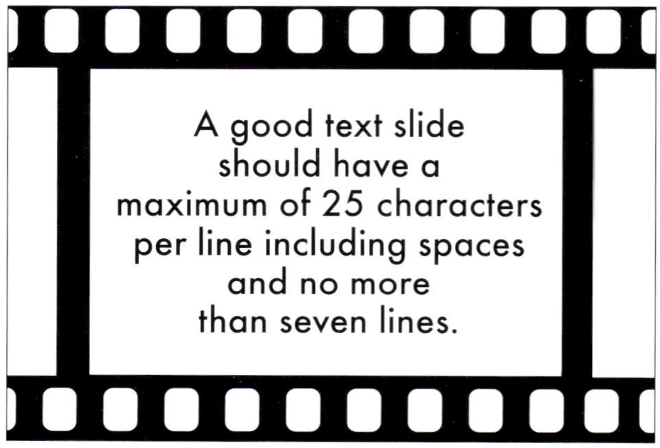

Fig. 10.5c A cardinal failure of many text slides is too much text on the slide.

Font size
Much research has been done to determine the size of type needed for good legibility. The height of the letters should be at least 3% of the height of the image.

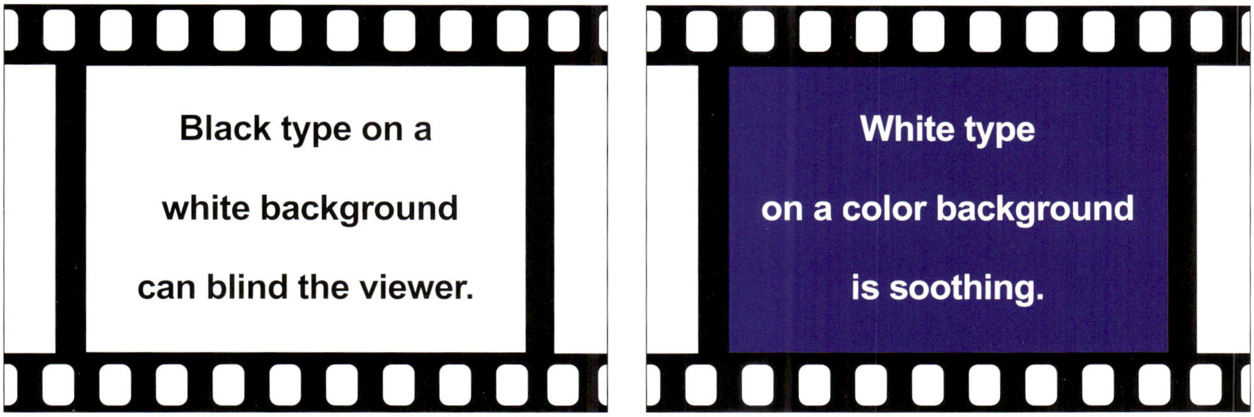
Black type on a
white background
can blind the viewer.
White type
on a color background
is soothing.

Fig. 10.6 If the background of a text slide is too bright it can blind the viewer (a). A white typeface on a color background is more soothing (b). Blue is a proven good color since the human eye is relatively insensitive to blue.

It is easier to remember a few rules of thumb according to which slides are perceivable with normal projection:

- If the text on the original can still be read when viewed from a distance equal to six times the width of the original, the text on the slide will also be legible. One tip is to place the original (A4 size) on the floor. If this can be read from a standing position the slide produced from it will also be legible.
- If the text on the slide can be read from a normal reading distance without any optical aids, then it can also be so when projected.
- The size of the type should be such that, when filling the entire image format, seven lines of text with no more than 25 characters (including spaces) can fit on the page. The same applies for computer generated presentations.

Titles should have the largest type size, with the rest of the text about 25–30% smaller. Any additional type sizes should be used only as an exception, and it is preferable to vary the text with upper and lower case letters.
Text can also be structured by varying the space between lines and by using indented text. The amount of text should be reduced by conscious use of meaningful concepts and phrases. If this is not sufficient, then the text should be divided into several slides.
The color of the type and the background play an important role in the legibility of a slide in addition to the size of type (Fig. 10.6 a–c).

Arrangement of text
Text should be aligned in relation to the side edges and the face lines of the title, logo and any graphical elements. Lists and longer text passages should be flush left; setting these flush right makes it more difficult to read text passages. Bibliographical data, however, can be set flush right.
Centering is advantageous only for short bits of text or titles.
Grouped style is generally not appropriate for text on slides, since the text is too short. If grouped style is justified, words must be hyphenated carefully to avoid large blanks. Logos, graphical elements such as lines and bars and sub-titles also reduce the amount of space for text, since this has to be arranged in accordance with these lines. Thus these should be reduced as much as possible to leave space for the text.
It is very important not to place text too close to the slide's edges. A "comfort zone" should always be left between the edge of the slide and text area to allow for subsequent framing.

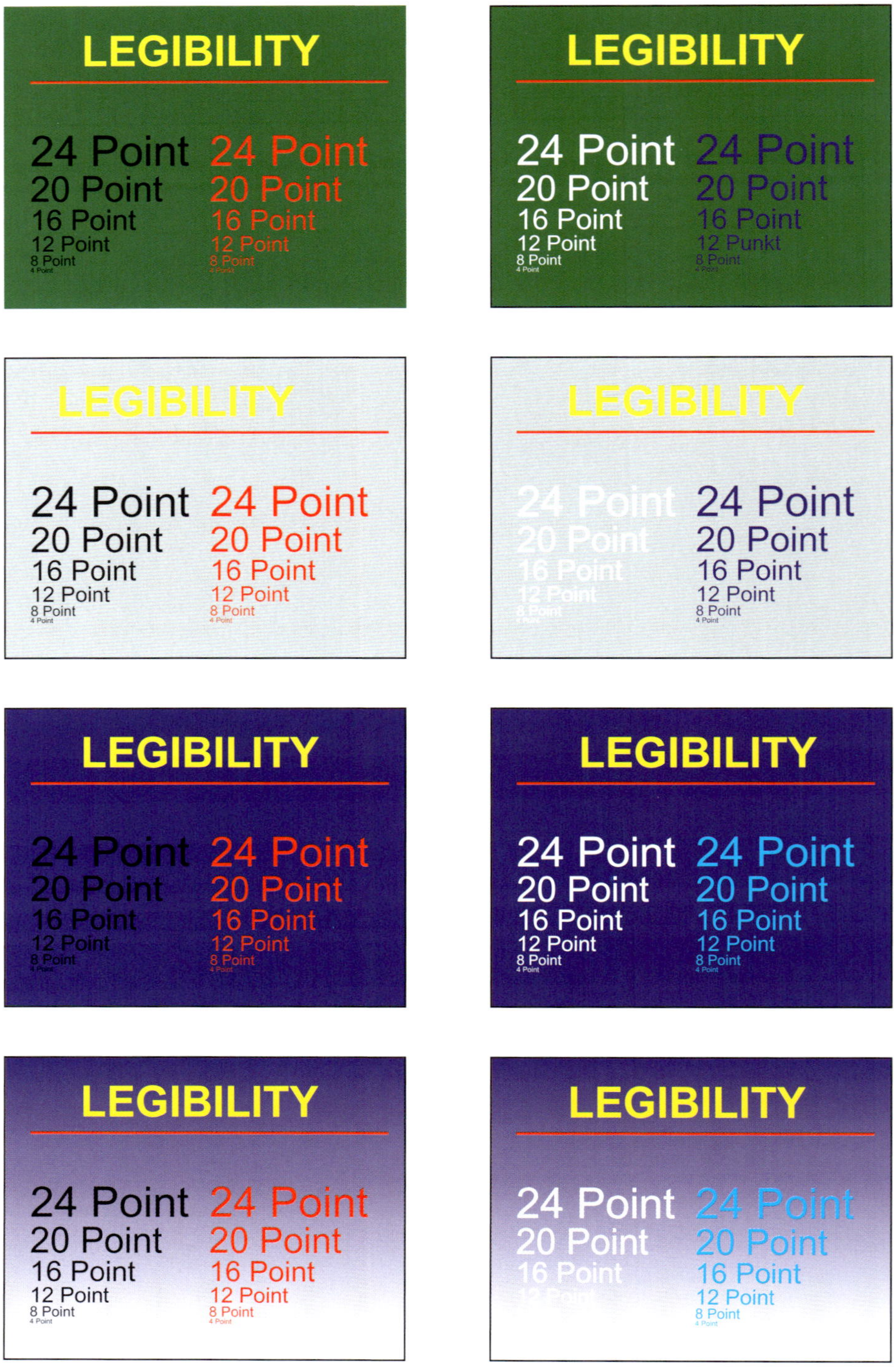

Fig. 10.6c Legibility of a typeface depends not only on its size but also on its color and that of the background. Typefaces should stand out from the background not only due to their color, but also to their brightness.

Color of type

Above all, the color of the type should contrast with that of the background, this being true not only for the color itself, but also for its brightness. It must also be kept in mind that different colors are focused at different planes. Thus red type on a blue background is not good, especially when they are equally bright.

A large mixture of colors, especially against a black background, should be avoided, because the viewer is quickly tired by having to focus on the various colors.

Suitable colors for text are white, yellow and bright blue, for example.

Blue text should never be used on a black background, or – even worse – black text on a blue background, since the eye is not sensitive to blue, resulting in too little contrast.

The complementary pairs of red-cyan and green-magenta should be avoided; on the other hand, the combination of blue-yellow is tolerable.

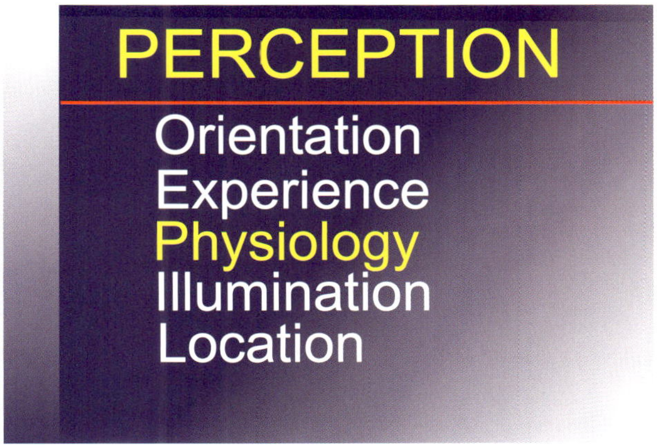

Fig. 10. 7 Text slides can structure a lecture and provide a thread for the observer (and the lecturer).

Marks

Marks such as bullets and other notation points help to arrange lists and thus graphically illustrate the weight of various points.

Many graphic programs feature a number of bullets; other suitable symbols can be found in symbol fonts such as "Wing Dings" under Windows.

Points, bullets, circles, squares, lines, arrows or checks are frequently used and especially suitable for lists.

Graphical elements should be used sparingly because they can easily make the image appear overloaded.

Sequences

Thematic summaries, lists, logical progressions, etc. can be grouped using sequential charts by adding each newest point; in doing so, the previous points are faded more into the background using color (for example, gray instead of white). This prevents the viewer from continuing to read and concentrates his or her attention more on the point being made.

If the entire structure of a lecture is to be outlined, all the points can be listed and the point under discussion emphasized through color (Fig. 10.7).

If overhead projection foils are produced, all the points should be listed and those which are still to be discussed should be covered up, thus obviating the need to change foils too frequently.

Logo and copyright symbol

Today, many companies and even university institutes speak of "corporate identity". This also entails a uniform appearance of text slides. It is doubtful, however, whether a university symbol should adorn each slide like a wine label.

It makes sense to limit the use of such logos to the title slide or to an introductory or concluding chart in the approved location. To repeat this on every slide wastes valuable space and distracts the viewer. Nevertheless, if the institute's logo must appear on every slide the lower edge of the image is the suitable place, also keeping in mind that its color should harmonize with the background to avoid attracting additional attention to it.

The same holds true for the copyright symbol,

which, if it appears at all, should be kept reasonably understated.

Image number, name of file
Retrieving the relevant data is simplified by adding image numbers or file path information. This is especially important for anyone who lectures frequently and has to keep track of a lot of charts.
Marking each image entails the same sort of problems as adding logos. It is more sensible to use the functions offered by many chart programs which allow the slides to be printed with its title and to dispense with a number which shows up on the slide.

10.2.3 Graphic slides: drawings and diagrams

Graphic slides clearly illustrate content and context, making them understandable at a glance (Fig. 10.8). Proportions of various values in relation to one another are particularly easily seen (or optically manipulated).
Tables with rows of barely legible columns of figures should be avoided and replaced with graphics, since such tables force the viewer to immerse him or herself before their content can be understood (Fig. 10.9). Drawings should also be simplified to the point that they can be perceived in the short time during which the slide is on the screen (Fig. 10.10).

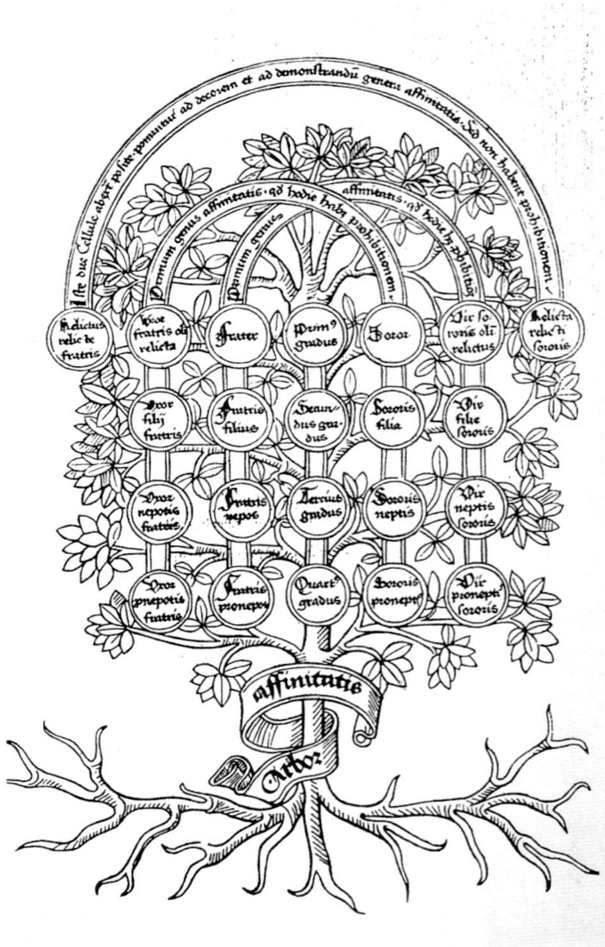

Fig. 10.8 Graphic slides can clarify contents and relationships. A classic illustration of this is a family tree.

General tips

Layout
Despite the fact that modern chart programs allow us to quickly produce a wide range of diagrams, we should keep in mind that they should be as simple and uniform as possible.
Anyone looking at charts must first learn to perceive even the simplest graphic. If the content of a lecture is presented using many types of graphics, the viewer is compelled to comprehend them each time a new one is introduced.

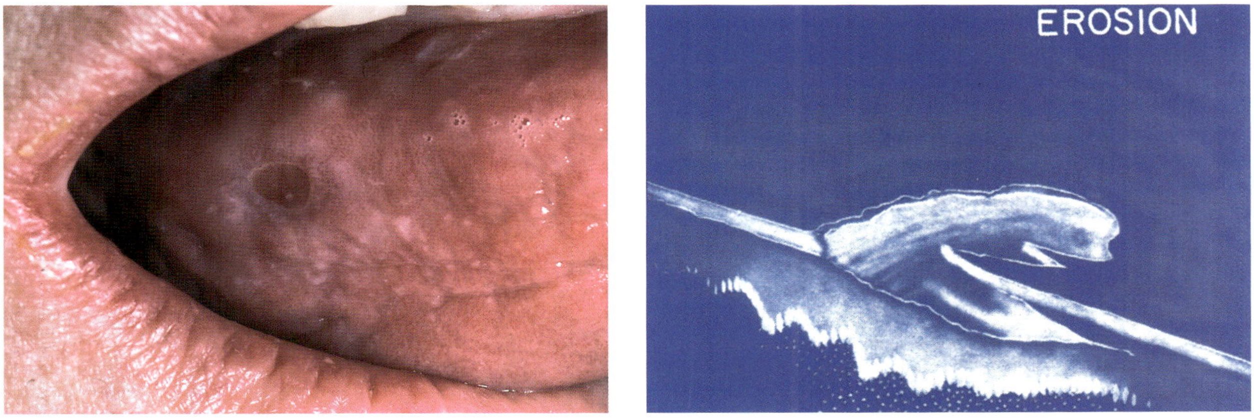

Fig. 10.9 Drawings often illustrate points better than do clinical images, since they simplify detail and thus are more schematic.

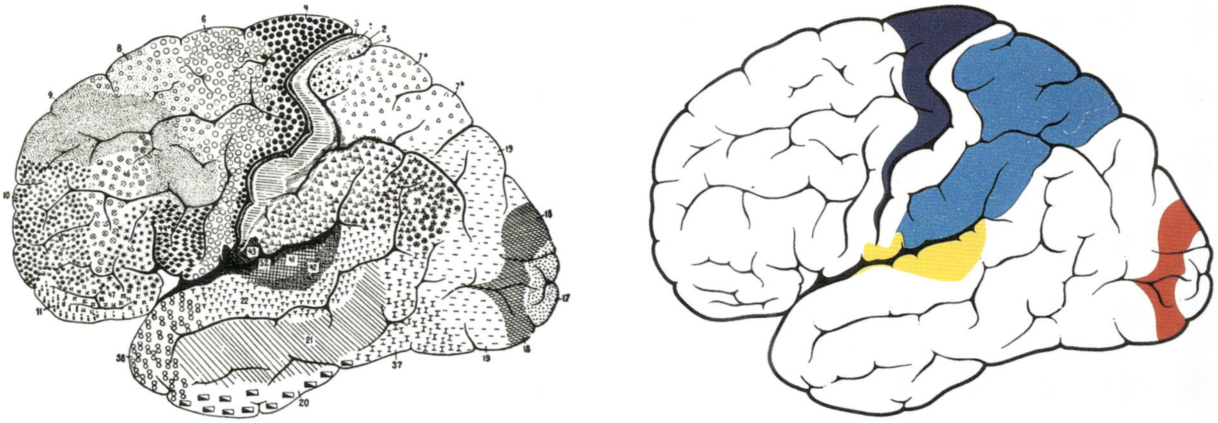

Fig. 10.10 Illustrations for books can be as complex as possible, since the time to examine them is not limited (a). For slide lectures such book illustrations should be simplified in keeping with the short time they are on screen.

Parts of diagrams

The x-axis (lower, horizontal axis) is the base of many graphics; for example, elapsed time can be represented, in accordance with the Central European convention of reading from left to right.

Values are generally placed on the y-axis (vertical axis). These include not only the title of the axis (for example, units of measurement) but the corresponding scale with a minimum and maximum.

The x-axis usually represents the value of 0. With percentage, the maximum is 100. The scale should be kept uniform to allow graphics to be compared. Gridmarks can improve the legibility of diagrams, especially if values are close together.

As in the case with a text chart, the title should be short and pithy; sub-titles can underpin the message (Fig. 10.11).

Values such as percentages, years, etc. should be written directly on the diagram if possible. Keys to parts are difficult to read and cause the viewers

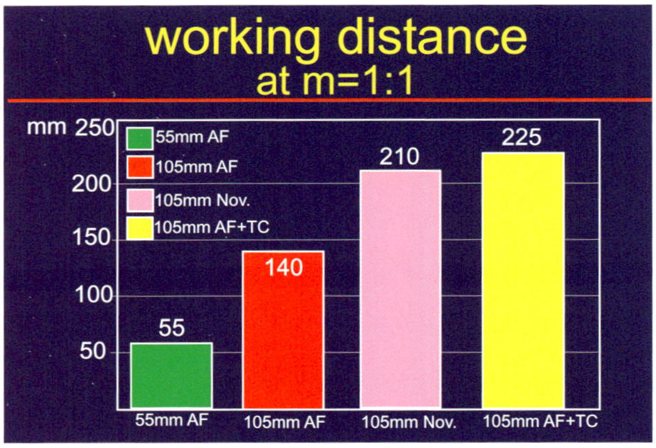

Fig. 10.11 Diagrams should have clear, simple text and be correctly labelled.

eye to flick back and forth between the list and the point in the graphic.
It is tempting to let colors get out of hand in a graphic, but these should be confined to a few easily distinguished ones.
Shading and patterns can be used effectively in graphics in black and white.

3D graphics
Many types of graphics can be presented so that they appear three dimensional, such as a circle cut up into a pie chart.
In principle, three dimensional presentation is more optically pleasing, but more difficult to read. In case of doubt, they should be left out.

Deviations
In scientific presentations it is obligatory that quantities to be measured are illustrated along with their deviation, whose mean value is presented as the result (standard deviation).

Types of graphics
• *Process diagrams (flow charts, critical path diagrams, structural diagrams)*
A frequently used type of chart which allows processes, structures and connections between different objects to be presented. Not suitable for representing numbers and changes between values. Special programs (Corel Flow, Visio etc.) are available for this.
Structural diagrams show the relationships between attributes or objects which have more or less the same value.
A critical path diagram shows processes or relationship of components.
The circle is a closed critical path diagram whose end point is also the beginning.
An interspersed diagram shows how partial values make up a larger value.

A flow chart is a special type of critical path diagram with standardized graphic elements which are in part also incorporated into a DIN norm. Suitable for computer or process sequences.
Another special form is the organizational chart, which is used in particular to show the relationship of personnel in a company. Aside from the most commonly used pyramid shape, it can be presented in a horizontal structure if the hierarchy is not to be strongly emphasized.

• *Bar graphics (block diagrams, bar charts, horizontal bar diagram)*
Frequently used type of diagram with which numbers and quantitative data are represented through horizontal bars. Less suitable for chronological sequences.
Text can be added to horizontal bars more easily than to vertical ones.
The individual bars can be separated from each other by spaces, or not (stepped bars). They can overlap or be represented as grouped bars with which data from one object can be represented.
A deviation bar chart shows the deviation from the zero point.
In contrast, a comparison bar chart or pair of bars with two series of data with the same scale to the

left and right of a zero line (age pyramid). By placing the grouped bars on top of one another instead of next to each other a component bar chart is created.
Changing this into 100% creates a 100% bar chart diagram and a good alternative to the circle diagram as it is much better for comparisons over time.

• *Column diagrams (vertical bar, column charts)*
Frequently used type of graphic to represent comparisons in concepts and size through bars vertical to the x-axis. Not suitable for non-quantitative information and very large amounts of data.
Variations are stepped bars, either grouped or overlapping, to show deviations and comparisons, as a component stepped bar and as a 100% bar diagram.
Column diagrams are better for showing growth than bar diagrams. Care should be taken that the ordinate always begins at 0 and that the columns and the spaces between them are always the same width.

• *Line diagrams (line charts, x-y diagrams, line graphs)*
Continual developments, series of numbers, fluctuations, trends, etc. are represented by line diagrams in which the connections between the points are linear. Overlapping and stepped diagrams are also possible.
Values which are far apart can be represented logarithmically.
In index line diagrams the data is linked to an initial point whose value is set at 100.
Three dimensional representation creates a band diagram, which is more difficult to read, however.

• *Curves*
Constant quantitative relationships can be shown by using curves. They can be derived from flattening a line diagram or from a mathematical function. They help avoid zig-zag curves and clarify trends.

• *Area diagrams (area charts, band charts, area graphics, zone diagrams)*
These are special forms of the line diagram in which the area between the base line and the data line is filled or emphasized through color.
It appears to be more impressive, but is frequently more difficult to read than a simple line diagram.
Very suitable for showing developments; data series which are similar or overlap are problematical.
As in the case with column diagrams, area diagrams which are overlapping, layered or have been converted into 100% are also possible.
In zone diagrams, only the area of difference between two data lines is filled in with color or a pattern (e.g. visualizing difference between profit and loss).
If possible, text should be placed within the areas.
Colors should become lighter from bottom to top.
If zones overlap the curves with the lowest values should be placed to the front.

• *Circle diagram/pie chart (sector diagram)*
Frequently used type of graphic to show partial values which always add up to 100%. Unsuitable for time sequences and to show many single values.
The sections in the circle are arranged according to size, generally starting from the 12:00 o'clock position. Since the human eye is not good at assessing areas the values should be placed next to the areas. This type of chart is effective only if the values differ clearly from each other.
Two circular diagrams next to each other show values at various times. It is better to use the column diagram for longer time sequences. Changes in a basic totality can be expressed in proportional circular diagrams, although only large increases or decreases only can be clearly seen.

Individual values can be emphasized by taking them out of the circle.
The three dimensional version creates a pie chart out of the circle; this pie should be neither too flat nor too steep (angled at about 50-60 degrees).

• *Spider charts (polar coordinates, radial networks, vector diagrams)*
Spider charts are especially good for showing deviations of a number of attributes in relation to several specifications. Spider charts are inappropriate for units of measure and time sequences. Spider charts for instance are well suited for illustrating the characteristics of various composites in relation to dental enamel or other desired value vs actual value comparisons.
Characteristics, dimensions and values should be placed to the outside next to the individual streams. The individual lines should be clearly distinguished from one another and limited in number.
A chart showing desired values vs actual values can also be produced as an area chart.

• *Table diagrams (line-column-graphic)*
Special form of table whose legibility is optimized by selecting a few important values and presenting them graphically in improved form. Suitable for short pieces of information, but not for long columns of numbers.

In addition, there are a number of other special forms of graphics which are not presented here.

• *Manipulations*
Distorted presentation of information by changing the basic structure of a type of graphic in order to emphasize certain information or relativize changes.
No data is distorted, but the viewer of the graphic is deceived, and thus such manipulations should be avoided.
For example, if a value is missing within a series of data (e.g. the results for a year), the place for this data should be left empty. "Abnormalies" are frequently presented in shortened form, thus falsifying the result, since the data next to it are optically more distinguishable. Differences between various values can be intensified if entire parts of a scale are left out or the scale does not start at 0. With column graphics attention must be paid that the columns have the same width. Narrower columns appear overall to be smaller than wider ones. With circular graphics it should be noted that brighter segments appear larger than dark ones, even if they are actually the same size. Positioning a certain segment of a pie chart in the foreground can increase its significance.

10.2. 4 Combining text, graphics and real images

Text or graphics can be enhanced by illustrations, which can include clip art from graphics programs, freehand drawings and photographs.
The combination of image and text or image and graphic can make a slide visually more attractive. However, care must be taken that the actual message of the slide is not compromised by the addition of an illustration, since this automatically attracts the viewer's eye.
The image should not be overloaded, which can easily happen if too many graphic elements or illustrations are used.
Illustrations are apt for text slides which appear relatively empty, that is, which have very little text on them (Fig. 10.12). Simple images are preferable, since they can easily be recognized and interpreted and also only take up a small amount of computer memory.
Real images take up a lot of memory, even when they are integrated into a slide at a relatively low resolution.

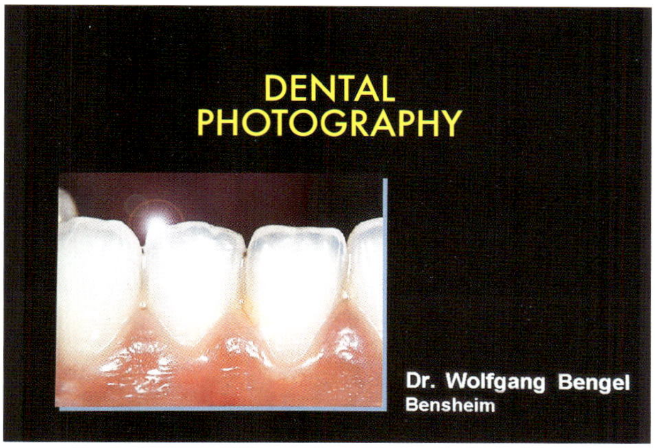

Fig. 10.12 Example of a combination of image and text.

10.3 From Original to Projection

The original which has been produced according to the above criteria must be turned into something which can be projected. This is done by:

- ✓ Producing the slide using photographic techniques
- ✓ Producing a slide by use of a color film recorder
- ✓ Screen photography
- ✓ Producing overhead projection viewfoils
- ✓ Computer presentation

10.3.1 Producing slides using photographic techniques

Producing text slides using photographic techniques is now a thing of the past. Only three of the photographic techniques which were once commonly used will be described here. These are simple to apply, but achieve professional results.
In each case the starting point is an original with black type on a white background. The larger the original the less it has to be enlarged for projection. For this reason, the originals should be at least DIN A5 format and preferably DIN A4. In this instance, too, a standardized approach leads to quicker and more uniform results. A laser printer is the ideal way of producing these, as it achieves high resolution results. Ink jet printers can also be used, but the sharpness of the print-outs is not as good. However, this is noticeable only if individual words are photographed to fill the frame and projected on a large scale. Even better resolution than with laser printers can be achieved with letters which can be rubbed on, such Letraset®, which however are distinguishable only in the case of extreme enlargements (Fig. 10.13).

The recommendations in Chapter 7 should be followed in photographing the originals.

Ektagraphic HC Slide Film

Kodak Ektagraphic HC Slide Film allows "black and white" slides to be produced as white type on a deep black background (Fig. 10.14). The text subsequently can have a color underlay or can be colored in. A guideline for exposure for a DIN A5 or DIN A4 original and using daylight balanced lamps from Kaiser is a setting of f/8 and a shutter speed of 1 second.
Processing: Development in Dokulith 1+3 for 2 minutes, stop bath SB-1a for 10 seconds, fixing in Kodak Rapid Fixer 1–2 minutes, 10 minutes wash under running water.
Special pens or transparent retouching dye is then applied to the dried film. A simpler method is to make a sandwich slide with self-adhesive color sheets.

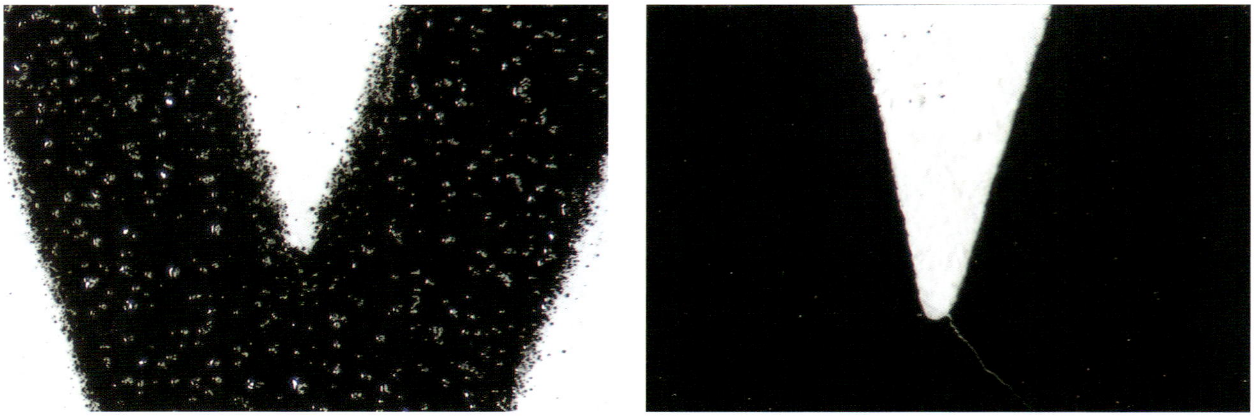

Fig. 10.13 Part of the letter "V" magnified 50 times (a) from a laser printer, (b) from a rub-on letter. The ragged edge of the laser print is noticeable under extreme magnification.

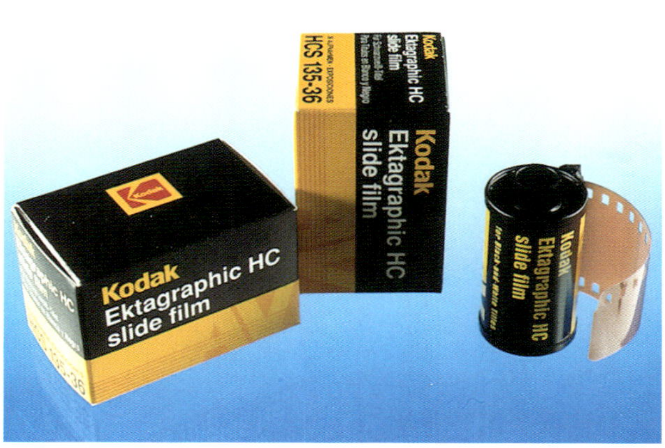

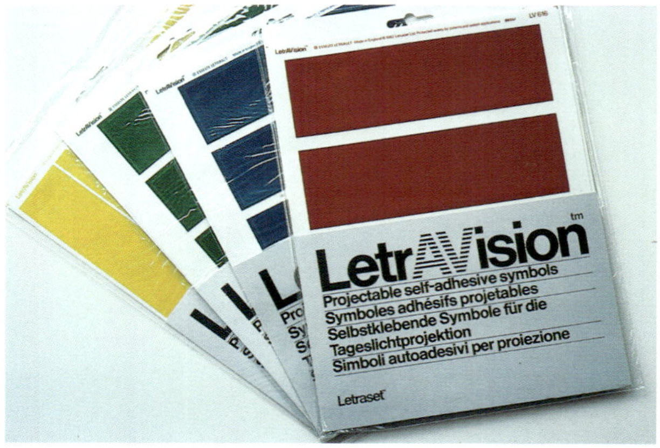

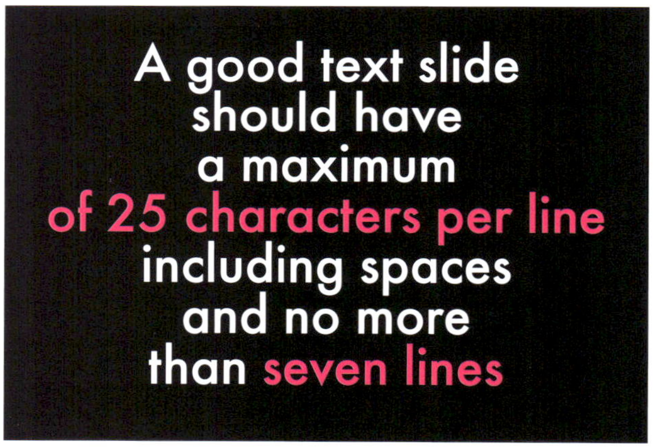

Fig. 10.14 Ektagraphic HC slide film (a) can be used to easily produce brilliant text slides; self-adhesive sheets (b) can add color (c).

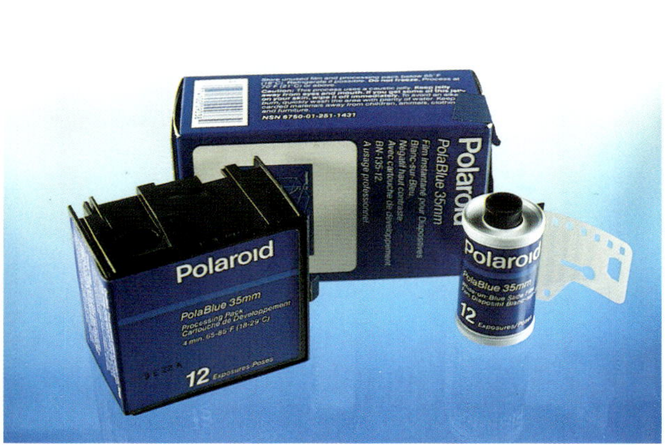

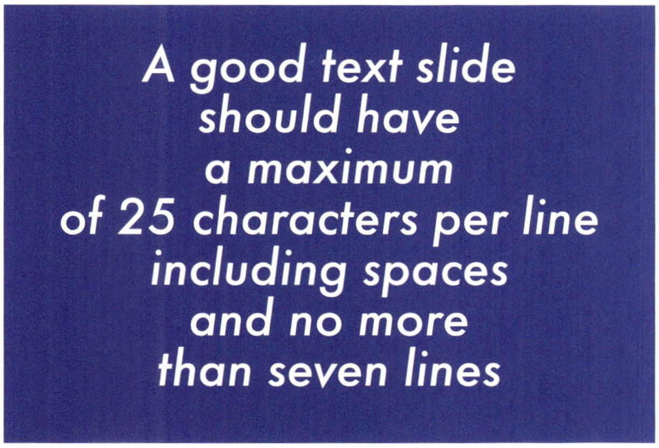

Fig. 10.15 PolaBlue film (Polaroid) (a) allows production of "blue slides" (b) in just a few minutes.

PolaBlue Instant Film

The PolaBlue auto process slide film from Polaroid permits last minute production of "blue slides" (Fig. 10.15).

A guideline for exposure for a DIN A5 original and using daylight balanced lamps from Kaiser is a shutter speed of 1 second and f/5.6 to f/8 (an exposure bracketing in $^1/_2$ stops is recommended, since the film has a very small exposure latitude).

Development is done using the Polaroid Autoprocess system and takes 4 minutes.

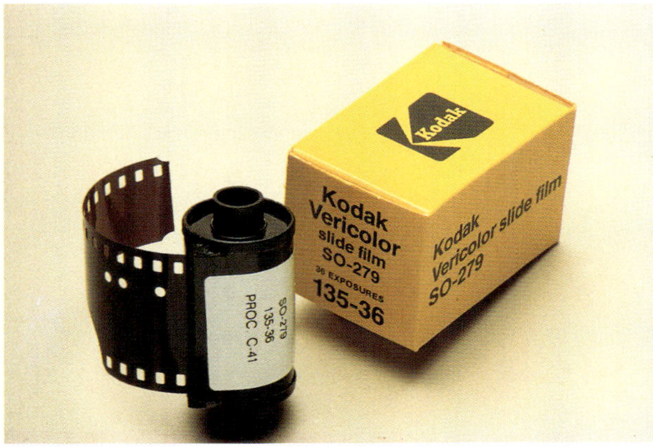

Fig. 10.16 Vericolor slide film SO-279 offers many ways of producing color text slides photographically.

Kodak Vericolor Slide Film SO-279

Kodak Vericolor Slide Film SO-279 offers the greatest latitude in producing slides using photographic techniques. It also allows production of "blue slides" as well as (even multi-colored) "blue slides", slides with any color font, as well as precise color gradations (Fig. 10.16). Guidelines for exposure for originals from DIN A4 to DIN A7 and illumination with four opal lamps of 75 W each are an aperture of f/8 and shutter speed of 2 seconds (with orange filter).

The film was originally designed to produce color slides from color negatives. Thus it reproduces colors as complementary (under consideration of the orange negative mask) and reverses the brightness.

When an original with black type on a white background is photographed through an orange filter and the Vericolor film is developed using the conventional C-41 process, the result is a blue slide with white type (Fig. 10.17). A red filter over the lens results in a cyan colored background. Individual lines can have different colors if strips of transparent color sheets are placed on the originals. Using a graduated filter on the lens results in graduated brightness of the background (Fig. 10.18 and 10.19).

Figures 10.20 a and b demonstrate the process of producing text slides using photochemical techniques and computer generation.

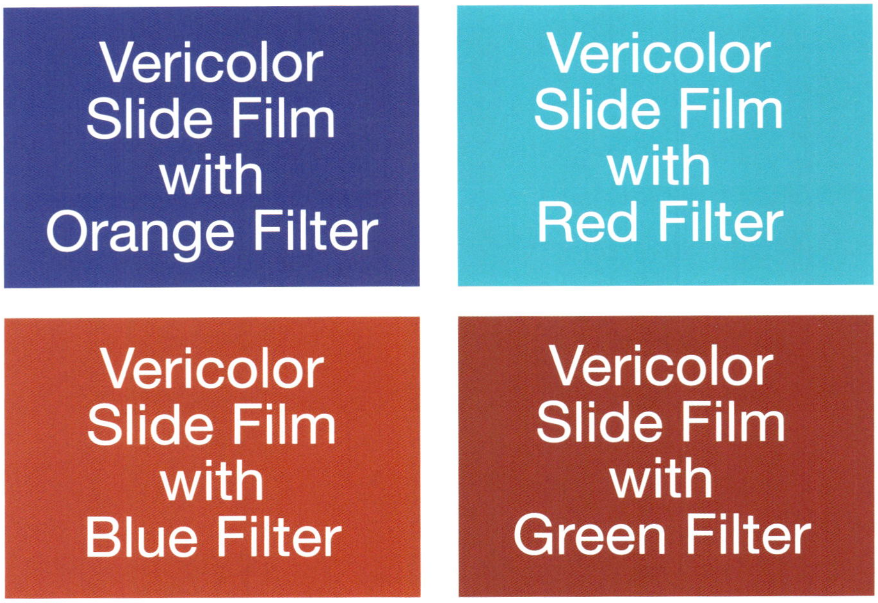

Fig. 10.17 If originals with black type on a white background are photographed with color filters, the resulting text slides have white type against various color backgrounds (a–d).

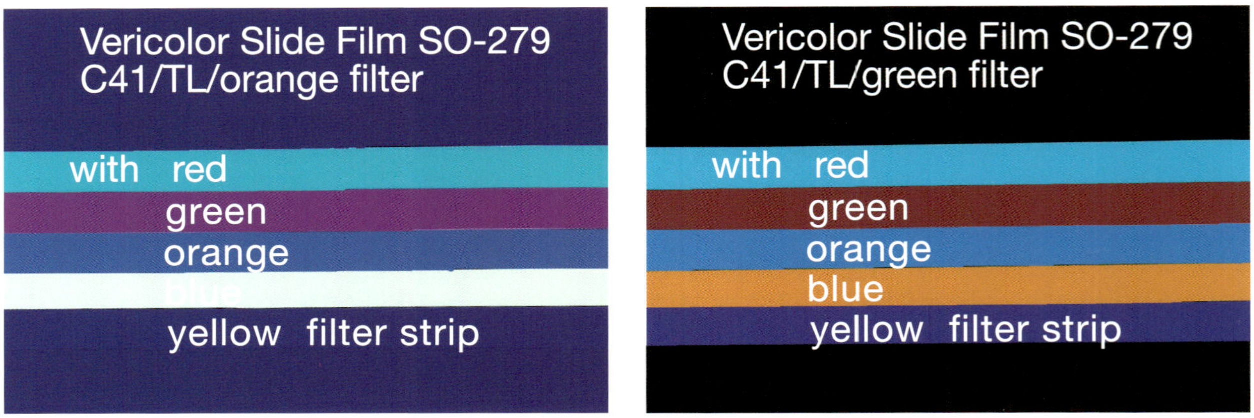

Fig. 10.18 Color strips placed over the original when photographed allow color to be used for emphasis. Vericolor Slide Film SO-279 C 41/KL/Orange filter

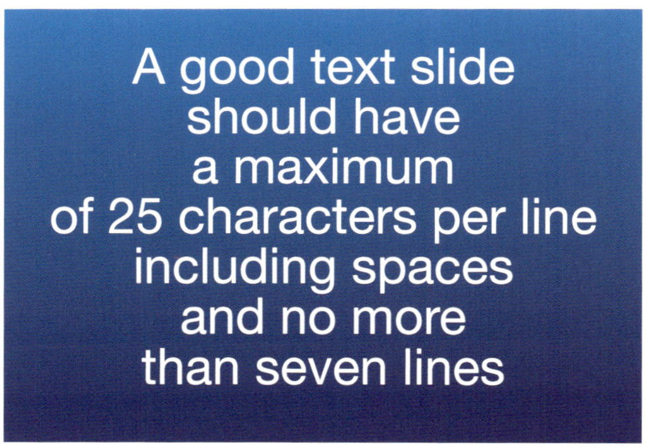

Fig. 10.19 A graduated filter on the camera produces color gradations of the background.

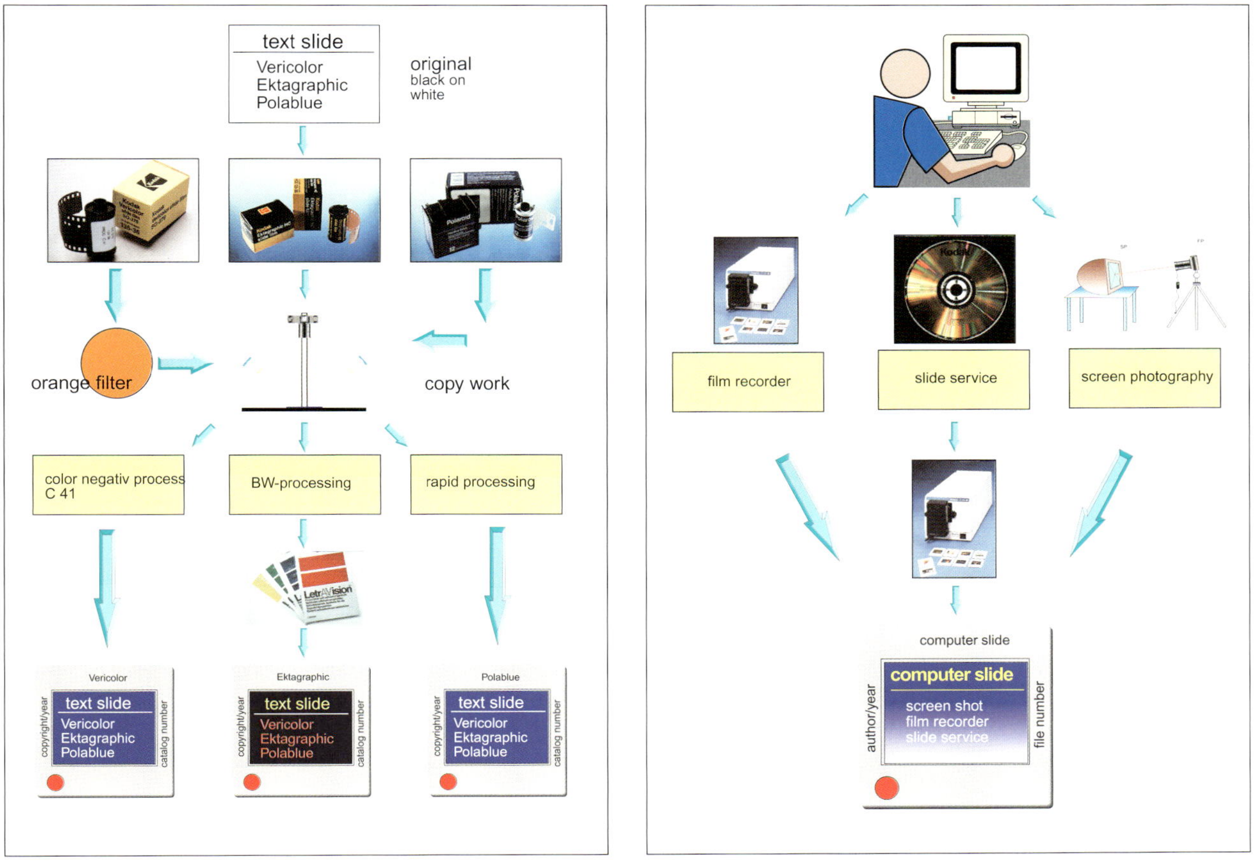

Fig. 10.20 There are many ways in which to produce text slides for lectures using photographic techniques. Three methods still being applied today are schematically illustrated here (a). The current method today is to produce slides on the computer (b). There are various ways in which to achieve good slides for projection.

10.3.2 Computer generated text slides

Computer generation of slides is the norm today. It is possible to change the typeface, color, background etc with just the touch of a button.
The most frequently made error is the overuse of such possibilities, resulting in overloaded, all too colourful slides which are difficult to perceive. Thus it is especially important to adhere to the guidelines for producing good slides.

Software for producing slides
Computer programs for producing presentations are appearing on the market every day. The rapid upgrading of older versions of existing programs makes the choice even more difficult. Proven and widely used programs include:

- ✓ Power Point
- ✓ Corel Draw
- ✓ Astound
- ✓ Harvard Graphics for Windows

Production using a color film recorder
If the desired outcome is a high quality slide which demonstrates neither lines nor stair-stepping even with large scale projection, then a film recorder is

a necessity. Such a film recorder is connected to the PC and records the image created on the screen on conventional color slide film at high resolution in keeping with the data on the slide (Fig. 10.21).
If the photographer does not have his or her own film recorder, it is possible to provide the data to a service bureau on a diskette, CD or via the Internet for recording.

Film recording in essence is like photographing a screen. This is done by using a special cathode ray tube which projects the image on the film's surface into an attached 35 mm camera. The exposure generally is aimed at producing a resolution of 4K (4000 lines), although better systems produce 8000 lines.

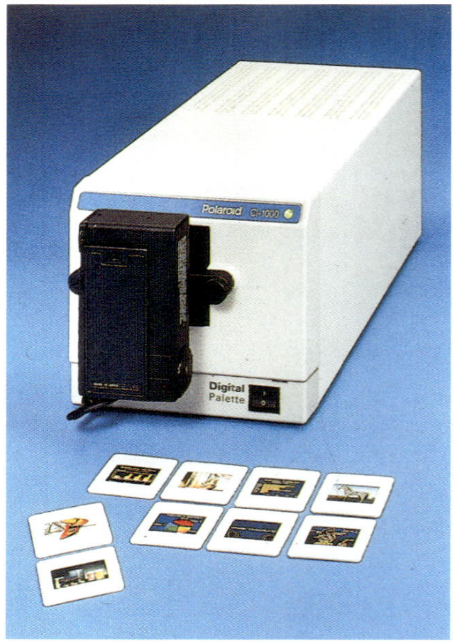

Fig. 10.21 Film recorders are indispensable for achieving optimal results for computer generated slides (Photo: Polaroid).

10.3.3 Monitor photography

Photographing the image on a monitor is a very quick and inexpensive way of producing "computer slides". If the characteristics of an image on a screen are kept in mind, the results of photographing today's 17 or 19 inch monitors with small shadow mask diameters can not be distinguished from professionally produced slides at a normal viewing distance. However, two things must be kept in mind when photographing an image on a monitor: the curvature of the monitor and its use of lines to build up an image.

Monitor construction

In principle, a monitor is a glass tube out of which air has been pumped; its lightly curved surface is coated on the inside with a layer of phosphorus. A beam of electrons is passed across this layer in lines, with the intensity of the beam determining the brightness of the resulting points of the image. Color monitors have three phosphor compounds in the screen which are separately excited by three electron beams. A shadow or slit mask is placed in the path of the electron beam close to the screen, allowing discrete control of individual picture elements via the electron beam. The smaller the holes in the mask, the greater the number of picture elements and the less they can be seen by the naked eye. Shadow mask sizes of about 0.26mm are common today.
At least 50 images per second must be produced to achieve a flicker-free image with fluent movement. In order to reduce the amount of data required, television images are transmitted as half images which are interlaced.

Technical requirements for photographing monitors

These properties of how an image is produced determine the way in which a screen can be photographed.
Since 1/25th of a second is needed to produce the complete picture (Fig. 10.22) (the first half image in 1/50th of a second, the second half image in the second 1/50th of a second) the shutter speed must be greater than 1/30th of a second (between 1/15th and 1/25th of a second for moving images). Shutter speeds shorter than this

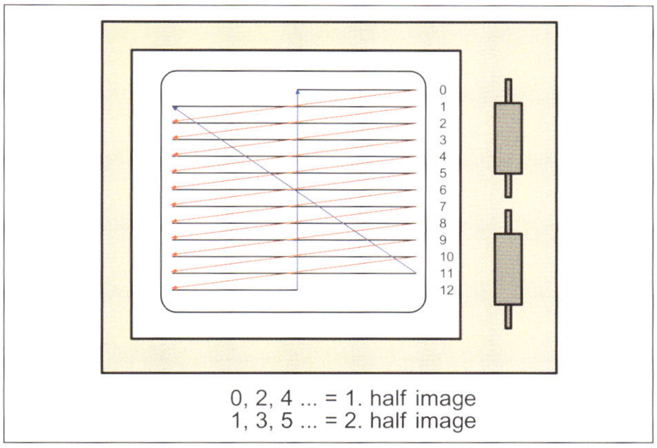

Fig. 10.22 The image on a screen is composed of two half images which are perceived as a single image by our lazy eyes.

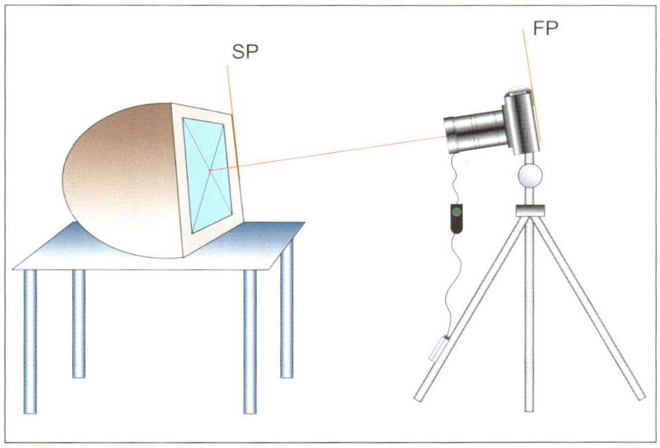

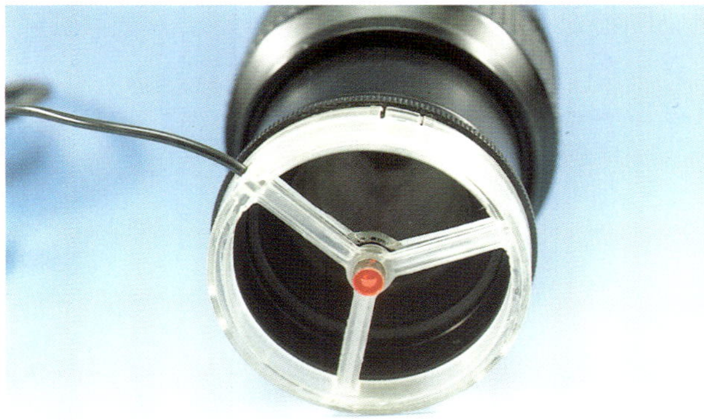

produce an incomplete image with horizontal black stripe. Longer times can be used for static screen images. Thus it means that no rapidly moving subjects can be photographed and that the camera must be mounted on a tripod.

The curvature of the screen can cause vertical and horizontal lines to appear bowed outwards. Newer flat-screen monitors cause no problem in this regard. In order to avoid the problem of curved lines in an image, a telephoto lens should be used (135mm to 200mm). The longer the focal length of the telephoto lens, the less the image will appear distorted due to the screen's curvature. It is important that the optical axis of the lens be perpendicular to the place on the monitor which is in the middle of the viewfinder. An adjustment system (Kaiser Fototechnik) is very helpful; using this, the mirror image of a diode in the middle of the lens is aligned with the diode's point of light on the screen. (Fig. 10.23).

The room should be darkened to avoid reflections from the room lights or the windows onto the

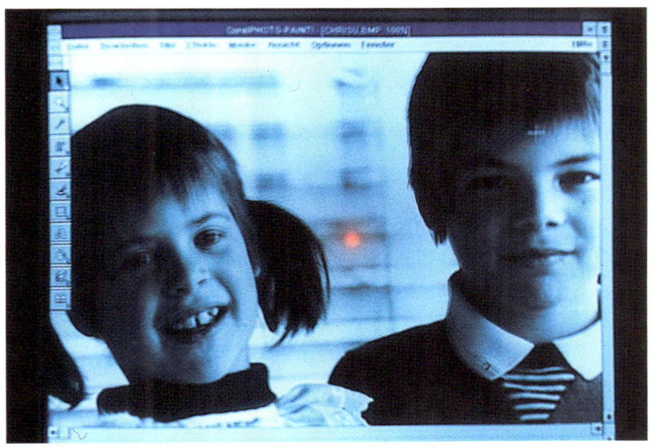

Fig. 10.23 To achieve optimum results the camera should be exactly perpendicular to the screen surface. The Kaiser adjustment system serves this purpose well (a). An LED in the middle of the lens (b) can be used to place the lens exactly in front of the screen (c). This reliably avoids distortions from the curved screen.

screen. The monitor should be adjusted for optimal contrast and color saturation.
Medium and high speed films can be used, since the resolution is determined by the raster of the TV image. Use of a cable release is recommended.
Monitors have a higher color temperature than daylight (about 6000K to 7500K); higher quality monitors allow this to be adjusted. Using a filter such as a KR3 filter, for example, can thus improve the results. Such filters are available from photographic suppliers.

The pictures show practically the same raster as that of the shadow mask which has been photographed. However, this raster is obvious only if the observer is standing very close to the screen when the image is projected.
When slides are projected the observer frequently notices that this raster effect improves image sharpness and contrast.
In order to reduce the negative effects of the raster structure as much as possible, the image should fill the monitor screen fully. The larger the monitor screen and the higher its resolution, the better the photographic result will be. Most programs for producing slides permit menus and tools to be switched off to allow the entire screen to be used for the image.

Hints on slide projection
Showing 35mm slides for instruction and lectures is currently the most widely used type of illustration which also achieves the best possible image reproduction.
The two types of projection are rear-screen projection (rear projection onto a screen) and front projection onto a slide screen.
Walls which are matte white and have diffused light emission have the advantage of allowing observers who are sitting further to the side to see the images without difficulty. Specially designed screens, for instance, pearl ones, are better suited for long, narrow rooms.
Viewing distance should be between two times and six times the size of the image. Tables show how to choose the correct focal length for the lens of the slide projector.
Extraneous light, such as that from undarkened windows in the room or from walls which reflect light from the screen, reduce image contrast.

10.3.4 Producing overhead projector transparencies

Transparencies for overhead projectors can be made by different methods.

Laser printers
Color laser printers work in the same manner as do black and white laser printers. Integrated raster image processors (RIP) separate the image to be printed into the four basic colors of yellow, magenta, cyan and black.
A laser beam projects the image onto a revolving image receiving ribbon. The first color toner is transferred to the location. The first partial image (e.g. the yellow one) is transferred to the drum and the toner cleaned off the ribbon. This process is repeated with the other colors. Finally, the complete image is transferred from the developer drum to the paper and fixed using heat and pressure.

Inkjet printers
There are two types of inkjet printer: fluid inkjet printers and solid ink printers.
In the case of **fluid inkjet printers**, two different techniques are used to squirt ink out of the jets.
With **thermal inkjet printers** heat elements are activated which heat the ink in fractions of a second, releasing ink dots (Canon: bubble jet process; Hewlett Packard: inkjet process).
Piezoelectric inkjet printers spray the ink droplets via a piezo multiplayer element which presses on a membrane and distributes the ink (e.g. Epson: Stylus Color) (Fig. 10.24)
Solid ink printers employ the phase change method. The four basic printing colors are contained in solid form in wax based color tubes. When needed, they are changed into liquid, printed on the paper and then pressed flat.
Generally inkjet printers require the use of special paper, since the depth of penetration of the colors

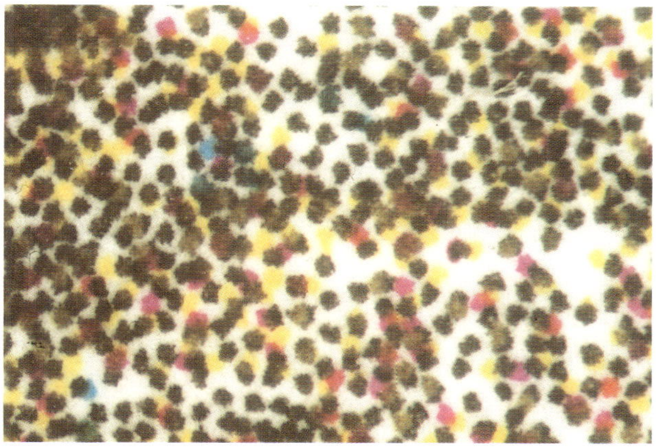

Fig. 10.24 Inkjet printers are high performance and cost-effective printers which today can also print out photo quality images, despite the fact that the image is comprised of numerous dots of ink, as shown in this 50x magnification from an image.

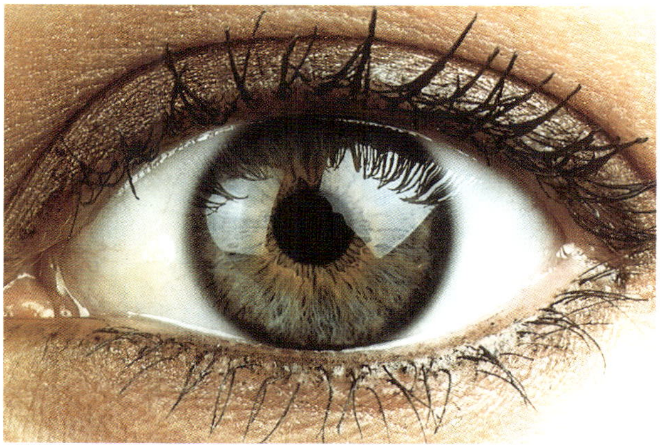

Fig. 10.25 Thermal dye sublimation printers currently produce the best results. The resulting prints can not be distinguished from those produced by photo chemical means.

into the paper is important. If the ink is diffused too much on the surface of the paper the colors appear matte, while too little diffusion does not allow the colors to adhere sufficiently.
When printing transparencies about 5–10 minutes should be allowed for drying so that the ink does not smear.

Thermal transfer printer
This technique seems to be becoming less prevalent. These types of printers print the colors on the paper using melted wax.
The thermal transfer method employs a wax coated ribbon, which is made up of consecutive films of cyan, magenta and yellow (CMYK ribbons have black as well). During printing the heating elements melt the wax layer and thereby transfer the colour onto the paper.

Thermal dye sublimation printers
Although they are still relatively expensive, thermal dye sublimation printers currently produce the best results. The melted wax is transferred in a gaseous state (skipping the liquid phase = sublimation) to the specially coated paper and produces a chemical reaction. The amount of color is controlled by the temperature of the printer head (Fig. 10.25).

10.3.5 Screen presentations

Images on screen can be projected using special techniques which will replace conventional slide projection. This has already happened in presentations for small groups at seminars and meetings. Using these techniques for larger groups still results in inferior image quality, at the moment. But image quality of the beamer improves very fast.
These techniques are described here only in general.

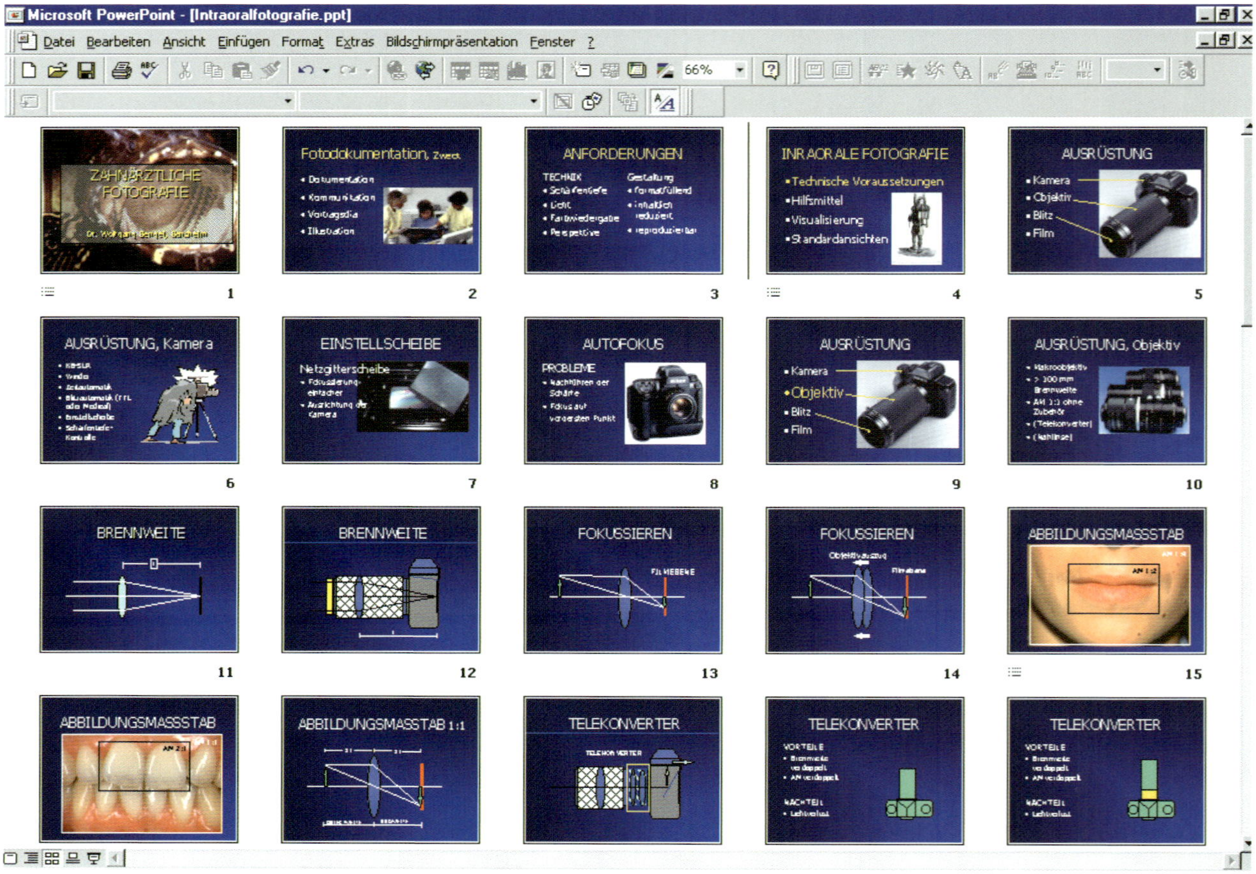

Fig. 10.26 The future of presentation technology is computer presentation.

Advantages of screen presentations

- Image elements can be animated, not only drawing attention to the presentation in general, but can be used very effectively to make important points, improving didactics of a presentation. These allow dynamic developments and relationships to be presented with a great deal of finesse, bordering on possibilities of animated films.
- Sound and video can be added
- The layout of entire series can easily be changed
- Individual "transparencies" can be added from existing presentations at the touch of a button
- Storing and archiving presentations is much easier. No need to "re-archive" slides after a lecture, with the associated problems.
- The lecturer's logistical problems are greatly reduced. No more need to carry around bulky slide trays; he or she now brings the presentation along on CD if the presentation means are available at the lecture hall (Fig. 10.26).

Disadvantages of screen presentations

- Image quality is still inferior to that of a slide presentation. Screen resolution is still the limiting factor, although with improved technology this will improve.
- Dependence on complex technology, with compatibility problems, still prevalent. Presentation equipment still not available in all higher learning facilities. These disadvantages should abate with time. Every lecturer is aware that even slide projection can have its problems.

It can be assumed that in the coming years screen presentations will augment and eventually replace conventional slide projection. Thus today it makes a great deal of sense to use both technologies in parallel if the projection of clinical slides, which is currently still of superior quality, is required.

Tips for producing screen presentations

✓ Adherence to basic guidelines for producing originals (see above)
✓ Sparing use of colors (not too many)
✓ Sparing use of animation. Not every title has to be introduced with a double somersault.
✓ Scan images (e.g. clinical images) only at a resolution of 72 dpi or 82 dpi in order not to increase the data file of the whole presentation unnecessarily.
✓ Use standard programs (e.g. Power Point, Astound) to avoid compatibility problems at the lecture site.

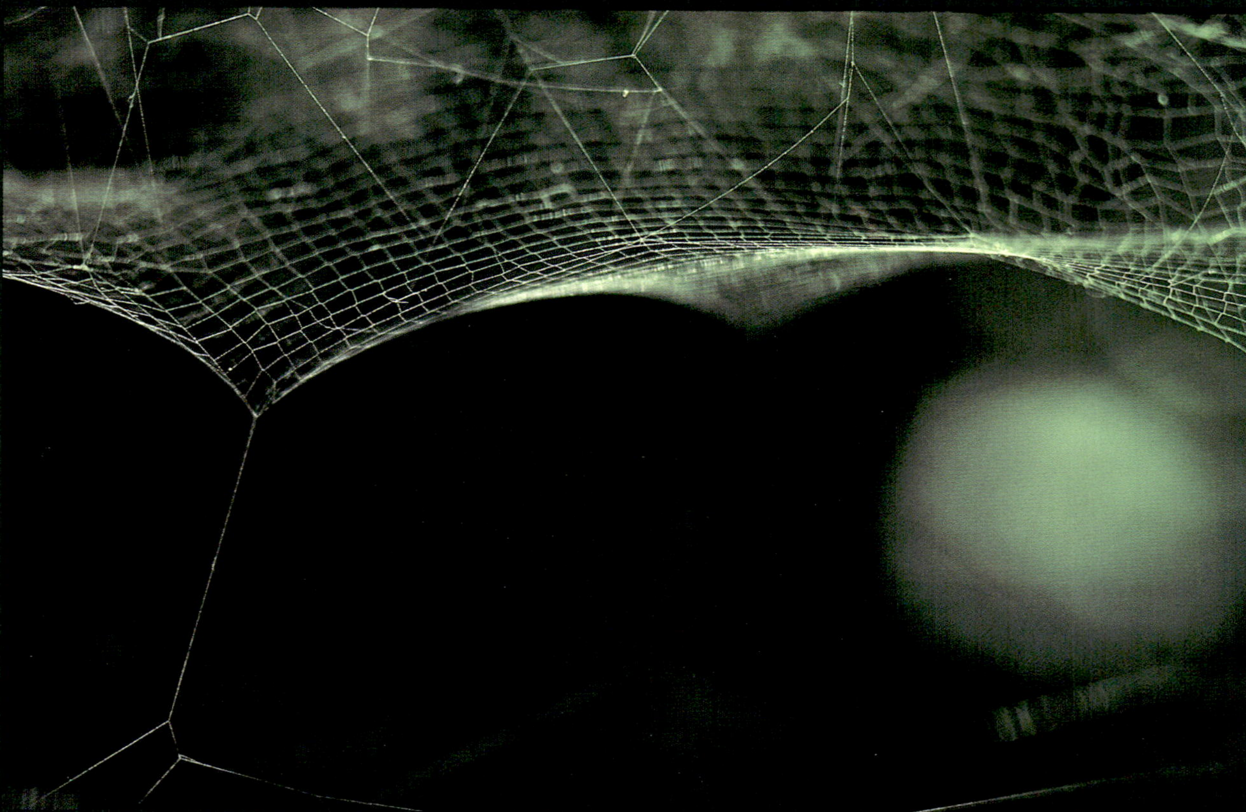

11 Storing and Archiving Your Photographs

When it begins to take longer to find a picture than to file it, the photographer should seriously consider how to organize the archive.

There are three requirements for such an archive:

✓ Protection against damage
✓ Rapid access
✓ Expansion

There is no such thing as the ideal archive. Its set up and organization should be governed by:

✓ Type of images
✓ Number of images
✓ Diversity of image content
✓ Purpose of images
✓ Accessibility
✓ Cost

◄ Diffusion is not limited to the atmosphere and the particles contained in it. Fine structures such as this spider web, which resembles the roof of the Olympic Stadium in Munich, disperse the light and become luminous structures, especially against a dark background.

11.1 Storing Your Photographs

11.1.1 Unframed images

Negatives and unframed slides can be stored in binders. Each page accommodates seven strips of film with six images, that is, enough for one film. It is useful to store a contact print with the negatives (Fig. 11.1).

11.1.2 Framed images

In general it makes sense to have slides mounted when they are developed. Only those which are required for later use in presentations are put in glass mounts.

Advantages of glass mounts:

✓ Protection against physical damage
✓ Protection against dust
✓ Slide is in a perfect plan position for projection
✓ Slides do not "pop" during projection, requiring no subsequent focusing
✓ Allows irrelevant areas of slides to be masked off

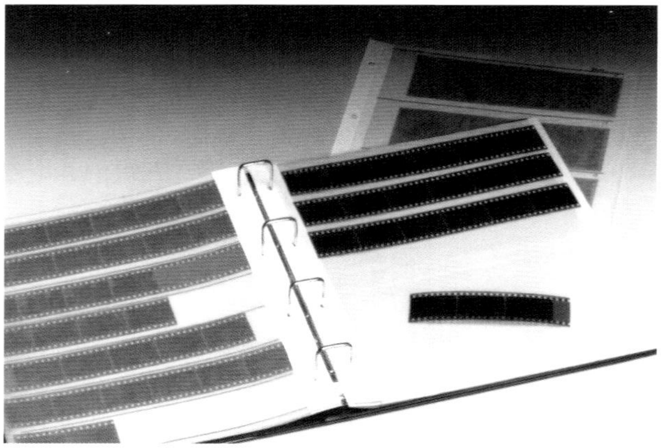

Fig. 11.1 Transparent sheets for ring binders are available for storage of negatives or unmounted slides. (Photo: Kaiser)

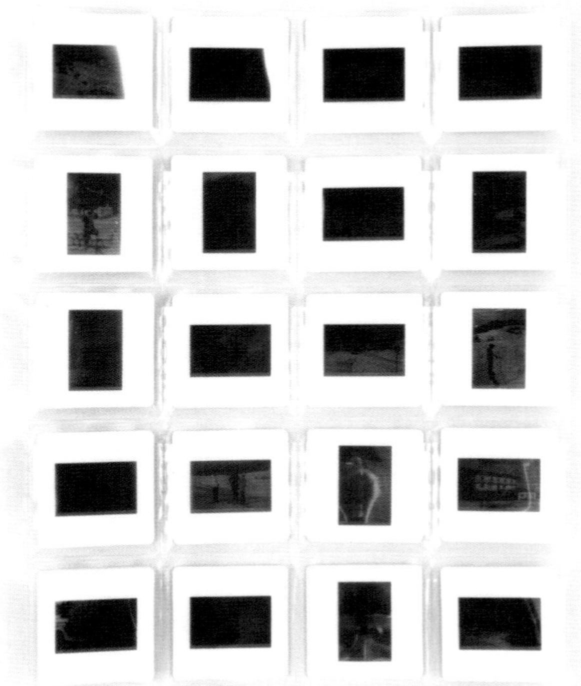

Fig. 11.2 Plastic transparent sleeves for unmounted slides can be stored in ring binders. Preferably, the type for hanging files should be used as they do not distort the sheets. (Photo: Rowi)

Disadvantages of glass mounts:

✓ Possibility of Newton rings
✓ Water of condensation creates dark areas during projection
✓ Emulsion can be attacked by fungus and bacteria
✓ Greater cost
✓ Heavier weight

Possible damage of images due to fungus and bacteria is reason enough to store slides which are not required for presentations without glass mountings.

There are many ways of storing images.
Clear plastic sheets which can accommodate 20 35mm slides can be stored in ring binders or hanging files (Fig. 11.2). The latter are preferable since there is no distortion due to weight.
Flat plastic boxes in which the laboratory supplies the developed slides save a lot of space and cost. These boxes can be stacked and can be labelled. Unfortunately, these present difficulties in accessing images easily and quickly since the boxes are closed. Nevertheless, this system is useful in storing duplicates or less important images.
Clear plastic slide cassette systems which open up are available from various photographic suppliers (e. g. "Journal 24" from Archivtechnik Kunze, boxes from Abodia). These store 24 slides (Fig. 11.3). These cassettes are labelled on the back and stored on shelves or in special archive cabinets (Fig. 11.4). It is easier to find an individ-

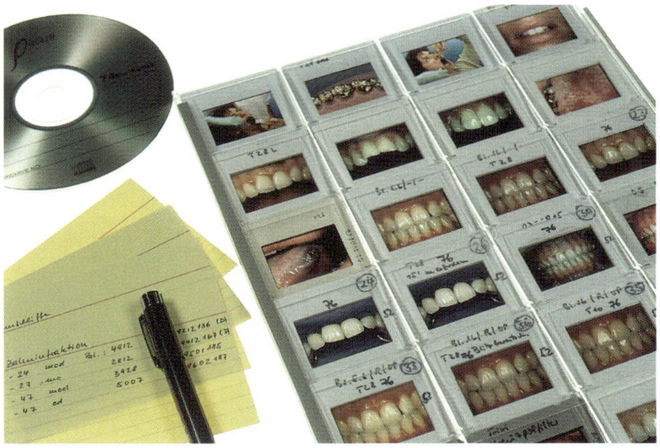

Fig. 11.3 Journal 24 is a proven archive system which is also available from Abodia in a similar form. Each cassette holds 24 slides.

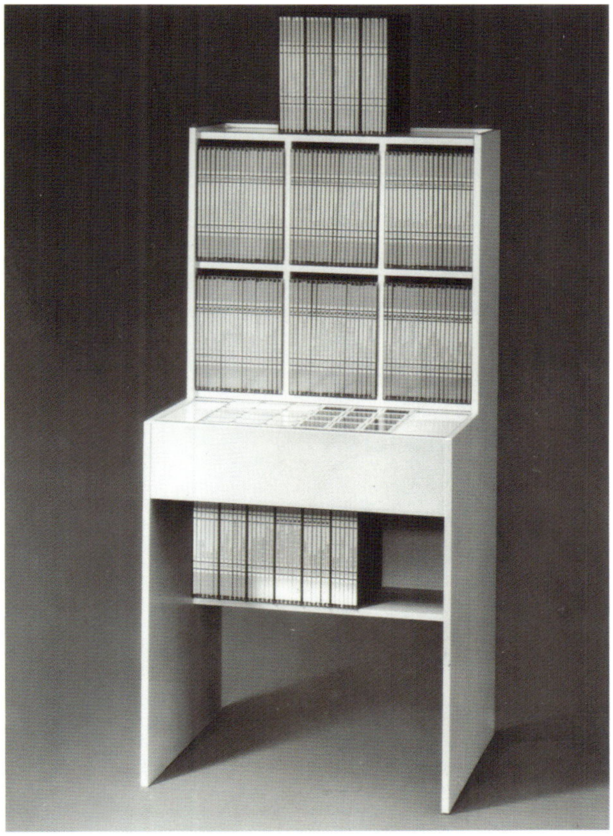

Fig. 11.4 The individual archive cassettes are stored on shelves or in special archive cabinets. (Photo: Archivtechnik Kunze)

Fig. 11.5 If the plastic cassettes are reproduced on a light box, an "archive cassette" for a lecture or slide series can be produced. This allows an overview of a maximum of 24 x 24 = 576 slides.

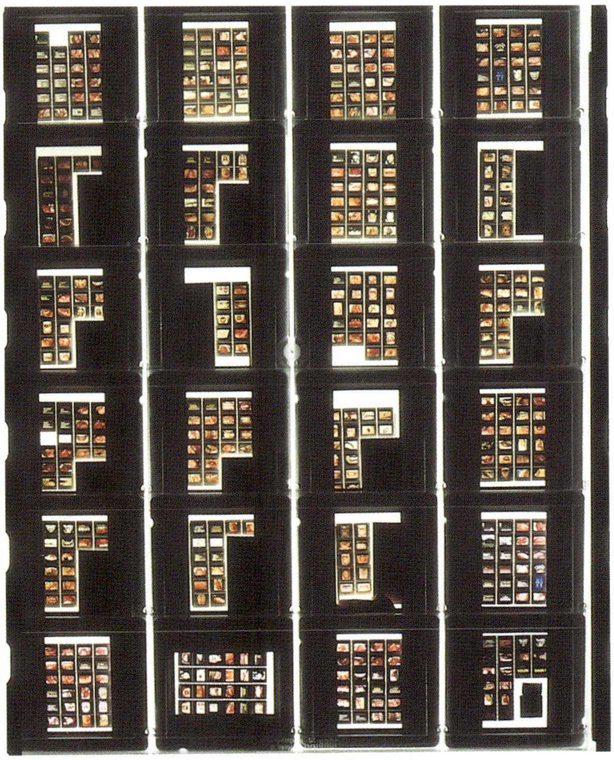

ual image if a photograph of each cassette is taken. If all of these "archive slides" are stored in a box, their total is 24 x 24 = 576 images, though they have to be viewed with a magnifier (Fig. 11.5).

Slide series which are ready for projection can be stored in universal or carousel slide trays. However, these do take up a lot of room and make it difficult to update the series.

There are many types of filing cabinets available. Cabinets with drawers without any light box system can accommodate many slides but require systematic filing because the slides can not be seen. Some slide storage cabinets with a lightbox have horizontal frames in drawers for slide storage (Fig. 11.6). However, for larger collections, a system which allows slides to be stored vertically is preferable; the slides can be viewed against a vertical light box. Each rack can hold up to 200 slides,

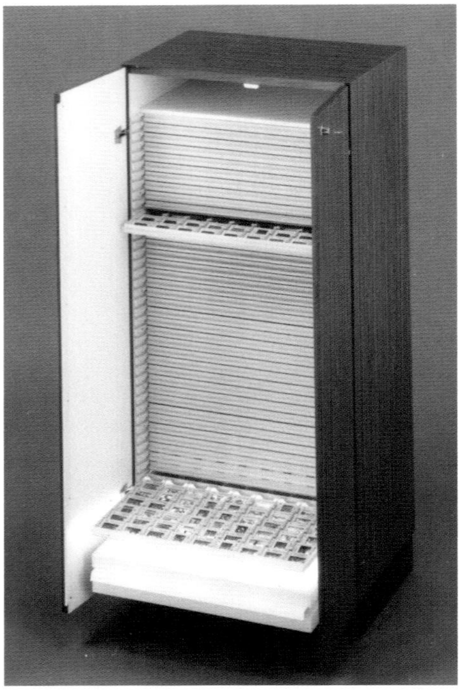

Fig. 11.6 Filing cabinets with horizontal racks permit images to be sorted according to subject. However, filing cabinets with vertical racks are easier to use and offer more room – see Fig. 11.7. (Photo: Abodia)

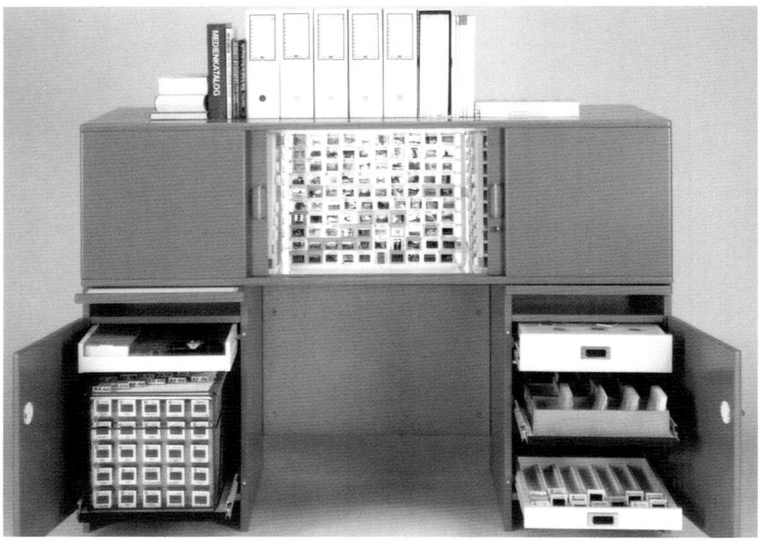

Fig. 11.7 Filing cabinets with vertical racks are to be recommended. Such a cabinet can contain over 10,000 images, sorted according to subject. The lower section can be organized according to preference, e.g. for duplicates, a card filing system or slide mounting equipment. (Photo: Abodia)

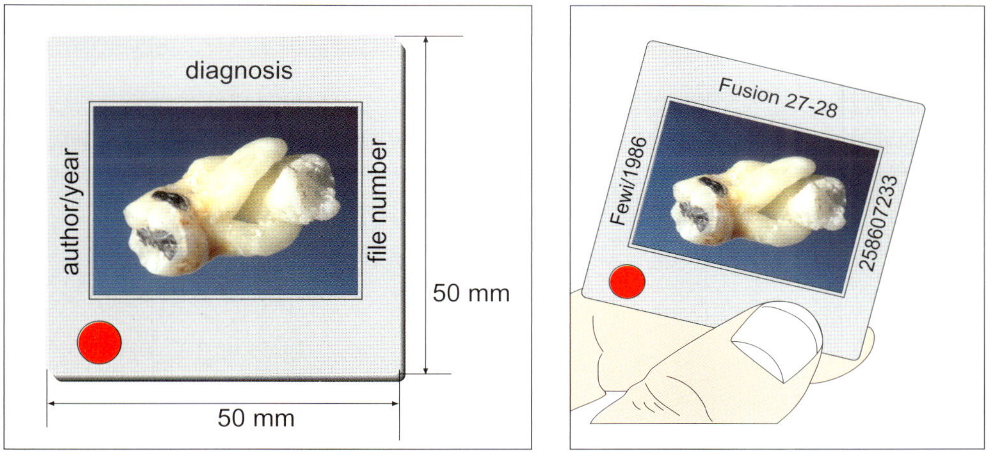

Fig. 11.8 Slides can be marked according to DIN specifications (a) or according to the user's own system (b), though this should be strictly adhered to in order to avoid creating a "mass grave" for images.

and according to individual designs, the upper part of the cabinet alone can hold 12,000 slides (Fig. 11.7). The lower part of the cabinet can be arranged according to individual preference, accommodating duplicates or organizational aids, for instance.

The advantage of these types of filing cabinets is that the images can be stored according to categories, permitting individual slides to be more easily found, since the photographer has an overview of a particular subject.

Each slide must be marked. DIN 108 specifies that this information must include the title of the slide, copyright, year and catalog number (Fig. 11.8a). Figure 11.8b shows how this would look. The catalog number indicates the file number of a filing cabinet (here 25), the position number of the image and details about the date on which it was taken (8607). The title contains the diagnosis. A red dot shows the correct position of the slide in the series for projection.

11.2 Organizing and Filing Your Photographs

The structure of the archive depends essentially on the number of topics and images. The most important consideration when setting up a new filing system is that it must be expandable. There is nothing worse than having to reorganize an existing archive.

Basically, images can be stored in sequence and then retrieved using a computerized system or even file cards. These methods are generally used for large picture archives. For our purposes a mixed system is recommended. For larger slide collections the basis is a slide viewing system (e.g. from Abodia) in which the slides can be found, stored according to subject. Ideally, the originals remain there, and lectures, publications, etc. illustrated only with duplicates or, even better, with a "second original", or electronically with scanned slides. The slides in such a cabinet with a viewing system can be filed in sequence in drawers.

Complete series or lectures can be stored in archive boxes; these can be easily accessed and

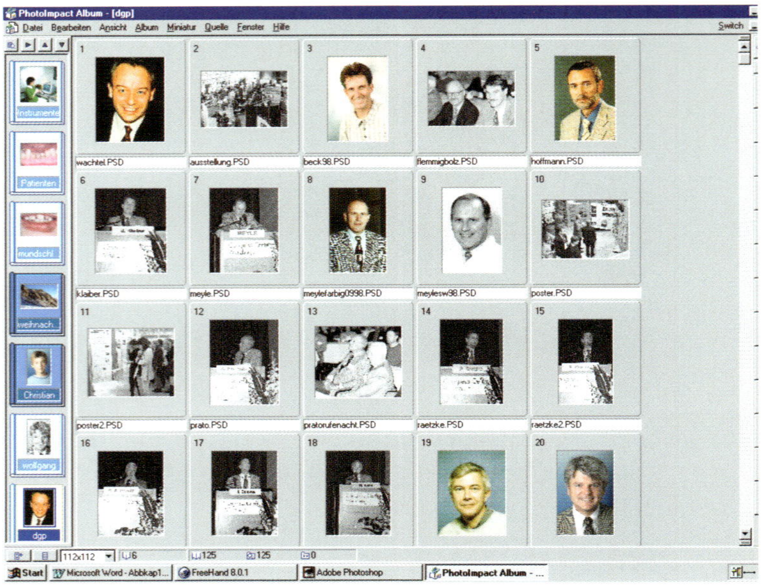

Fig. 11.9 Many reasonably priced image retrieval systems are on the market, some of which are modules of image editing solutions, such as PhotoImpact.

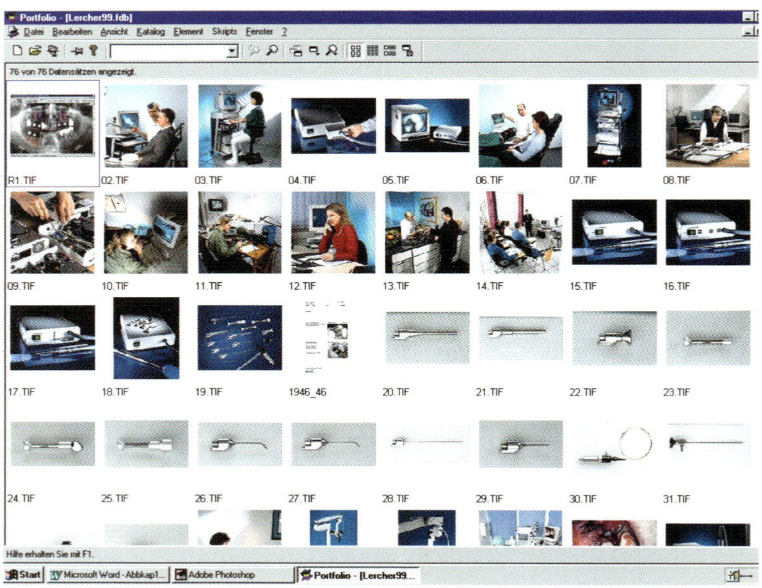

Fig. 11.10 Generally professional image retrieval systems – such as Portfolio from Extensis, shown here – also produce thumbnail images of the originals, which allow the images to be retrieved and selected visually.

permit changes to be made to such series without effort. When images are resorted after lectures or when slides are being put into slide trays the condition of the slides can be checked and any new ones added.

Slides sorted according to topics can be found again without difficulty and allow the most suitable illustration to be selected. However, this should be done with the aid of a card catalog or computerized archive system. There are many such computer filing systems on the market and standard software programs such as Access allow the user to create his or her own databases.

When building up a new archive, consideration should be given to whether all the images should be scanned in, either by the user or a service bureau, and then stored electronically (CD-ROM, Photo-CD, DVD). Programs allow images stored in this way to be very easily accessed, since they are stored not only using key-words, but also as "thumbnails," that is, small images which do not take up much computer memory (e.g. Foto Station, Portfolio, album-function from PhotoImpact, etc). There are many low cost programs for this purpose available on the market today (Fig. 11.9 and 11.10).

Since the trend is toward digital imaging, it makes good sense to consider such a storage system from the outset. However, it must also be borne in mind that even with these systems – regardless of whether CDs or DVDs are used as a storage medium – that technology will continue to progress and images will have to be transferred to new media. Regardless of how images are stored, the archive should be "tidied up" from time to time, since our expectations change and too much "dead wood" should not be hoarded. Always keep in mind the fundamental adage: the most important and cheapest aid to archiving is the waste paper basket.

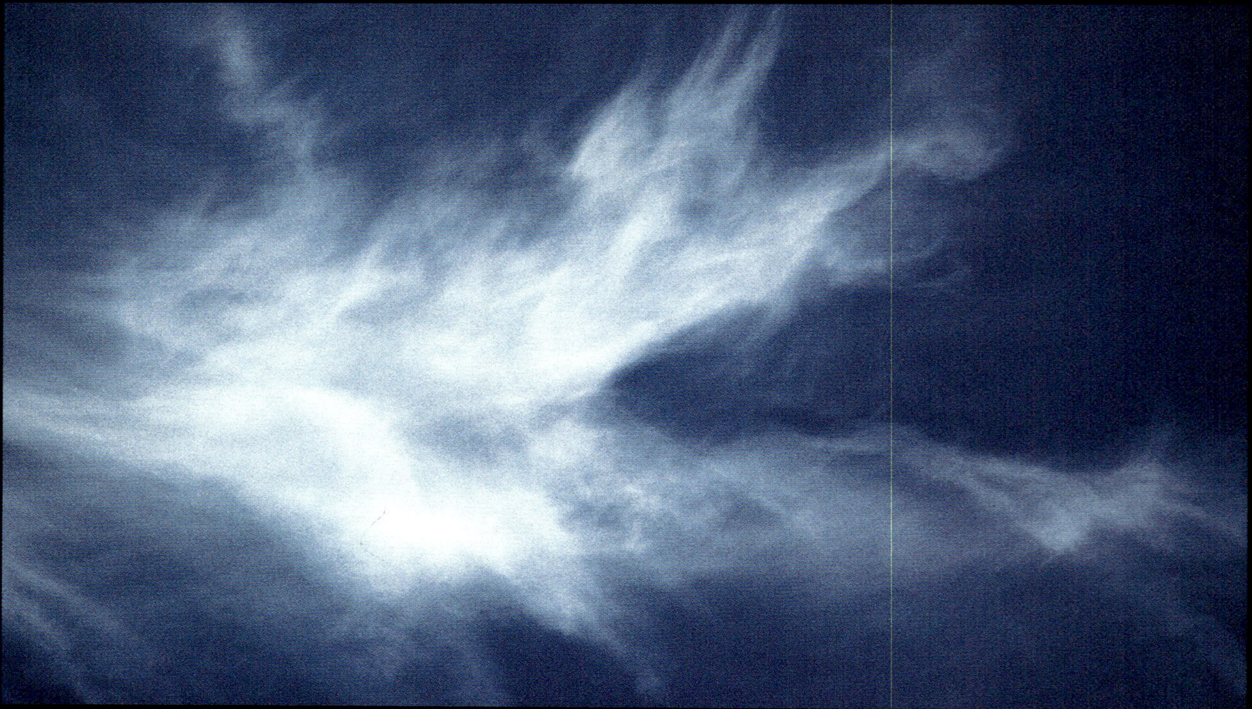

12 Digital Photography

The increasing use of computers in dental practices makes us wonder if it were not better for images to be made and stored electronically right from the start. This would eliminate the photo laboratory and make images available immediately. Intraoral video cameras have been increasingly used in the past few years, allowing the production of electronic images. These images can be archived relatively easily. However, their image quality is still fairly restricted, being suitable for a good screen image or for print quality up to about the size of an instant picture.

Another disadvantage of such video systems is that many of them produce relatively distorted images, as they are taken with a wide angle lens.
Video cameras are not the answer to achieving image quality comparable to that of conventional photography. For this, digital photographic cameras must be used.
The following presents the basics of digital cameras and describes a number of current systems, with no intention of completeness, since the development cycles in this field are too rapid.
The aim of this overview is to aid the potential user in making a decision as to whether to buy a digital camera and if so, which one.

◄ Light from the sun is not polarized, that is, it vibrates in all directions across the direction of travel. If it hits light molecules it is scattered and up to 60% of the light is polarized. Unlike many animals (e.g. bees) we can not directly see polarized light. If however we look through or photograph through a polarizing filter the influence of the polarization becomes obvious. Since most of the blue light from the sky is polarized practically every scene under an open sky is covered in a "blue veil". A polarizing filter eliminates the polarized portion of the light and thus the blue cast, increasing color saturation: the sky appears deep blue and the image has greater depth.

12.1 Basic Technology

12.1.1 Image capture

In digital cameras an electronic component (CCD-chip or CMOS sensor), placed in the position where conventional cameras have the film pressure plate, converts the light falling on it into an electrical signal. This process can be broken down into individual steps to make it more understandable. In reality, these individual processes occur in parallel and simultaneously.

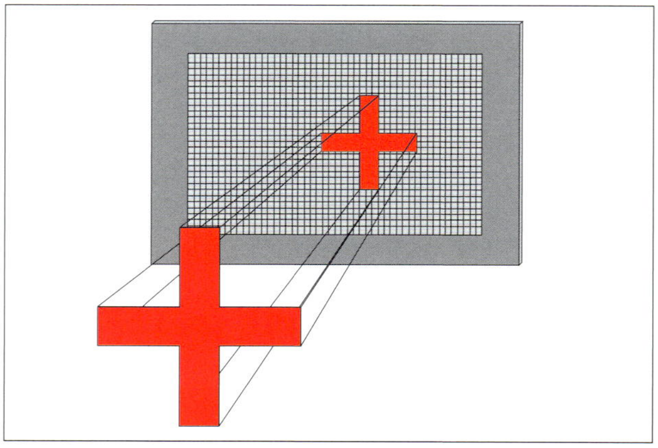

Fig. 12.1 The image projected onto the CCD chip is rastered into millions of pixels.

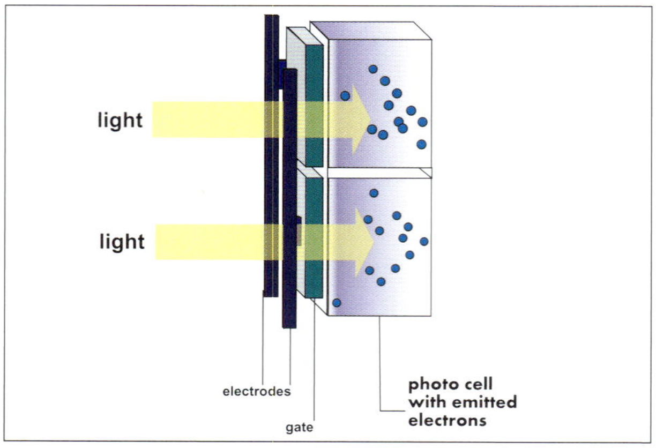

Fig. 12.2 The photo cell emits electrical signals in relation to the amount of light striking it.

- Rastering of the image into pixels
- Determination of pixel brightness
- Conversion of analog to digital
- Adding information about color

Rastering of the image into pixels

First, the image is converted into individual pixels. The greater the number of these, the higher the resolution of the image and the sharper it appears to us. Good digital cameras raster an image into about 3-5 million pixels (picture elements = pixels) (Fig. 12.1).

The rastering is done by the CCD chip which is comprised of about the same number of CCD elements (about 3-5 million). The image is projected by the optical system onto the CCD chip. Each CCD element can convert the light striking it into an electrical current.

Thus in the first instance the number of CCD elements determines the image quality: the greater the number of CCD elements, the better the image quality.

Determination of pixel brightness

A CCD element is comprised of an electrode grid and a silicon layer; certain area sensors also have color filters in front of them.

The energy of the light falling on the CCD element releases electrons in the silicon layer which are bundled by a current on the gate. The brighter the light signal the more electrons are released. (Fig. 12.2).

Thus each CCD element produces a signal which is proportional to the amount of the light reflected off the object and which strikes the single CCD element. This weak electrical signal is first produced as an analog current voltage.

The brightness of a pixel can therefore be expressed as the strength of the current which can be measured when this pixel is accessed.

Voltage levels are useless to a computer and thus the analog voltage value has to be converted into computer-readable form, that is, digitized. This is performed by the analog-digital converter.

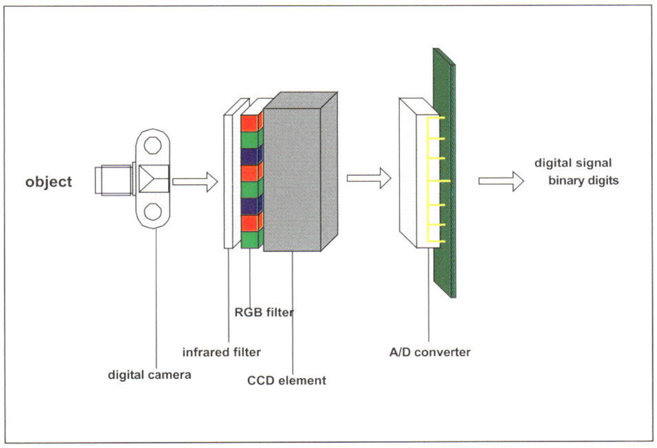

Fig. 12.3 Functional diagram of digital photography: rastering of image, conversion into electrical signals and subsequent digitization.

Analog-digital converter

An analog-digital converter converts the infinitely variable voltage value into a limited number of discrete digital values (Fig. 12.3). In the simplest case this means current = yes = 1, no current = no = 0. Such a converter can distinguish only between black and white. For text recognition or line drawings this alone would already be sufficient.

If images with grayscales have to be entered on the computer detectors have to be used which can distinguish these minimal differences in brightness. An important criterion for the quality of such digitizers is the number of brightness values they can distinguish.

In addition to resolution, which is determined by the number of pixels and is used to describe the so-called pixel resolution or - better - "structural resolution," there is also a grayscale or color resolution, which describes the ability to discriminate grayscale or color. In addition to the quality of the lenses or sensors, an important factor is the analog-digital converter. Its resolution is expressed in bits (bit depth).

A computer stores numerical values as a series of zeros or ones.

The smallest unit of information which a computer can process is called a bit (bit = binary digit). A bit has either a value of 0 or 1.

If four bits are used to code a numerical value, 16 different values can be clearly represented.

0000	0001	0010	0011
0100	0101	0110	0111
1000	1001	1010	1011
1100	1101	1110	1111

These can represent, for example, the numbers 1 - 15 or gray levels or other values.

A byte equals 8 bits.

A byte can represent 256 (=2^8) different sequences of zeros and ones. These can be the numbers of 0 to 255, 256 characters, or, for example, 256 gray levels.

A kilobyte (kB) equals 1024 such units of information. A megabyte is equal to 1024 x 1024 or 1048576 bytes.

A digitizer with a 4 bit resolution can thus convert the analog signals produced by the photo sensor into 16 digital values, allowing 16 gray levels to be distinguished.

Relationship between resolution in bits and grayscale resolution:

Resolution in bits	numbers	gray levels
4	0-15	16
5	0-31	32
6	0-63	64
8	0-255	256

The better the resolution of the analog-digital converter the greater the number of gray levels can be distinguished.

How many gray levels are needed to convert a halftone into a computerized form without significant loss of quality?

Aside from the scientific assessment of the image, the human eye is the yardstick, which can distinguish a resolution of about 2% difference in grayscale. That means about 64 gray levels can be distinguished. Thus a 6 bit resolution is sufficient in principle, but to compensate for any possible errors, an 8 bit resolution is generally used.

At this point the image consists of about 3-5 million pixels which vary in brightness from one another.
Now color has to be added.

Color information
A color image has information about color as well as about brightness. The CCD elements (photo sensors) are only able to measure the intensity (brightness) of the light. Different wavelengths (colors) can not be registered.
To record color information a trick is used. Color information is stored by using filters which divide colors into red, green and blue, generally done by using mosaic filters (Fig. 12.4). These consist of a regular mosaic of small green, blue and red filters which are placed in front of a CCD sensor. This is done by applying them to the protective glass of the CCD chip. Of the filters, 50% are green, since the green information also provides the signal for luminance (brightness); 25% are red and 25% are blue filters.
These small filters do what color filters always do: they let their own color light through and block the light of the complementary color. This means that the CCD element with a red filter only measures the brightness of the red part of the light, the neighboring "blue CCD element" only the blue portion, etc.
The image data of a 3 megabyte chip at this point is 3 million bytes. Each byte contains information about the position, brightness and color information about a basic color of the particular pixel.
The missing color information of the individual pixels (e.g. the brightness of the green and blue portion of a "red CCD element") are added by the computer through interpolation by the neighboring pixel values. Thus the amount of data is increased. The image data, which was 3 megabytes, is now suddenly 9 megabytes. The electronic image loses brilliance and sharpness through this process of interpolation and thus must be subsequently enhanced, e.g. through electronic sharpening. It must be kept in mind that only the color information is interpolated, and not the physical resolution.
For a photorealistic image up to almost size A4 printed off on an inkjet printer 9MB is sufficient. If the image is to be printed in offset printing at 300 ppi (pixels per inch), this amount of data is sufficient for about 13 x 18 cm (see table).
The heart of the camera, the CCD chip, thus above all determines the image quality, but also the price of the camera. If relatively inexpensive video chips are used the resulting images are often unsatisfactory. Lights appear to be overlaid with white and shadows not differentiated ("swallowed up"). Hence good CCD chips offer a color depth of more than 8 bits per color channel.
The current development trend for digital cameras

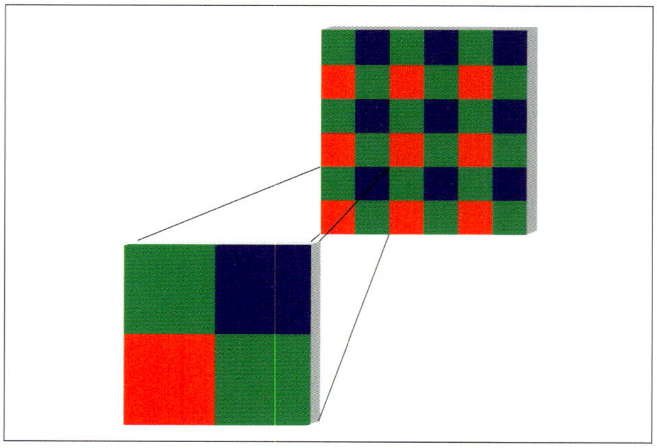

Fig. 12.4 A mosaic filter allows only its own color through, so that each CCD element only registers the brightness information of "its" color.

Resolution	Number of pixels	Data in MB	Output size in cm at 180 ppi	Output size in cm at 300 ppi, 60 screen
email-mode	320 x 240	0.2	–	–
VGA	640 x 480	0.9	9.03 x 6.77	5.42 x 4.06
XGA	1024 x 768	2.25	14.45 x 10.84	8.67 x 6.5
SXGA	1280 x 1024	3.75	18.06 x 14.45	10.84 x 8.67
UXGA	1600 x 1200	5.5	22.58 x 16.93	13.55 x 10.16
EXGA	2048 x 1536	9	28.9 x 21.67	17.34 x 13

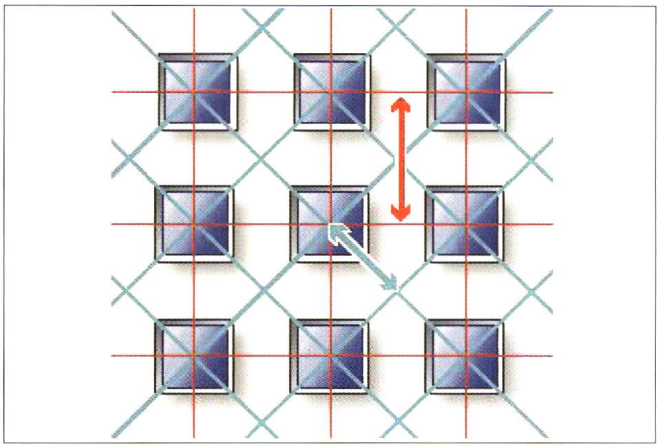

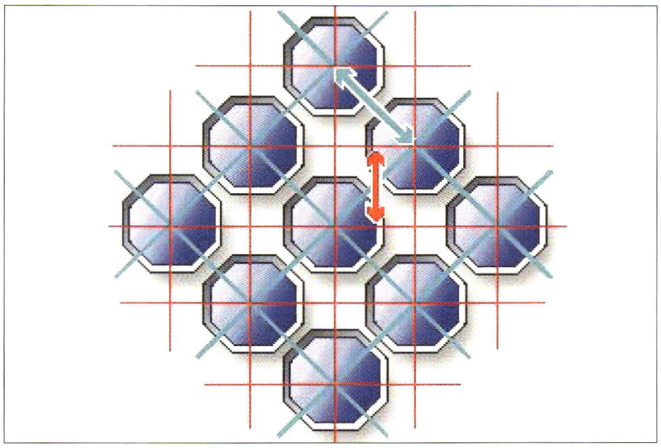

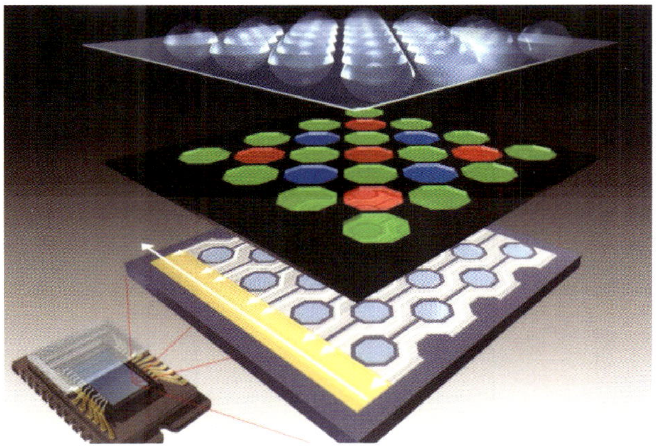

Fig. 12.5 The SuperCCD technology (c) is aimed at greatly improving resolution. Unlike conventional rectangular CCD elements (a), the light sensitive sensors on the SuperCCD are octagonal (b). This allows the individual elements to be placed closer together. Resolution, light sensitivity and contrast are increased (Photo: Fujifilm).

is the appearance of new models at least every six months; these differ from the previous models in particular in that the CCD chip offers yet another million pixels. Moreover, innovations in CCD chips are occurring which promise further developments.

In conventional chips the individual CCD elements are arranged in a rectangular pattern. In the so-called SuperCCD chip (Fuji) the individual cells are rotated at 45 degrees and are also octagonal (Fig. 12.5). Thus more individual elements can be fit in each area. The pixel intervals are reduced by about 30%, since the data conductors also take up less room. The advantages are better resolution of the chip in horizontal and vertical direction, greater light sensitivity and better contrast. The first digital SLR to use the SuperCCD chip was the Fuji FinePix S1.

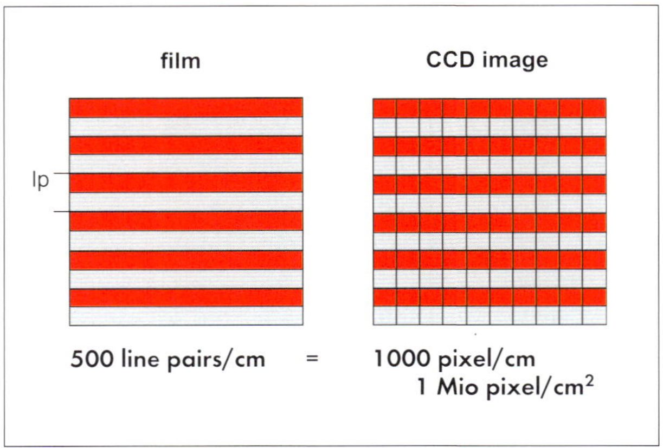

Fig. 12.6 The resolution of film translated into electronic terms. A resolution of 500 line pairs per cm corresponds to a resolution of 1000 pixels/cm. This results in a resolution of over 8.6 million pixels for the overall area of a 35mm slide or negative. This corresponds to more than 20 MB per individual image.

If a comparison is to be made between the performance of the new "Super CCD" and that of conventional chips, the comparison should not be made between the number of CCD elements (pixels) but between the amount of image data. The "4.3M" on the front of the FinePix 4700Z from Fujifilm does not mean that it has a 4.3 mega pixel chip, but that 4.3MB of image data (not interpolated) are provided by a 2.4 mega pixel chip.
Another technology, which JVC terms "6 Mega Pro Mode" projects two images onto the CCD chip in quick succession. The second image is shifted by one pixel (pixel shift technology). Thus a 3 mega pixel chip is to produce an image quality comparable to that of a 6 mega pixel camera, however, only with static subjects.

CMOS (complementary metal oxide semiconductor) technology is an alternative to conventional CCD chips. One advantage of CMOS chips is that the entire circuitry is built-in, whereas a conventional chip has up to six supporting chips, each with its own energy supply. A CMOS chip requires only about 1/10th of the current as that of a CCD chip.
The surface of the chip has light sensitive transistors; at the input and output terminals are digital signals only. The camera manufacturer needs only to build the camera around the chip (optics, power supply, storage). Production of such CMOS chips is far less complicated and thus significantly less expensive than that of the complicated CCD chips. Hence we can expect that CMOS technology will take over from CCD technology if the image quality is expected to remain the same.
The "gold standard" in terms of resolution continues to be 35mm film. A good 35mm image has more than 500 line pairs (Lp) per cm (Fig. 12.6). Translated into the language of digital technology, a line pair corresponds to two pixels. Hence 500 Lp correspond to 1000 pixels per cm or 1 million pixels per cm^2. With a total area of about 8.6 cm^2 per slide this means about 8.6 million pixels per slide. This produces more than 20MB of data per slide. In comparing image quality, digital cameras have as a yardstick this resolution of current 35mm slides or negatives.

12.1.2 In-camera storage

Aside from the CCD chip other electronic components determine the quality of the various cameras. Image data are first stored in RAM (random access memory) and then in the camera's internal storage (Fig. 12.7). Their capacity and processing speed determine the rate at which pictures can be taken in succession. Generally, amateur cameras allow two or three pictures to be taken in a row before the camera's computer has to process them. Top grade professional cameras such as the Nikon D1 H or the Canon EOS 1D can take up to 8 images per second and up to 21 images in high speed burst mode. Naturally this requires far more sophisticated electronics than required in amateur cameras.
There are also differences in data formats. Many

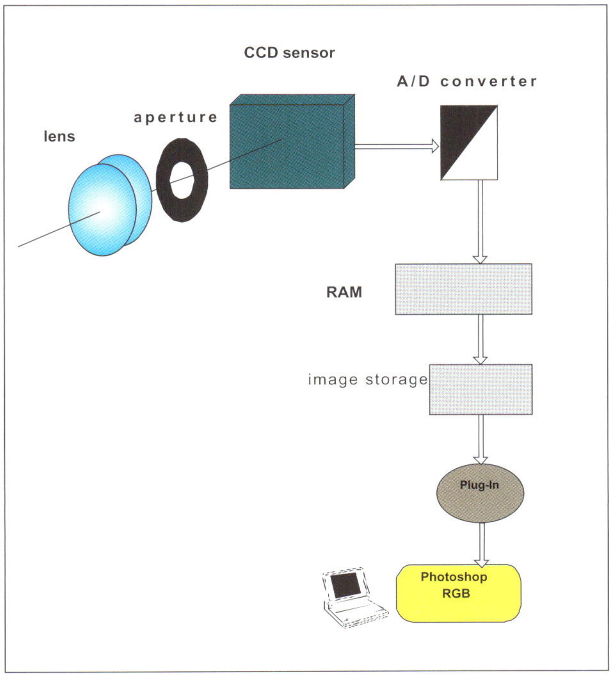

Fig. 12.7 Functional diagram of digital photography

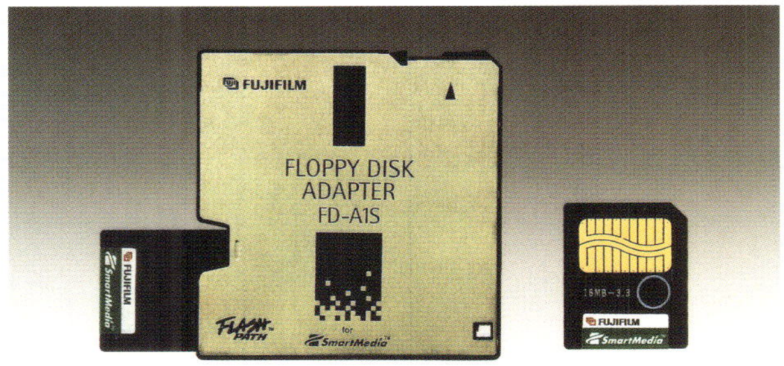

Fig. 12.8 The SmartMedia card is widely used as a storage medium in digital photography. (Photo: Fujifilm)

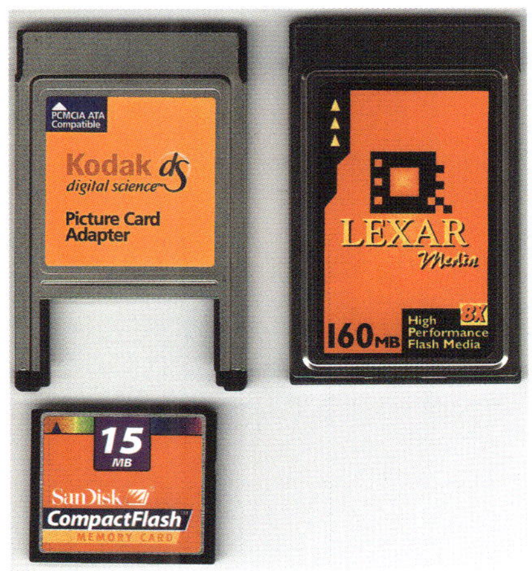

Fig. 12.9 The CompactFlash card currently has a higher storage capacity than the SmartMedia card, though they do not have the capacity of PC cards (right).

cameras allow the user to select the storage format. Most allow images to be stored simply in TIFF format or in JPEG format with various compression levels in which image data, and thus image quality, are lost.
Storage media range from 1.4 inch diskettes to other removable hard drives. The most common storage media are:

SmartMedia cards have the advantage of being small and light, thus being well suited to small amateur cameras. Currently their capacity ranges from 8 to 64 MB, with the trend being toward greater capacity (Fig. 12.8). PC card adapters are available for the PCMCIA slot for SmartMedia cards, and FlashPath adapters for the floppy drive. SmartMedia readers allow image data to be quickly downloaded to the computer via the USB (universal serial bus) connection.

CompactFlash cards are more robust and faster. Currently they have a capacity of more than 300MB, although the trend here too is toward greater capacity (Fig. 12.9). A 1 GB CF card has been mooted. They can be downloaded into laptops via simple card readers or PC card adapters. Some cameras offer both options: SmartMedia cards and CompactFlash cards. At the moment CF cards are used more often.

PC Cards are currently being used only in professional digital cameras. They interface with laptops

via the PCM-CIA slot or via special card readers in the PC. They have a capacity of several hundred MB.
The memory stick is a new storage medium which is currently found only in Sony cameras.
Some Sony camera models have a commercial 3.5 inch diskette as a storage medium, thus making downloading completely simple. Nevertheless, this design is a cul-de-sac in technical development terms due to the limited capacity of the diskette and ever increasing image resolution.
It is doubtful if another design will prevail, namely that of writing image data directly onto a small special CD-ROM (Sony MVC-CD 1000) using the camera's own CD writer. Before purchase of such a system, the user should weigh up how many high resolution images can be stored on a particular medium. It is also important to ascertain whether the controller of the memory cards is located on the card itself or in the camera. If it is on the storage medium itself, then these are future-proof and will allow the highest capacity storage media to be used.

The *IBM Microdrive* is a relatively new storage medium. It is a miniature hard drive which has a CompactFlash interface, that is, can be used in any system which can accept CompactFlash cards. Although this storage medium weighs only 16g it can store up to 1 GB, and the smaller version up to 340MB. If large image capacity storage is required and no notebook or PC is available for "intermediate storage," then such a Microdrive can be used. Its disadvantage is high cost and high energy consumption of this rotating medium.
The IBM Microdrive stores data magnetically, but the iD-Photo system has a magneto-optical memory. Advantages are greater data security, longer life of the stored data, and above all, lower cost. An MO medium should last 30-100 years - aside from the problem of whether MO media will still be in existence then - and allow more than 1 million operations.
The iD-Photo has a 6 x 5.5cm case and has a 730MB capacity, with plans for over 1GB.

12.1.3 PC connections

At the very latest, when the camera's own storage medium is full, the images have to be downloaded onto a computer. There are various means of doing this. Data transfer can be done via cable, without a cable or via the camera's own storage medium.

Image transfer via a cable to the computer's serial port is relatively slow, and should be done only when no other option is available. Transfer via universal serial bus (USB) is much faster and can currently be performed at 1.5 megabit/second. Improvements can be expected relating the speed of USB data transfer. Professional cameras offer image transfer via SCSI interface or via the fast IEEE 1394 FireWire interface.

Aside from special applications, it is more sensible and practical for clinical photography to use the camera as stand-alone and not interfaced with the computer.
Some models allow data to be transferred via infrared (IrDA interface, IrDA = Infrared Data Association). Image transfer via radio is still new; via the "Bluetooth Technology" which was introduced in 2000, this can be done at distances of up to about 10m.
Data transfer via the camera's own internal memory cards (see above) is unproblematical.
Professional cameras such as the Kodak DCS models or the Nikon D1 have PC cards or CompactFlash cards which can be inserted in the PC card slot of notebooks or a card reader. They are accessed like a hard drive (Fig. 12.10).
Adapters are recommended for storage media of amateur cameras. Economical PC card adapters are available for SmartMedia cards and CompactFlash cards. They can be connected via the PC card slot of notebooks or via card readers.
For some cameras a special software is necessary which will allow image transfer to the computer.
Some professional cameras offer Photoshop plugins, allowing images to be imported via the commands "File, Import".

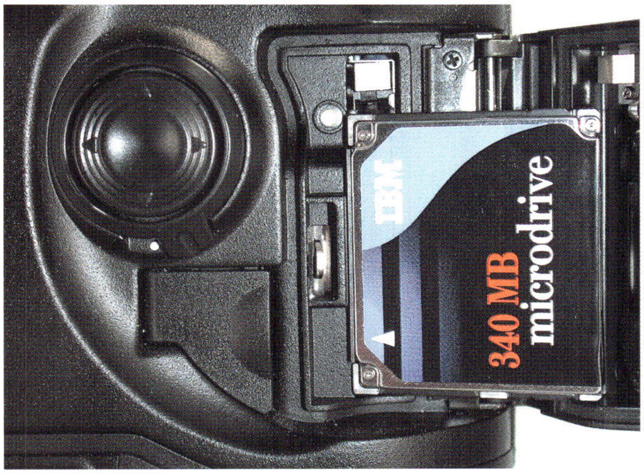

Fig. 12.10 The IBM microdrive is a removable storage medium for some professional systems.

12.2.1 Amateur cameras

Amateur cameras cost between $ 500 to $ 1,500. Though these once differed from professional cameras in their image resolution, top amateur camera models today also have CCD chips with a resolution of about 3-5 million pixels.
The main disadvantage of amateur cameras for dental photography is that their capability for close up photography is very limited. Though most of them have a macro setting, this is for wide angle photography. The other disadvantage is that as a rule they are rangefinder cameras which exhibit parallax at close range.

12.2 Camera Systems

The market has been flooded with digital cameras since Photokina 1996 at the very latest. Hence it is difficult in a book to present a complete and up to date survey of the market as the technical development cycles of these products is extremely short.
With this in mind I will concentrate on cameras which can be used effectively for dental photography without striving for completeness. The cameras can be loosely divided into amateur and professional systems.

Olympus C 2500 L

Camera type: digital 3x zoom SLR with integrated lens (Fig. 12.11)
Lens length: 26mm-110mm equivalent to 35mm
CCD chip/resolution: 2/3 inch CCD with 2.5 million pixel CCD
Subject-to-camera distance: standard: 0.6m – infinity; close-up 0.3m –0.6m; super close-up 0.02 –0.6m
Storage: SmartMedia cards and CompactFlash
Image storage: TIFF (uncompressed) and JPEG
Image transfer to PC: data input and output (RS 232C), video output: PAL
Power: 4 x AA NiMH batteries, optional: AC adapter
Features: center weighted integral and spot metering, up to five images in a burst.

The Lester Dine (USA) company has adapted a ring flash/side flash combination which also permits intraoral photography given that the lens is suitable.

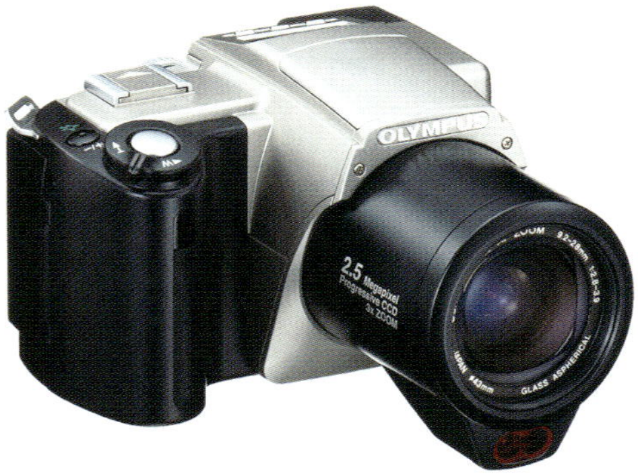

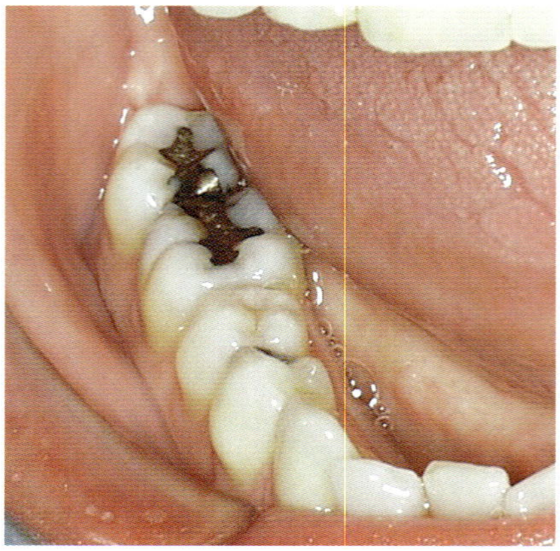

Fig. 12.11 The Olympus C2500L is currently not a leader in terms of resolution, but has advantages over other amateur cameras because it is an SLR (a). The Lester Dine company has adapted a macro flash for the digital camera. Although this does not result in extreme reproduction ratios, it still produces usable views (b). (Photo b from Lester Dine).

Olympus Camedia E-20N

Since September 2000 the Olympus company has been producing a digital SLR camera with an integrated zoom lens and a 4 mega pixel chip: the E-10. This camera is halfway between an amateur and a professional camera. Now the E-20N is available with a 5 mega pixel CCD-chip.

Lens: Olympus lens 9 – 36 mm 2.0 - 2.4, ED Glass Aspherical Zoom Lens, equivalent to 35 - 140 mm lens on 35 mm camera. Optional 0.8x (wide) 1.45x, 3x (telephotos)

Image sensor: 2/3 in. CCD solid-state image pick-up 5.0 Megapixel (effective) 5.2 Megapixel (total CCD resolution)

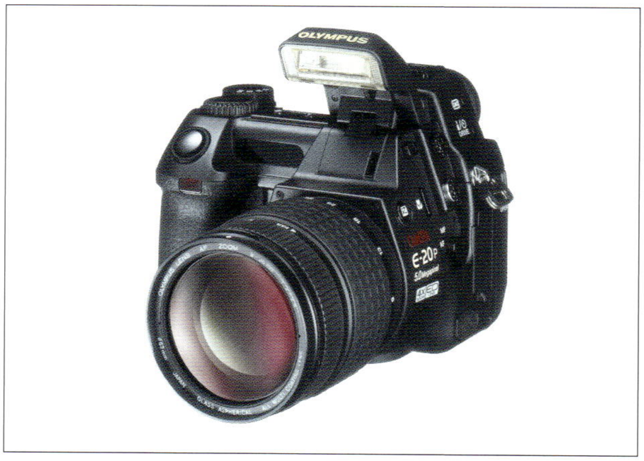

Fig. 12.12 Olympus Camedia E-20 N, a digital SLR with 5 million pixels (Photo: Olympus).

Recording modes: Still image: EXIF, JPEG (DCF: "Design rule for Camera File system"), TIFF (non-compress), DPOF support RAW (16 bit per color), with Photoshop Plug-in for RAW 10 Bit A>D Converter

Sequence: 2.5 frames per sec. up to 3 frames TIFF; 4 frames RAW IS mode: 4.5 frames per sec. to 7 shots in PS JPEG mode, 1 second shot to shot

LCD panel: 4.5 cm / 1.8 in. wider angle color TFT LCD monitor with 114,000 pixels (made from low-temperature poly-silicon), brightness adjustment is possible. Adjustable 20, 0, 90 Degrees (click stops) 95% accurate area-view of subject.

Exposure control: Programmed auto exposure, Aperture priority, Shutter priority, +/– 3Ev by 1/3EV steps exposure compensation. Auto Bracketing: selectable from 1/3EV, 2/3 EV and 1EV; 3 or 5 images. Aperture priority: Wide F2.0 – 11, Tele F2.4 – 11.

Removable media card: 3V (3.3V) SmartMedia™ Card. One 32MB card including Panorama function is supplied with camera. 3V CompactFlash™ Type II (Flash Memory-Micro Drive supported).

Outer connectors: DC input terminal, Data input/output terminal (RS232C), USB interface. Video Output terminal (NTSC), external flash PC terminal, Hotshoe (FL-40TTL).

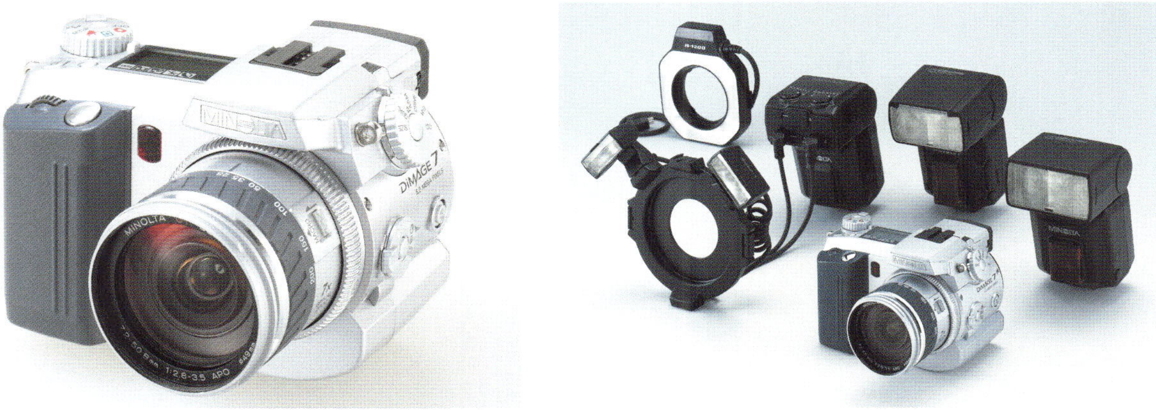

Fig. 12.13 The Minolta Dimage7 (a) was the first 5 megapixel consumer camera to reach the market. It is compatible with a variety of accessories, for example macro flashes (b). (Photo Minolta)

Minolta Dimage7

The Minolta Dimage7 was the first consumer digital camera with 5 million pixels reaching the market (Fig. 12.13).

Lens: 7x optical zoom lens equivalent to 28 - 200 mm lens on a 35 mm camera. The macro setting produces sharp images when the subject is as near as five inches from the lens. Aperture is f/2,8 - f/3,5.

Viewfinder: Viewfinder (LCD) with a visual resolution equivalent to about 120,000 pixels. The variable position viewfinder can be tilted up to 90 degrees.

Operating speed: Start-up time approximately 2.6 seconds. Shutter-release time lag: approximately 0.13 second. Capturing interval: approximately 0.9 second. Playback loading interval: approximately 0.2 second.

Dedicated external flash: Very interesting for dental photography is the possibility to use external macro flashes as macro twin flash 2400 and macro ring flash 1200. For both the macro flash controller is necessary.

Recording medium: CompactFlash card Type I and Type II. IBM Microdrive (170MB, 340MB, 512MB, 1GB).

Power: Four AA Alkaline or four AA Ni-MH batteries. Use of Ni-MH batteries is recommended.

Nikon CoolPix 5000

Camera type: digital rangefinder camera with 5 megapixels (effective).

Focal Length: 7.1 - 21.4mm (35mm camera format equivalent: 28–85mm)

Storage Media: Type I and Type II CompactFlash(TM) cards and the IBM Microdrive.

Sensitivity: ISO equivalent approximately 100, 200, 400, 800, or Auto (auto gain to 800)

Interface: USB 1.1 Interface

Power Sources: One rechargeable Nikon EN-EL1 lithium-ion battery supplied; MH-51 charger supplied; 6V 2CR5/DL245 lithium battery available separately; Nikon MB-E5000 battery pack available separately with 6 1.5V LR6 (AA) batteries; Nikon EH-21 AC adapter/charger available separately (Fig. 12.14).

Fuji FinePix 6900 Zoom

Camera type: digital rangefinder camera, optical viewfinder.

Sensor: 6.0 Million Pixel File (2832 x 2128) using Fujifilm 3.3 Million Octagonal Sensor Super CCD System.

Lens: 6X Aspherical Zoom, f/2.8-f/11; 13 steps. (35 – 210mm, 35mm camera equivalent zoom).

Sensitivity: ISO equivalent approximately 100, 200, 400, 800.

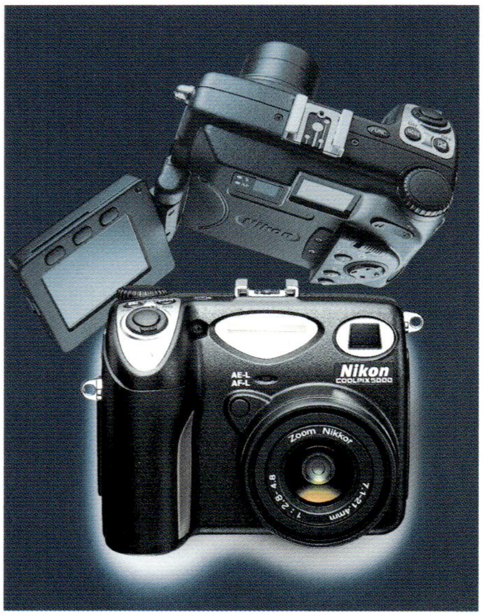

Fig. 12.14 The Nikon Coolpix 5000 has an image resolution of 5 million pixels (Photo: Nikon).

Manual Focus Control Ring on Lens.
Interface: USB port for fast computer file transfers.
Optional Lens Mounting Ring for use with 55mm Filters, 1.5x Telephoto lens or 0.79x wide angle lens.

Canon Powershot G2
Type of camera: Compact Digital Still Camera with Built-in Flash and 3x Optical Zoom Lens. Lens and Flash accessories available.
Image capture device: 1/1.8-inch Charge-Coupled Device (CCD) with 4 million pixels (effective)
Focal length: 7-21mm (35mm film equivalent: 34 - 102mm)
Focusing range: Normal AF: 70cm (2.3ft.) - infinity. Macro AF: 6cm (0.2ft.) (wide-angle) / 20cm (0.7ft.) (telephoto) - 70cm (2.3ft.). Manual focus: 6cm (0.2ft.) (wide-angle) / 20cm (0.7ft.) (telephoto) - infinity.
External flash: Use of following external flashes is recommended: Canon Speedlite 220EX, 380EX, 420EX, 550EX and Macro Ring Lite MR-14EX.
Storage media: CompactFlash (CF) card (Type I or Type II.
Image recording format: JPEG or CCD RAW.
Computer interface: USB.

Sony Cybershot DSC-707
Image capture device: 2/3 inch CCD with 5 million pixels (effective)
Focal length: 9,7-48,5mm (35mm film equivalent: 38 - 190mm)
Aperture priority (range): f2.0-8.0, 13 step.
Shutter priority (range): 30 ~ 1/1000, 46 step.
Still image format: JPEG, GIF, TIFF.
Connections: Video / USB Interface / AC Pwr.

Kodak DC 4800
Camera type: digital rangefinder camera, optical viewfinder
Lens length: 28mm - 84mm equivalent to 35mm
CCD chip/resolution: 3.3 mega pixel sensor
Subject-to-camera distance: 0.2 - 0.5m (close-up); 0.5m - infinity (normal)
Storage: CompactFlash
Image capture: four images at highest resolution, 16 images at lower resolution
Image storage: uncompressed in TIFF format, various compression levels in JPEG format
Image transfer to PC: USB interface via removable medium. Image transfer software supplied allows user to directly access images. The DC 4800 is designated an external drive.
Power: lithium ion battery pack, charger supplied
Features: metal case, three light sensitivities can be selected (ISO 100, 200 and 400), three apertures which can be manually set, various filter functions, additional flash synchronization connection for external flash.

12.2.2 Professional digital cameras

These are SLRs with interchangeable lenses which are either special designs or are based on existing professional camera models. For our purposes the main advantages are:

- Use of interchangeable lenses (suitable for close-up work, no distortion)
- SLR technology (image in viewfinder and real image the same)
- use of existing accessories (e.g. macro flash)
- rapid image capture
- large image storage (PC cards)

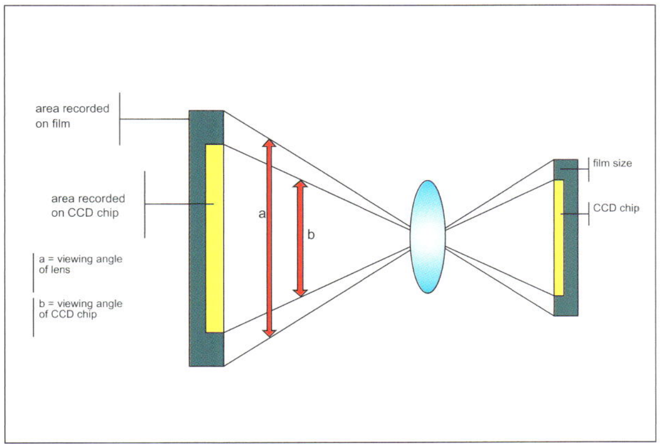

Fig. 12.15 Since CCD chips are presently smaller than 35 mm format only the middle portion of the image in the viewfinder is taken. This can be compared to using a telephoto lens instead of a normal lens. Thus this is referred to as a conversion factor, with which the lens used has to be multiplied in order to compare this to 35mm format.

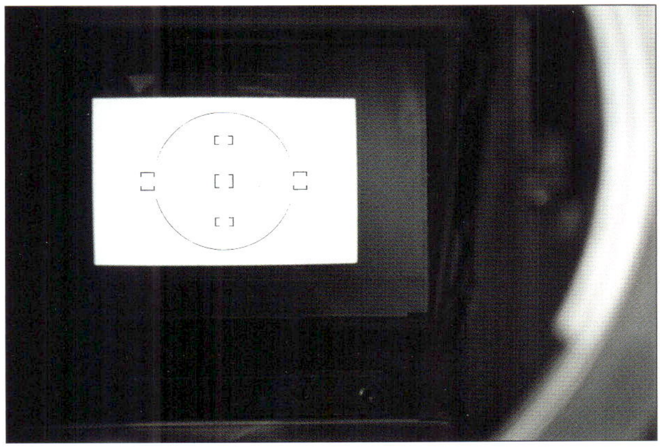

Fig. 12.16 View into a Nikon D1X showing the mirror image of the focusing screen with the five focus areas. The image area of the viewfinder image is smaller than the "normal" 24 x 36 mm area of the film.

However, these advantages do not come without a price, which starts at around $ 3,000.
There is one significant point about this camera type which distinguishes one from another: the factor of lens length. The lenses of these cameras are designed for 35 mm format (Fig. 12.15). The image projected by the lens onto the "film plane" strikes the CCD chip in digital models. The CCD chip is generally smaller than the 24 x 36mm format of 35mm cameras. This means that only the central part of the viewfinder image is recorded, which is indicated in the viewfinder by a frame (Fig. 12.16). This has the same effect as if an image were being taken with a longer focal lens. This is termed a "lens focal length conversion factor" by which the basic focal length has to be multiplied. This factor should be borne in mind in selecting a lens. If for example the camera has a conversion factor of 2 and the photographer wants to use a 100mm macro lens, he or she should select a 50mm macro lens. The lens conversion factor can be calculated by dividing the diagonal of the 35mm format by the diagonal of the chip. The larger the surface of the chip, the smaller the lengthening factor. Some systems use lenses designed for the APS system; in this case the projected image is adjusted to the reduced film format.

Kodak DCS series (DCS = Digital Camera System)

Digital SLR cameras based on Nikon and Canon bodies which have been on the market since 1991 and which had a strong influence on the development of professional digital cameras.
The cameras differ among other features in their CCD chips. Some of the DCS cameras ar no longer marketed, but still in use in clinics and dental offices and therefore sold second hand, e.g. the

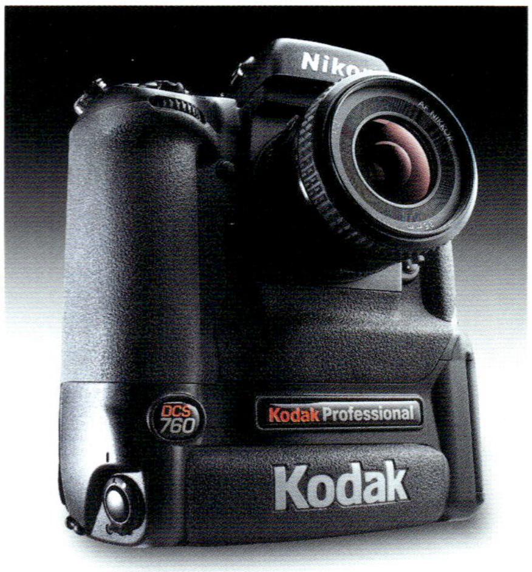

Fig. 12.17 The Kodak DCS 760 is a professional digital SLR camera which is based on a Nikon F5 (Photo: Kodak).

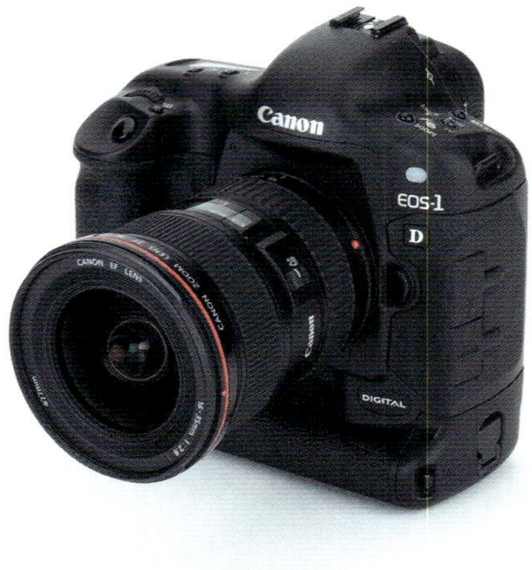

Fig. 12.18 The Canon EOS-1D – a professional digital SLR camera (Photo: Canon).

Kodak DCS 330, which was adapted from a commercial APS camera.
Interesting for dental photography is the Kodak DCS 760.

Kodak DCS 760

A 6 Mpixel SLR camera (data file size 18 MB). The camera is based on the Nikon F5 (Fig.12.17). Internal microphone for voice recording. Graphical user interface with Instant review, 1:1 focus check, spot densitometer, histogram. Large, bright color LCD panel for image analysis. Image storage: Dual PC card slots,Type II, III. IR filter included. Optional anti-aliasing filter. ISO Settings: 80 to 400.
As the camera is based on the Nikon F5, nearly the whole range of Nikon lenses and accessories can be used.

Canon EOS-D 30

Digital SLR camera in the "lower" price segment, therefore very interesting for the dental practice.
Imaging device: CMOS sensor with 3,11 million pixels.
Lens mount: The D30 uses all EF lenses without restrictions or limitations.
Viewfinder: Full-frame reflex type, coverage approximately 95% horizontal and vertical, 0.88X magnification and 20mm eyepoint.
Flash contact: Accessory shoe for EX-series Speedlites; PC socket also built-in on left side of camera body. For dental photography the Macro Ring Lite MR-14EX is of special interest, offering eTTL-metering.
The EOS D30 supports USB and NTSC/PAL Video Out.

Canon EOS 1D

Digital AF SLR camera with CCD sensor (approx. 4,15 megapixels) (Fig.12.18).
All Canon EF lenses are compatibel. The lens focal length conversion factor is approx.1.3 x of indicated lens focal length. The ISO speed range is equivalent to ISO 200 – 1600. External flash guns of the speedlite EX series can be used with eTTL-metering (for example the Macro Ring Lite MR-14EX). Interchangeable focusing screens.
IEEE 1394 fire wire computer interface. Image for-

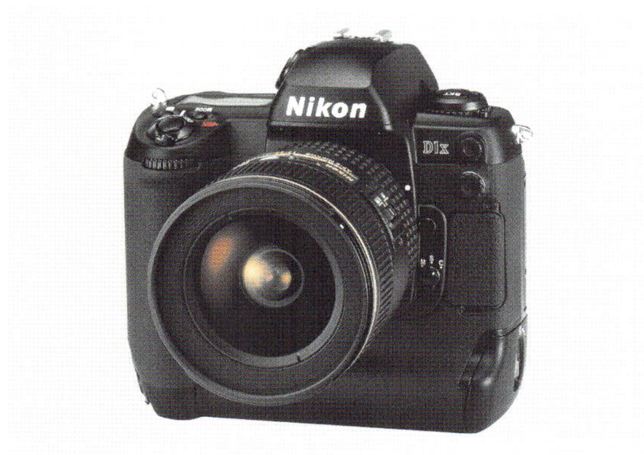

Fig. 12.19 Professional Nikon D1X digital camera. (Photo: Nikon)

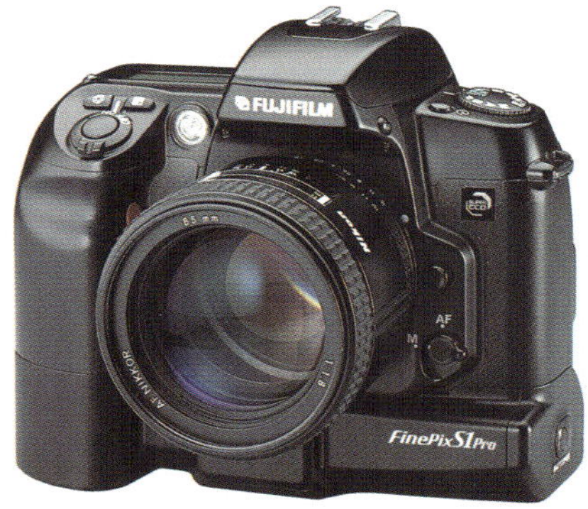

Fig. 12.20 FinePix s1 Pro: professional digital camera from Fuji based on Nikon technology. (Photo: Fujifilm)

mats are JPEG and RAW, 36 bit true-color, 12 bits RGB color.
Sound recording with the built-in microphone is possible (maximum 30s per recording). The WAV-file is attached to the image.
The power source of the camera is one Ni-MH Pack.

Nikon D1
2.7 mega pixel SLR camera which corresponds to the Nikon F5/F100 in terms of optics. Not a remake of the F100 but a one-off development. The Nikon bayonet connection allows access to over 80 Nikkor lenses. A lithium niobat lowpass filter is integrated which filters out infrared. Special features of the camera are: exposure control, high speed autofocus, shooting speed 4.5 images per second in series of up to 21 images in succession, fastest shutter speed 1/16,000th of a second, flash synchronization up to 1/500th of a second, shutter delay 0.05 second. Images stored on CompactFlash cards in 12 bit raw or 8 bit TIFF formats as well as three different JPEG compression levels. The CCD sensor is 23.7 x 15.6 mm, resulting in a lengthening factor of about 1.5 compared to 35mm format.

Nikon D1x
Digital SLR camera with 5.47 Mpixel CCD sensor (Fig. 12.19). Allows 3 frames per second, up to 9 consecutive shots. Improved color accuracy. Compact flash cards and IBM microdrive as storage media.
IEEE 1394 and RS 232-C computer interface. Lens conversion factor 1.5.

FinePix S1 Pro (Fujifilm)
Digital SLR based on Nikon F60 (Fig. 12.20). Has a 23.3 x 15.6 mm "SuperCCD" with 3.4 million pixels. The SuperCCD chip is aimed at producing the image quality of a 6 mega pixel camera.
Nikon lenses with F mounts can be used. Lens conversion factor 1.5. Takes 1.5 images per second at maximum of five images. Shutter speeds between 30 sec and 1/2000 sec. Image storage on SmartMedia and Type II CompactFlash and Microdrive. Camera has USB connection and video output.

Minolta Dimage RD 3000
2.7 mega pixel SLR using Vectis series lenses (Minolta APS system) (Fig. 12.21). The 2.27 mega pixel resolution is achieved by two 1.5 mega pixel CCDs onto which the light is directed by a prism.

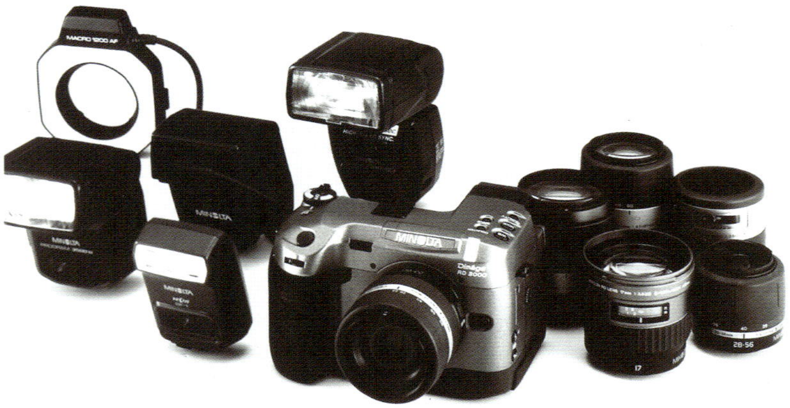

Fig. 12.21 Minolta Dimage RD3000, a digital SLR adapted from APS technology.

Both partial images are rejoined using a special algorithm. Lowpass filter integrated which reduces infrared, thus reducing color aliasing and improving image quality.
An integrated intermediate lens used in combination with Vectis lenses permits image capture without lens lengthening.
The V3.5/50mm macro lens and the 1200 AF-N Macro Flash are particularly interesting for our purposes.
Storage medium is a CompactFlash card.
Image compression: TIFF (uncompressed), as well as JPEG formats in three levels.
Data transfer is also possible via a SCSI interface.

Contax N Digital

The Contax N Digital is the world`s first digital SLR camera with a 24 x 36 mm CCD sensor (6 megapixel). That means that no lens focal length conversion factor has to be kept in mind. The full range of Carl Zeiss T* lenses can be used. As the digital camera is based on the Contax N1, the N Digital offers nearly all basic functions of the N1 (Fig. 12.22).
The N Digital can write in several formats, including JPEG (3 compression ratios) RGB-TIFF, and RAW formats. The N Digital uses the Compact Flash type I and II and the IBM Type II Micro Drive. The camera is equipped with a computer interface for high-speed Firewire (IEEE1394) image transfer.

The speed range is ISO50 to 1600 equiv. (1/3 step). The display panel on top of the camera gives information about: exposure counter/self-timer counter/exposure A.B.C sequence/fine focus A.B.C. sequence/bulb time, focus frame selection, exposure compensation (when exposure compensation dial is in green position), drive indicators, battery status (shooting mode), aperture, shutter speed/film speed/camera customized functions.
The rear LCD panel informs about: exposure counter, recording format, white balance, digital function customized setting, memory card cover indicator, battery status (playback mode).
As power source four AA-type Ni-MH rechargeable batteries are used; alternatively an AC power adapter.
For dental photography the Makro-Planar T* 100mm F2.8 is recommended.

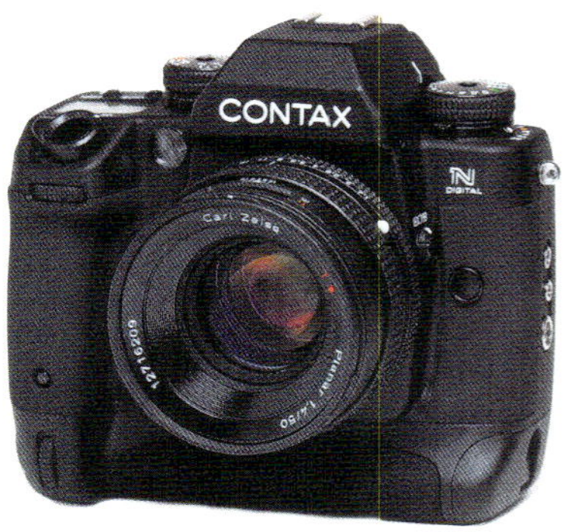

Fig. 12.22 Contax N Digital – the first digital SLR camera with a 24 x 36 mm CCD sensor.

12.3 Selection Criteria

It is not easy to make a decision about purchasing a camera with so many available. A decision should be made in steps, with the initial one being the choice between a digital or conventional SLR. The advantages of a digital camera are that images are available immediately and in digitized form, as well as being of relatively high resolution. If digital images are not required immediately the alternative is to photograph the images conventionally and then digitize them (e.g. 35mm scanner, Kodak PhotoCD). The purpose of the images can also weigh in the decision. If only slides are needed, then conventional photography is preferable. An intermediate step using digital images is then not sensible.
If a digital camera is chosen then the decision must be made between an amateur or professional model. Serious photo documentation which is to produce the same quality as that of conventional photography can be achieved currently only with professional digital systems. Due to their limited capability for close-up photography (viewfinder parallax, insufficient reproduction ratio, image distortion in close-ups) amateur cameras can not be considered for high quality photo documentation. However, they can be used to augment conventional photo documentation for special applications.
Once the decision has been made whether to purchase an amateur or professional digital camera individual technical points should be weighed up in the final analysis. The most important of these are covered in the following.

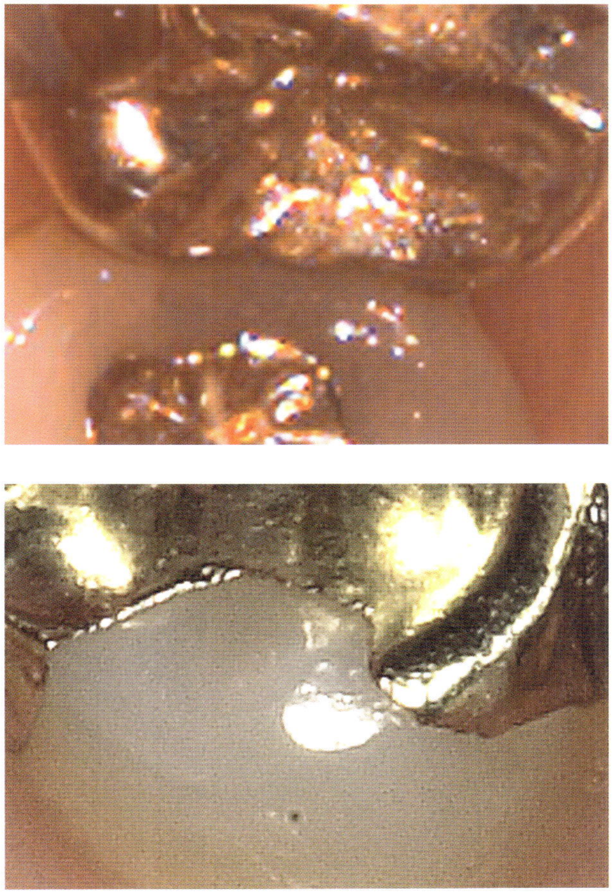

Fig. 12.23 Blooming is the "overflow" of electrons onto the neighboring CCD elements, which can be recognized from the false colored pixels (a). Short circuit switches in modern camera chips are designed to make this problem a thing of the past. (b) shows an enlargement of an image taken with a Nikon D1. No blooming is evident.

CCD chip
In addition to resolution, which has been covered in the above, other factors also play an important role in image quality. Dental photography in particular has the problem of strong reflections from highly reflective surfaces (highlights). In digital photography these produce effects such as blooming and aliasing. Blooming is the "overflow" of electrons of the individual CCD elements into the neighboring ones. This occurs in very bright, high contrast areas. In an image this can be seen by colored false pixel on the edges of highlights which are also too large (Fig. 12.23). Modern CCD chips have short circuit switches which prevent the overflow and thus the blooming. Other CCD chips have LOD technology (lateral overflow drain). A sort of overflow channel, like that of a swimming pool, prevents the overflow of electrons into the neighboring CCD elements.

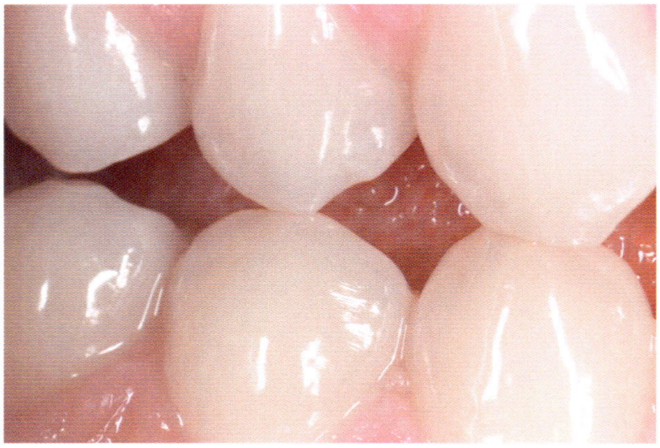

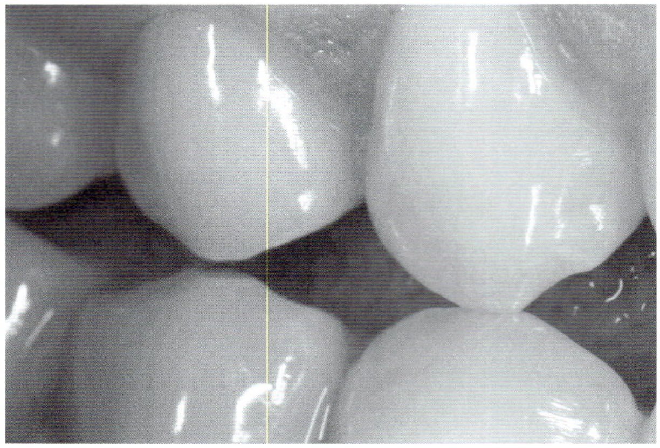

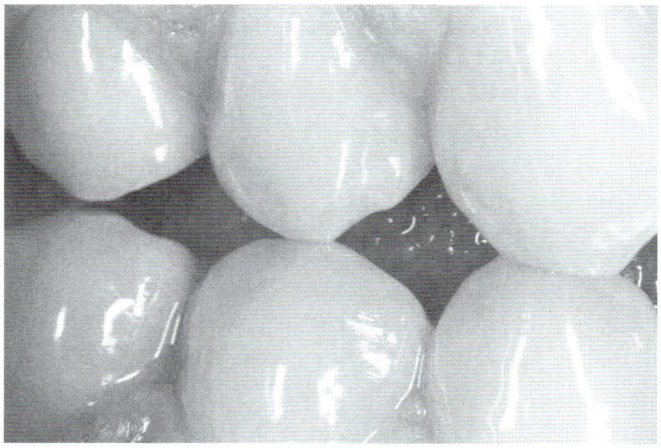

Fig. 12.24 Older CCD chips were characterized by low sensitivity in the blue channel. This can be checked by separating the image (a) into its individual components. The image of the green channel (b) appears much cleaner than that of the blue channel (c). Here noise can be clearly seen which affects image quality. Modern sensors have no noise in the blue channel.

Aliasing is a jagged effect occurring on diagonal lines. At greater magnification it is also possible to see colored false pixels which adversely affect image quality. Anti-aliasing filters prevent this and improve image quality.

Old CCD chips were characterized by their low sensitivity to blue (Fig. 12.24). The electrical signals had to be increased, which resulted in stronger noise (comparable to increased graininess in silver halide photography). Today, blue sensitivity is supposed to be as high as red and green sensitivity. This can easily be proven using image manipulation software by comparing the individual color channels.

Noise can be eliminated in the following manner: select the Lab mode (Image – Mode) and change the a and b channel using the unsharpen function with a Gaussian blur filter on both images. The degree of blur should be selected so that the contours are still recognizable but the noise is eliminated. Finally, go into an overall view and change the image into RGB mode.

While the present trend is for an increasing number of pixels, the actual size of the CCD sensor has only changed in expensive professional cameras. This is due to the very costly production of the sensors. These are produced from silicon wafers which are coated in various steps. A certain number of CCD sensors can be produced from a wafer. If larger sensors are to be produced, fewer of these can be gained from a silicon wafer. The fewer the sensors produced from a wafer, the higher the rejection rate due to impurities which can occur even in spite of clean room conditions. Thus the costs

rise almost exponentially if larger chips are produced. A chip twice the size costs eight times more to produce. Thus manufacturers seek a compromise between quality and cost.
The current trend of putting more and more CCD elements (pixels) on almost the same size chip necessarily means that the pixel size and the space between pixels are being reduced. This requires the use of higher performance lenses in order not to negate the advantages of the larger number of pixels by bad optical quality.
The resolution of a lens, like that of a film, is measured in line pairs/mm. Very high quality 35 mm lenses are able to achieve 70 to 100 Lp/mm. At 70Lp/mm this means that the lens can render a maximum of 140 pixels per mm. This corresponds to a pixel distance of 0.007 mm (7 µm). Modern digital cameras have 1/1.8 inch CCD chips with approximately 3.3 million CCD elements. This results in a "pixel distance" of 4 µm. In other words, 250 CCD elements are found on a length of 1 mm. To render these separately requires a high quality lens which can resolve at least 125 Lp/mm.

Chip size	Number of pixels	Pixel-distance	Required resolution
1/3 inch	0.8 million	5 µm	100 Lp/mm
1/3 inch	1.3 million	4 µm	125 Lp/mm
1/2 inch	2.1 million	4,4 µm	113 Lp/mm
1/1,8 inch	3.3 million	4 µm	125 Lp/mm

Thus it can be seen that the chip size greatly influences the image quality indirectly via the quality of the lens.
A smaller CCD element also has the disadvantage of being less light sensitive than a larger one. This is compensated for by slightly increasing the current on the CCD elements. This not only increases the light sensitivity, but also the background noise, which in turn adversely affects the image quality. From this discussion it is evident that increasing the number of pixels per CCD chip soon or later reaches its limits. CCD chips with a larger surface and the same size elements would significantly improve image quality. However, as already noted, this is far more costly. Thus manufacturers try to improve image quality using other measures (Super CCD, pixel shift technology [see above])

Image compression
In addition to various compression levels (mostly JPEG), there should also be the possibility of storing uncompressed images.

Image capacity
Determine the number of images the camera's internal medium can store at the highest resolution.

PC connection
It is preferable to have removable storage media which can be read either directly or via adapter by a notebook or via a reader by the PC. If a cable interface is used IEEE 1394 or USB connections are recommended. Transfer via cable or serial port is too time-consuming and not recommended for the dental practice.

Camera power supply
Determine whether commercial batteries or battery packs or expensive special batteries are used. Modern battery systems without a memory effect are preferable.

Shutter delay
Lengthy shutter release delays make working with digital cameras difficult and ruin many an exposure. Ideally, the delays should not exceed those of conventional SLR cameras.

Energy management
Digital cameras consume a lot of energy, mostly due to the LCD display. It should be determined whether this display can be switched off or not. It should also be ascertained before purchase how many images can be made on one set of batteries.

12.4 Work flow

Using a digital camera in the dental practice does not differ from employing a conventional SLR system. Although it is possible to connect the camera directly to the PC, image storage on the internal storage media has been proven. The camera is easier to manage and there are no annoying cables. Other practical approaches concerning the work flow are described.

Before using the camera a number of important points should be checked on the display on the back:

- Number of remaining images
- Battery status
- Storage medium in the camera?
- Type of data

After that, the images are taken just as they would be with a conventional camera. It is recommended that with digital cameras too several images should be taken in close up photography, since the depth of field is very shallow.
To transfer the images to a PC, the storage medium is removed from the camera and either placed in the PC card slot (notebooks) or into an external card reader.
Another possibility is to use a cable connection for fast image transfer, e.g. using a Firewire (IEEE 1394) interface.
Normally the image files are copied to a file of the archiving software (e.g. Fotostation, see below). This file can be named "New images" or similar. The archiving software normally allows a quick control of the results. Unsharp or otherwise spoilt images can be deleted. Keywords have now to be added to the files (for example: patient name, diagnosis etc.).
Using the drag and drop function the images are then copied into the image editing software (e.g. Photoshop). Here the images can be enhanced (see below). After this procedure the image files are stored in the final image archiving file, called for example "patient images".

The storage medium ist put back into the camera and formatted again to delete the data.

Other cameras, as the Kodak DCS 330 need a special image transfer software as a Photoshop plug-in.
The Kodak Software is accessed via FILE-IMPORT-TWAIN_32 in Photoshop. Generally the first step is to open the folder of the PC card in which the images are to be stored. A Contact Sheet appears which shows all the images as thumbnails (Fig. 12.25). If these are recognizable, individual images can be deleted at this stage. A preview function allows the images to be displayed at a larger size to examine them in more detail. Simple image manipulation functions allow images to be rotated, cropped (saves memory) and color corrected.
The images, which are automatically numbered by the camera, can already be renamed at this stage; notes can also be added. A column on the right side lists many different details about the images, including when taken, technical details, etc.
Images can be loaded into Photoshop singly or in total using ACQUIRE.
Another possibility is to load the original camera data onto the hard drive. This can be important for reasons of documentation, since the original Kodak data cannot be manipulated. This original Kodak data can be accessed with the same software as on the PC card.

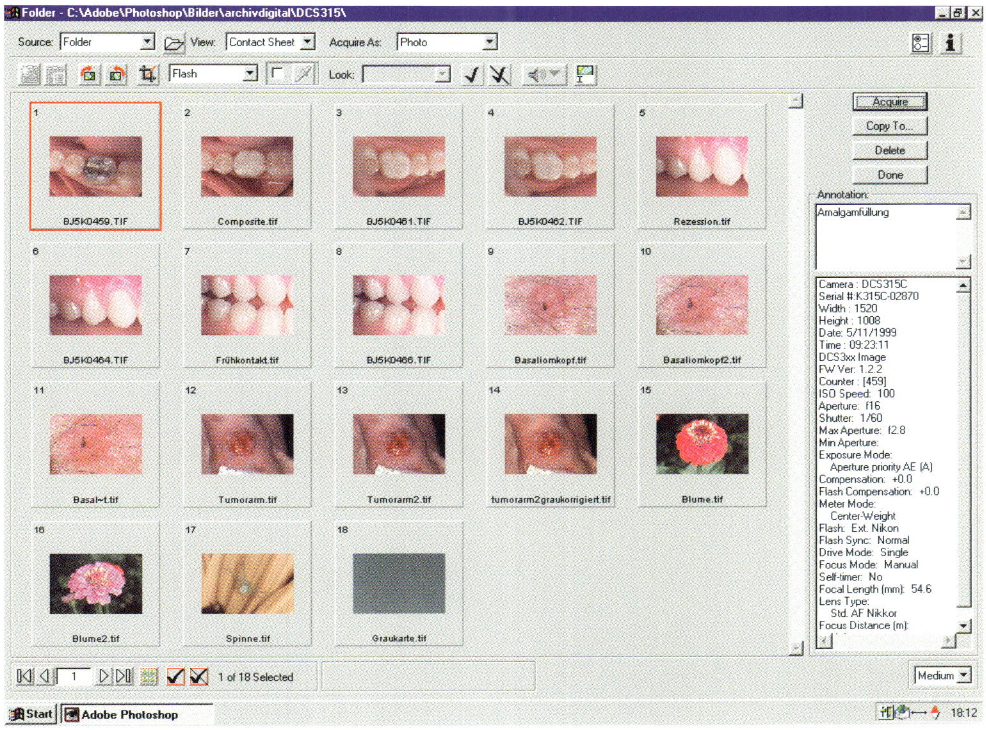

Fig. 12.25 Image transfer into image editing programs is sometimes done using special software, here, Kodak Twain Software as a plug-in for Photoshop. Even at this stage some corrections are possible and the technical details associated with the images can be checked.

12.5 Editing Images

Image editing measures can be divided into those which improve image quality and those which change their content. Details can be found in the handbooks for the various software programs. It has become common at conferences for the lecturer to declare that he or she has not manipulated the images. Although this was naturally possible to do before the age of digital imaging, it is now far simpler to do so.

Due to their technical characteristics it is necessary to make some enhancements to digital images. These can be done using practically any of the image editing software programs on the market. Standard professional image manipulation software packages such as Adobe Photoshop allow these improvements to be done quickly and automatically. The following procedure has proven useful:

- ✓ Align and crop image
- ✓ Brightness and contrast
- ✓ Color correction
- ✓ Sharpening

Align and crop images

Images which are not correctly framed can be aligned and superfluous pixels can be eliminated with careful cropping of the image. This reduces the amount of data and is done with the selection tool; rotation and corrections in perspective can be done with the "transform" command.

If the desired image size is known it is entered under "image size". The required transformation mode is bicubic.

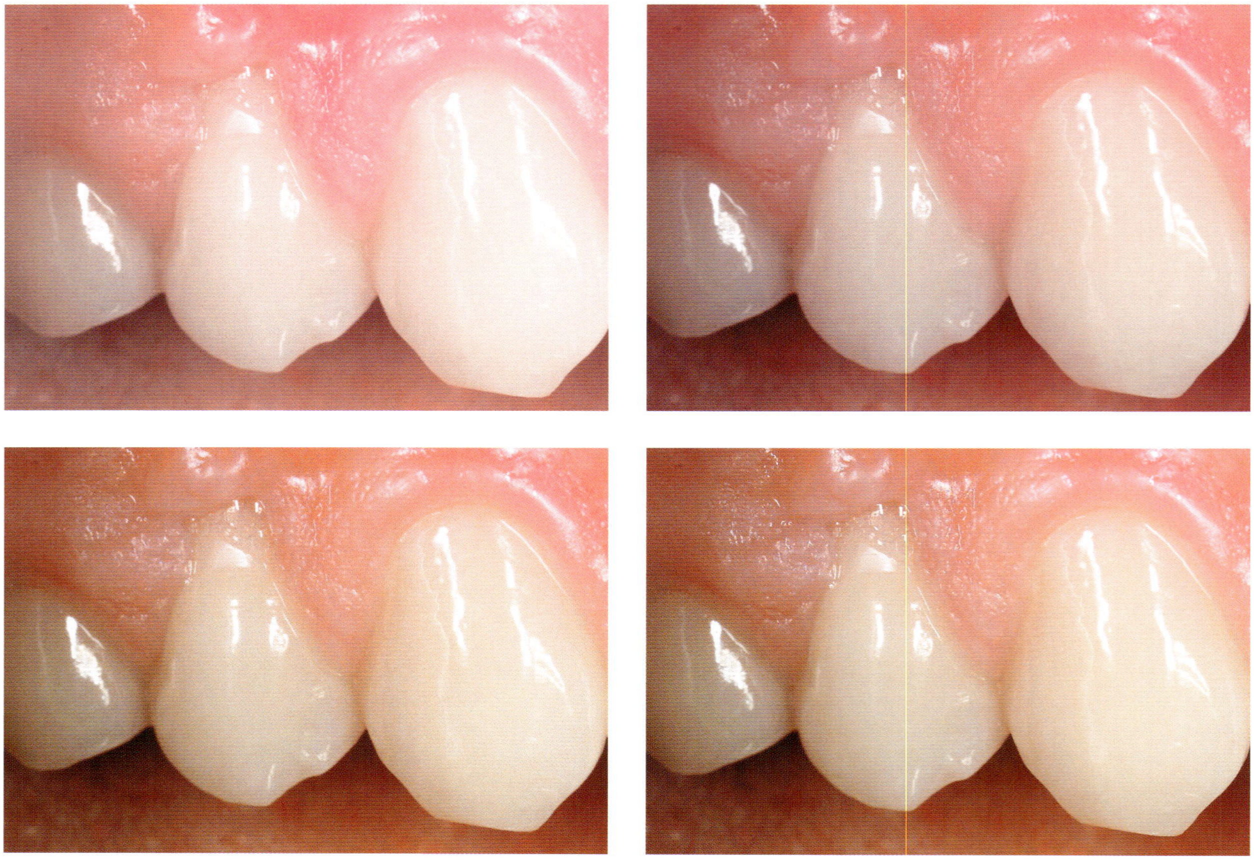

Fig. 12.26 Digitally produced images have to be enhanced. Starting with the initial image (a), brightness and contrast are corrected (b). Only then is color corrected if necessary (c). Finally, the image is sharpened.

Brightness and contrast

Since brightness and color influence each other, brightness and contrast corrections are undertaken first before any required color corrections. Various tools are available for this in the different software programs (Fig. 12.26a and b). In the "gradations curves" dialog box, first click on the brightest image area with the white pipette. This area is then altered to the values set in the pipette (C = 4, M = 3, Y = 3, K = 0). The black pipette is used in the same manner if there are image areas which are to be totally black. Finally, the image is set to neutral with the midtone pipette (each set at 127 in RGB mode). This type of global color correction should naturally be used only if there are truly neutral areas in the image. After that, the image brightness can be changed by clicking on the gradation curve in the middle and sliding it up or down. Instead of the entire image being simply brightened or darkened, which loses tone values, the gamma control changes the distribution of the tone values in the image without influencing the brightest and darkest area of the image. Slightly overexposed images should be corrected with a gamma value of 0.7 to 0.9 and slightly underexposed ones with a value of 1.1 to 1.3.

Alternatively, the overall tone value can be corrected using the command "tone value correction".

Color correction
Undesirable color casts can occur for instance if infrared filters are not used when images are taken. Such color casts can also be eliminated in various ways using the IMAGE – SETTINGS menu (Fig. 12.26c). A simple solution is found in the submenu VARIATIONS, which allows color, brightness and saturation to be changed using small preview images. Other options are "color balance," "selective color correction," and "color tone/saturation".

Sharpening
Sharpening of digital images is almost always necessary due to the interpolation process. This is true for images taken with the camera as well as for scanned images or those which come from a PhotoCD.
Most image acquisition programs have a sharpening function, although it is generally better to do this sharpening manually. Of course it is not possible to sharpen an image which is blurred or out of focus: the object is to increase the impression of sharpness in an image.
Simple sharpening can be undertaken by using the "unsharp mask" function, which emphasizes the image contours and increases the impression of overall sharpness.
Images such as portraits which have little data and large areas of color should be sharpened after conversion into Lab mode, when only the brightness channel is sharpened and the a and b channels are slightly softened (Fig. 12.26d). This creates continuous color areas and natural looking skin tones.
As a rule, images which are to be printed out by an inkjet or dye sublimation printer should be sharpened visually from the screen image. Images for offset printing can be more intensely sharpened.

12.6 Archiving Images

The subject of image archiving justifies its own treatment and thus is covered here only in principle. Some general hints are also found in Chapter 11. Basically it is possible to use special programs for dental photography offered with intraoral video cameras for this purpose (Dentron, Dürr, NewTech, Integra Medical etc). There are also general image archive programs available which are based on database programs (e. g. MS Access) or ones which are aimed at professional picture libraries for print media, such as Fotostation, Portfolio, Extensis, Cantus Cumulus) (Fig. 12.27). For a smaller number of images, database modules from standard image editing software are available, for example the Album module from PhotoImpact or amateur programs such as PhotoRecall or PhotoCat. There are also good Shareware programs available for image archiving.
It is recommended that in archiving images they be stored in RGB format. The CMYK color model is smaller and discards colors which it can not display. Lab format too is only of limited suitability.
For image archiving TIF or JPEG formats are recommended. Data archiving formats specific to the various image editing programs are to be avoided.
It makes sense to use the data information which can be stored with the image independently from the catalog program.
Since images are very memory-intensive it is recommended that they be regularly downloaded, for example, by burning them onto a CD-ROM. These CD-ROMs should be numbered and not labeled with text (instead of "parodontitis" it should be marked for example 00025). The image CD is then downloaded into an archive program, which normally generates thumbnail images, and then stored on a PC. It is also possible to add keywords and notes to the images. Images can be retrieved via the keywords and visually via the thumbnails.

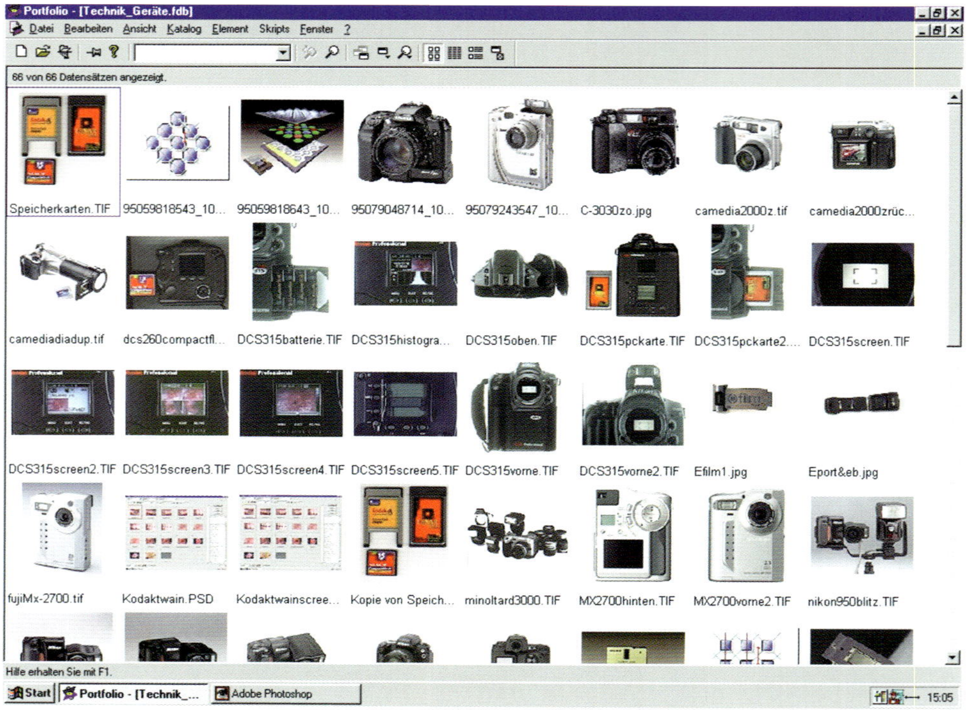

Fig. 12.27 Screen shot from a professional archive program (Portfolio from Extensis), which can easily accommodate large amounts of data.

12.7 Printing Images

If the dentist wants to give his or her patient an image to keep, it must be printed out. Economics dictate that in the practice this is generally done on inkjet printers, which are currently able to achieve photo-quality prints. The printers themselves are remarkably inexpensive, although the ink cartridges themselves are fairly costly.
Even better results can be achieved with thermal dye sublimation printers (e.g. Kodak Digital Science® 8650 or Olympus P-400) which, however, are still relatively expensive. Prints produced on these can no longer be distinguished from those produced photo chemically (e.g. Ilfochrome process) and exhibit absolute photo quality.
Fuji offers a printer which prints images using themo-autochrome technology; its format is limited to A6 (100 x 148mm), though 2, 4 or 16 individual images can be printed on one sheet. This process requires special paper in which color layers are sandwiched between the base and protective layers. The colors are released through heat and high quality photo realistic prints are produced.
Laser copies produced on photo paper are an inexpensive and high quality alternative.

12.8 Dental Imaging

Digitally produced images are amply suited as a basis for simulation of the results of treatment on a PC ("Dental Imaging"). Chapter 13.8 discusses this topic in more detail.

Conclusion

Digital cameras have the advantage of producing images which are both digital and immediately accessible. Quality is rapidly approaching that of conventionally produced images and for most applications the images' digital origins are no longer evident. For this reason, digital images are suitable for immediate data transfer, e.g. to send to a dental laboratory or to a colleague. They can also be immediately downloaded and stored in the software programs used in the practice.

If the same high quality image documentation is required for digital imaging as for conventional documentation, then the system of choice is professional digital SLRs with interchangeable lenses. Currently these are in the same price range as that of intraoral video systems. These systems can be regarded as being technically mature and suitable for routine applications in the practice. The downside of the advantages of digital imaging is the higher level of technology – camera and peripherals.

Amateur digital viewfinder cameras and SLRs without interchangeable lenses have only limited application for documentation or as adjuncts to conventional photography.

A cost-effectiveness analysis should be undertaken before purchase of a digital camera system and alternative solutions should also be weighed. Increasing use of computers in dental practices will mean digital documentation will become the standard in future. It makes good sense to look at these media today.

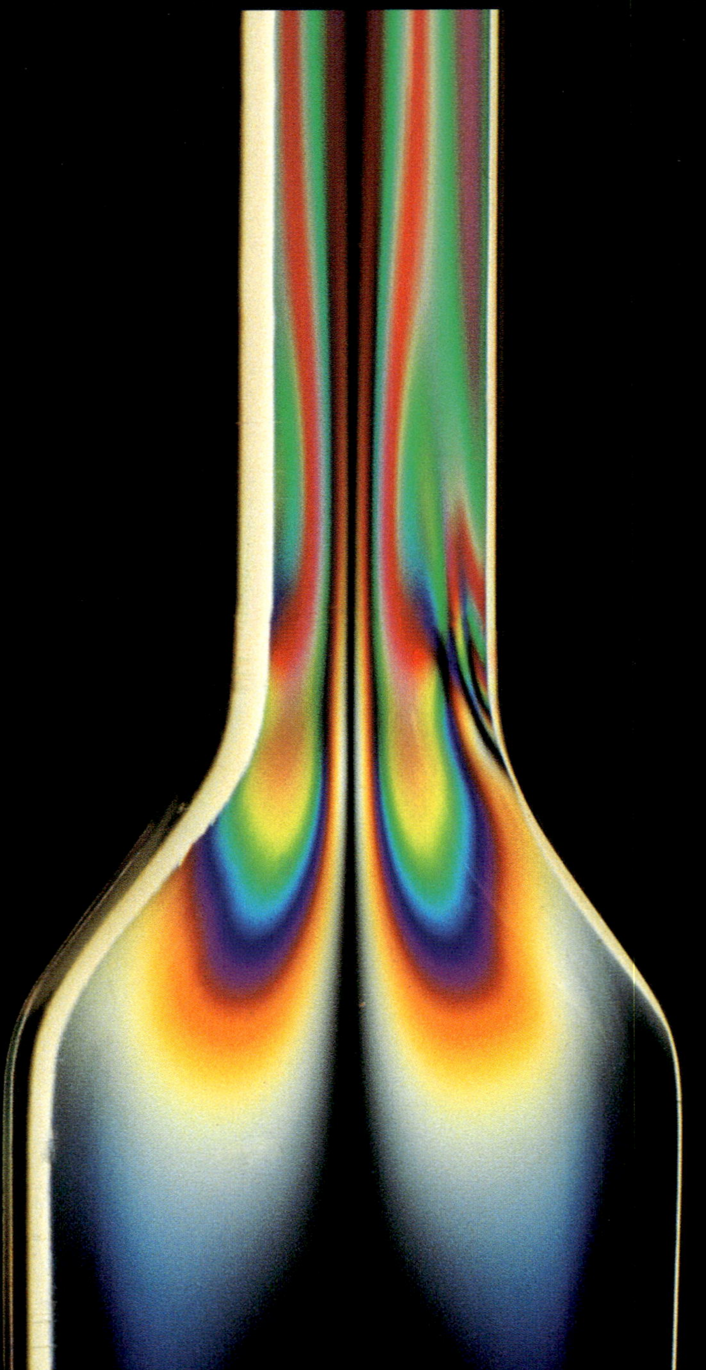

13 Intraoral Video Systems – Selection and Use

In March 1987 Fuji Optical Systems demonstrated a prototype of an intraoral video camera to the American Association of Dental Schools. The "DentaCam" was initially designed only as a teaching tool, but was shown at a dental convention in California the following year. This presentation marked the breakthrough for a new type of dental equipment to improve communication, diagnosis and documentation.

Today there is an almost confusing number of producers of such video systems. For this reason the following discussion makes no attempt at presenting a complete picture of the market, but is aimed only toward helping the potential user to make an informed decision in the purchase and application of such systems. Given the rapidity of development cycles, this overview can only be considered a snapshot.

◄ If transparent objects made of plastic – like this toothbrush handle – have polarized light shined through them and are photographed using a second polarizing filter with a grid at 90 degrees to that of the first, the internal stresses of the plastic show up in colors of the rainbow. The internal stresses lead to molecule formations which make the plastic doubly refractive. The polarized light shining through is split in two components; the two partial waves demonstrate a phase difference which causes the colored bands.

13.1 Applications of Intraoral Video Systems

There are three basic uses for intraoral video systems:

- Communication
- Documentation
- Diagnosis

13.1.1 Communication

In our television age a live video image appears authentic to the patient and is therefore one of the most influential instruments of communication and motivation (13.1). For this reason it is very easy to involve the patient in the treatment planning. He or she will have a much better understanding of our proposals, since "whoever recognizes the problem will also accept the solution" (Fig. 13.2)
A video image also enhances direct communication with the dental laboratory when images are transmitted directly from the PC via Email or data transfer line to the laboratory.
Images taken with an intraoral video camera can also serve as the basis of dental imaging (see below). Care should be taken, however, that the lens does not distort the image. This is frequently the case with video systems, as they generally have wide angle lenses.

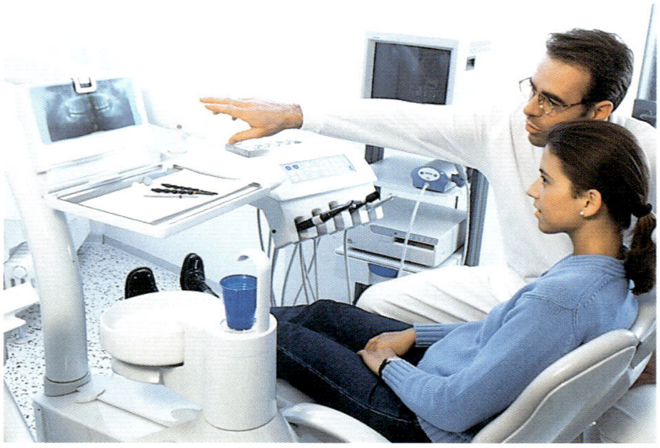

Fig. 13.1 The intraoral camera has become an integral and accepted piece of equipment in dental practices for patient consultations. (Photo: Dürr)

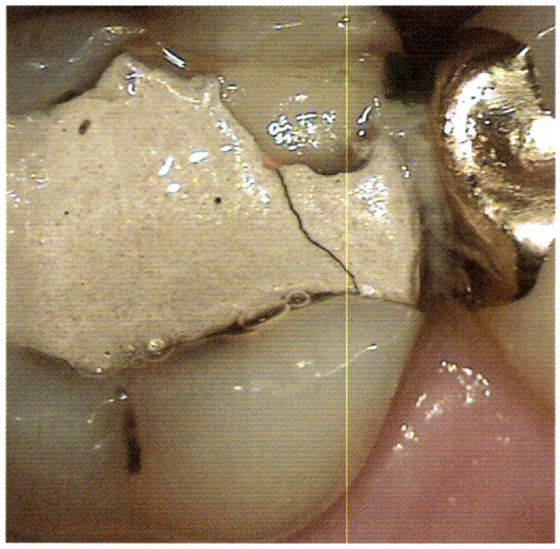

Fig. 13.2 There is no better means of demonstrating to the patient the treatment required than the intraoral camera.

13.1.2 Documentation

Documentation of the initial or intermediate stages of treatment is becoming increasingly important. This is done quickly and easily using video systems and archive software. The images are generally filed according to patient and can be retrieved. Documentation is useful for restorative work or periodontal surgery, but is also especially helpful in documentation of changes in the mucous membranes of the mouth which can be stored for comparison.

The limiting factor here is image quality. Video images are good enough to be shown on a monitor but not for higher demands. If high quality images are later required for printing or publication then these should be taken using conventional film or a digital SLR.

Documentation of changes in the mucous membranes in the mouth is becoming increasingly important, and thus the selection of a system must take the color rendition of mucous membranes into consideration.

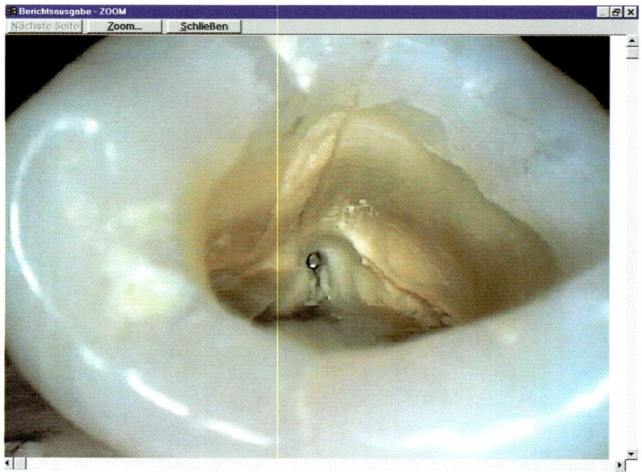

Fig. 13.3 Diagnosis can be significantly improved by the large magnification of the clinical image. (Photo: Lercher)

13.1.3 Diagnostics

Greater accuracy in diagnosis is possible due to the larger image magnification on the monitor (magnifications up to 40 - 100 times the size of the object are possible) (Fig. 13.3). Tooth infractions can be more easy recognized, marginal gaps are far more evident. Deficiencies in oral hygiene can be more easily detected and periodontal diseases perhaps detected earlier. There are also special adapters for microscopes (e. g. Dentron, Lercher, NewTech) which allow plaque to be displayed on

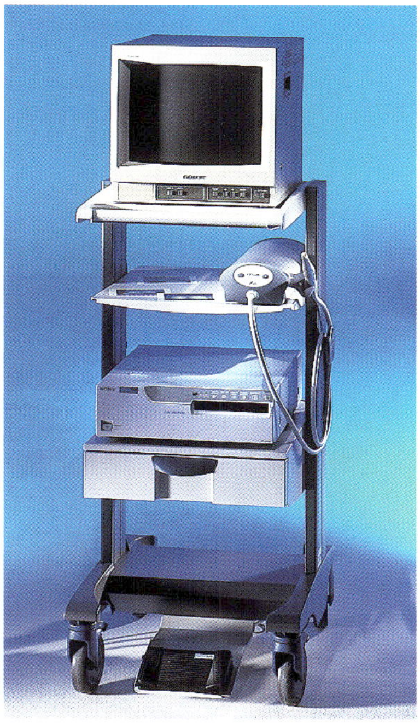

Fig. 13.4 VistaCam 2 as a video system in combination with a video printer. (Photo: Dürr)

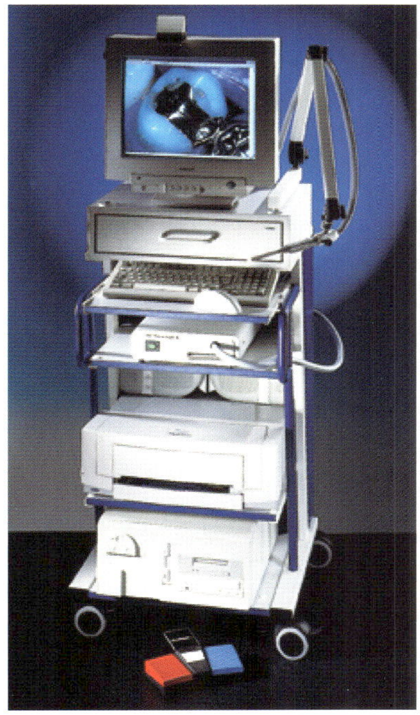

Fig. 13.5 Intraoral video system in a PC configuration. (Photo: Lercher)

the monitor. This is very impressive and instructive to a patient. A side effect of this is that many users of intraoral video systems have reported an improvement in treatment due to self-checking which is now possible. Anyone who has also documented his or her own work with a conventional camera has also discovered this.

One additional factor, which many manufacturers are keen to underscore, is that dental practices which use intraoral video systems appear to be particularly innovative. The patient has greater confidence in the professional competence because she or he can not readily differentiate between technical and dental competence. Nevertheless, this marketing aspect can sometimes have the opposite effect, at least in the interim, if this is emphasized without the necessary input from the dentist.

13.2 Technical Basics

An intraoral video system consists in the main of the camera itself, its associated electronics, a lighting system and a monitor on which the image can be displayed.

A video printer is a useful adjunct which allows the image to be printed out on paper. In many systems the printer also functions as a frame buffer which permits display of still frames (Fig. 13.4). Other systems have a separate internal frame buffer. The latter have nothing to do with a picture archive, but only have the function of "freezing" a moving image in order to discuss the diagnosis with the patient.

If the dentist wishes to save this image or digitally enhance it, an interface to a computer is necessary. Generally this is done using a "frame grabber card" which digitizes the video signal and makes it possible for the computer to read and manipulate. The result of such digitization is an image which can be stored using an appropriate archive program and enhanced using special imaging programs (Fig. 13.5) The CaddyCam (Dentron) uses another method. This stores the images as BMP files on a SmartMedia card which can be inserted into a reader which transfers the data to a PC.

13.2.1 Camera

The video camera itself consists of the lens, an integrated lighting system and a CCD chip, which is the technical heart of the camera. This electronic component converts light which falls on it into an electrical signal from which the monitor image is generated. This signal is a standard video signal, that is, it produces sufficient quality for a clear monitor image and printing out to about postcard size in an appropriate quality.

Mouth-mirror and endoscope cameras differ in design, with the latter including cameras with "universal lenses".

Mouth-mirror cameras have a mirror which is fixed to a video camera (Fig. 13.6). This permits intraoral subjects to be photographed. If the mirror is removed, extraoral images can be captured. One example of such a camera is the Dental Scout (Dentron) (Fig. 13.7). Mirror fittings are also available for endoscope cameras (e.g. from Lercher) (Fig. 13.8).

Endoscope cameras are designed like handpieces which have small lenses in the tips.

Three different types of camera can be distinguished according to the position of the CCD chip:

- ✓ Chip immediately behind lens
- ✓ Chip in intraoral part of the camera
- ✓ Chip in "handle" of the camera behind the optical system. Strictly speaking, this type of camera, as well as the mouth-mirror camera, are "extraoral" video cameras, since the image capture system is extraoral.

Variant 1: Location of the chip behind the lens has been largely abandoned. The required miniaturization is technically demanding and expensive; furthermore, such cameras can not be sterilized. Moreover, the front end of the intraoral segment was relatively large (Fig. 13.9).

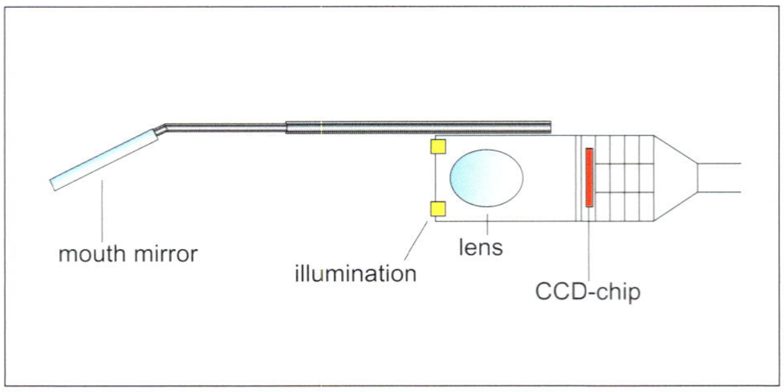

13. 6 Diagram of a mouth-mirror video camera.

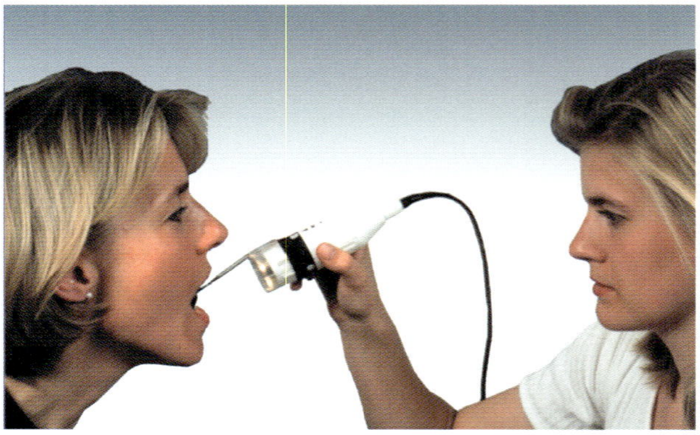

Fig. 13.7 The Dental Scout camera is in widespread use. (Photo: Dentron)

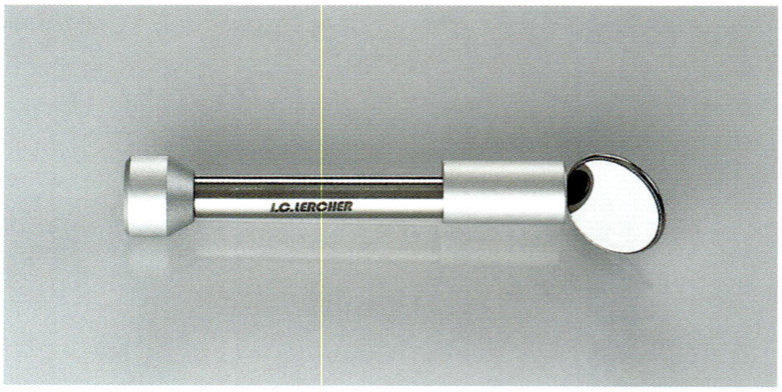

Fig. 13.8 Removable mirror fittings are also available for endoscope cameras. (Photo: Lercher)

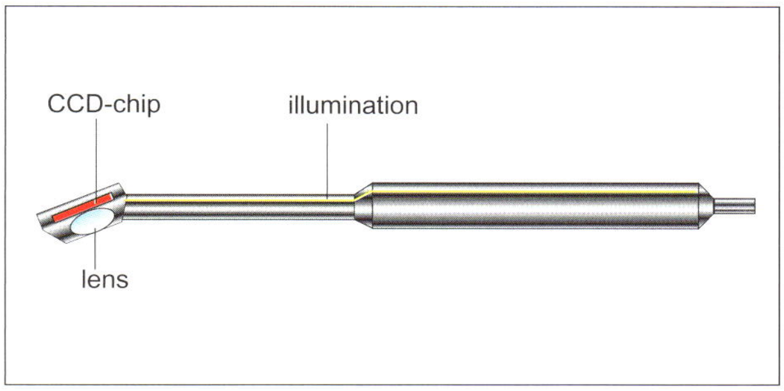

Fig. 13.9 Older design of intraoral video camera, with the chip in the camera head.

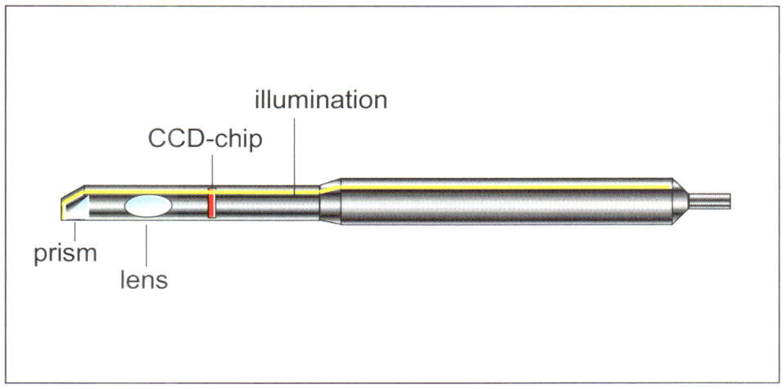

Fig. 13.10 Design of a camera with universal lens.

Fig. 13.11 Diagram of an endoscope camera. As in the case of the mouth-mirror video camera, the CCD chip is placed in the handle of the camera.

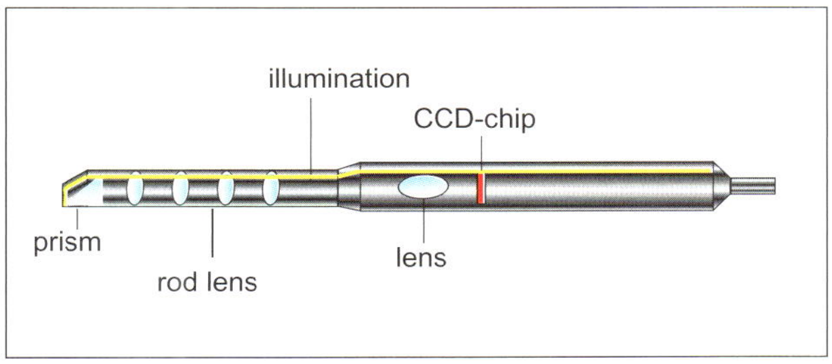

Variant 2: The positioning of the chip also causes problems with sterilization. Plastic coverings are often used to solve the problem. Cameras in this variation generally have universal lenses, which do not have to be replaced (Fig. 13.10). The drawback to these is lower image quality. What lens is able to capture good quality images from a few millimeters to infinity, ideally without distortion? Such cameras are thus aimed at more limited applications such as showing the patient aspects of his or her mouth. For many users this will be sufficient.

Variant 3: This has the advantage of interchangeable lenses and easy sterilization. Slender designs are possible. Image production is generally far better than with universal lenses, lighting is good and the images largely distortion-free. These systems, however, are also more costly (Fig. 13.11)

Mouth-mirror video cameras compared with endoscope cameras with universal lenses

Despite their greater apparent size, mouth-mirror video cameras have many advantages over endoscope cameras.

A dentist inexperienced in their use will find handling of the former relatively easy if he or she is versed in the use of a mouth-mirror. The image is steady since the mirror can be rested on the tooth. Mouth-mirror video cameras use a tele-macro-lens which takes the image in the mirror. This eliminates the problem of distortion which is endemic to wide angle lenses. Illumination is also provided via the mirror, the light from which is provided by the camera. This results in far more even lighting than is the case with many endoscope cameras which have the lighting system placed in the lens. Even small differences in the distance to the object can have a significant effect in the brightness of the image. The relatively large camera size does not necessarily mean that the camera itself is heavy. Used over time, it is more important to determine whether the whole system is easy to manipulate. Slender endoscope cameras with a long and heavy illumination system can be more tiring to use than a camera system which at first glance appears more bulky. In the end, mouth-mirror video systems are also easy to sterilize, since only the mirror itself is used intraorallly. It can be easily removed and sterilized.

On the other hand, endoscope cameras have significant advantages in image framing and magnification, which in the final analysis depends on monitor size. Mouth-mirror video cameras permit magnifications of up to factor 20, endoscope cameras to 40, and many as high as 100. Of course increasing magnification reduces depth of field, so that it makes these more difficult to manipulate.

Another advantage of endoscope cameras is their expansion capabilities (see Expansion).

Usage, ideally in the dentist's own practice, is the best way of making a fundamental decision on these systems.

13.2.2 Monitor

Flat-screen monitors with TFT technology are to be preferred to conventional monitors simply to save room. These can be easily integrated into a dental practice's working surrounding (Fig. 13.12).

Before purchase of one or even more of these type screens, it is recommended that the dental practice use these on a trial basis, since the light in the rooms can differ quite significantly. The ability to perceive the image depends greatly on the ambient light and the viewing angle. In general, it is recommended that monitors should be conveniently placed for diagnosis and patient consultation (Fig. 13.13).

Equipment from Planmeca, Ritter and KaVo for example demonstrate good integration of a monitor in a dental practice. Flat screen monitors should be able to turn, swivel and tilt in order to avoid reflections on the screen. The Ultradent Vision UV 5000 (Ultradent) is an interesting development. This is a 15 inch TFT flat screen monitor which can be turned and tilted. An integrated sensor allows it to be turned on without having to touch it; a hand movement also scrolls through stored images and switches from the computer to a video image.

In principle the monitor should match the performance of the camera. It makes no sense to connect an expensive camera which can resolve 500 lines to an inexpensive and lower performance TV monitor aimed at the home user market which perhaps resolves only 280 TV lines.

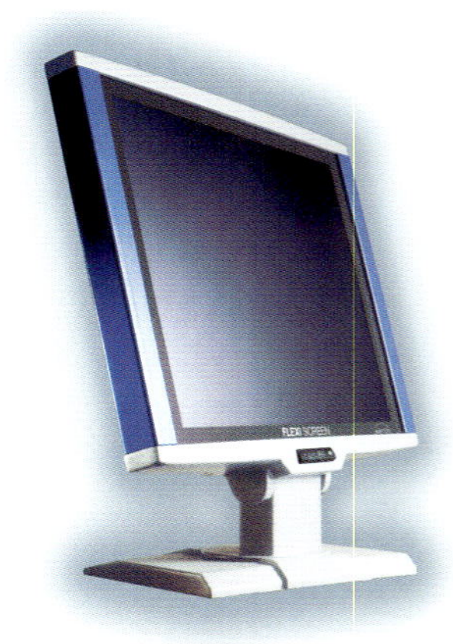

Fig. 13.12 Flat screen monitors are more easily integrated into dental units than bulkier monitors with tubes (Photo: NewTech).

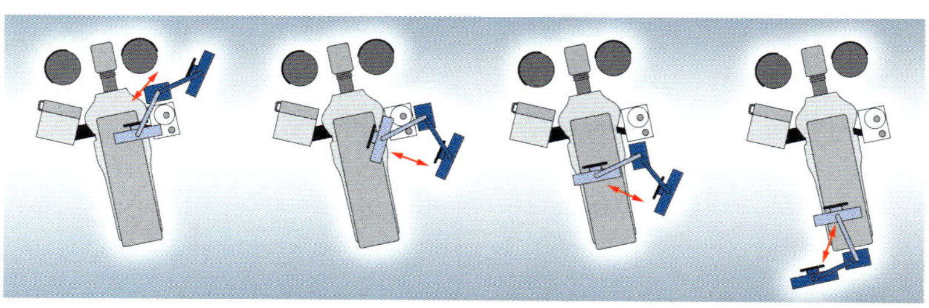

Fig. 13.13 The position of the monitor should be variable, so that all treatment situations can be addressed (Photo: NewTech).

13.2.3 Image quality/lighting/depth of field

The quality of the images depends most of all on the lens, the CCD chip and the lighting. Furthermore, differences in the signal processing electronics also play a role, although manufacturers are relatively circumspect on this point.

Frequently used image sensors are 1/4 inch CCD chips or 1/3 inch CCD chips which have an image resolution of about 480,000 pixels. An exception to this is the Satellite Scope DP-15 camera (RF System Lab/Japan) which has 760,000 pixels, according to the manufacturer.

In many camera-computer combinations the frame grabber card reduces the quality. High resolution video grabbers are much to be preferred over less expensive cards from the consumer market (Fig. 13.14).

Lighting not only influences color rendition but also the quality of the image. If the lighting source is weak and the object fairly dark the electronic signal has to be boosted. This reduces color saturation and increases noise, thus greatly degrading image brilliance.

As in photography in general, the depth of field depends on the aperture (and the reproduction ratio). A strong light source permits a small aperture and therefore generally results in a greater depth of field which eliminates the need to refocus. Some systems have an arc light (e.g. Reveal) which is better than the usual halogen lamps in terms of color temperature and amount of light. However, it does take a few minutes to warm up, since the light first has to reach operating temperature. Newly developed cameras have LEDs (light emitting diodes) as a light source.

Lighting can be uneven depending on where lights are located. Also, with some systems the lighting can vary substantially if the subject-to-camera distance is altered. With some systems there is room for improvement in the control curve which controls the brightness in relation to the camera distance and/or the reproduction ratio.

Some systems, such as the Dürr Vistacam2 have center weighted exposure metering and spot metering, which is designed to optimize lighting control according to the situation. In order to test these points the user should try videoing objects which

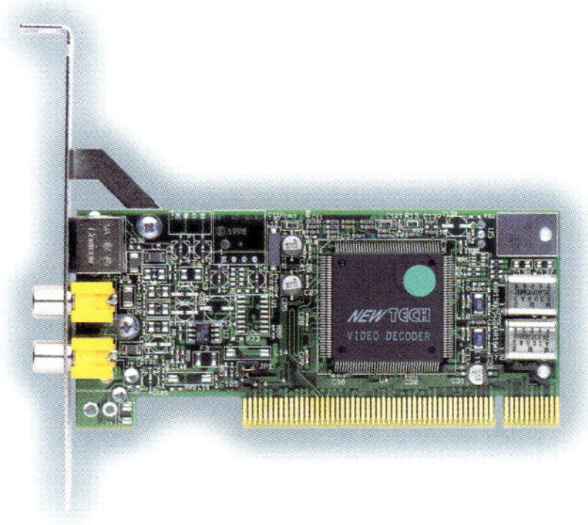

Fig. 13.14 The frame grabber converts the analog signal into a digital one. (Photo: NewTech)

present difficulties. The image brightness at various subject-to-camera distances should also be examined.

Image quality is also degraded by condensation on the surface of the lens which is caused by the moisture from the mouth collecting on the cold lens surface. Many cameras have special mechanisms (e.g. a small fan) to counteract this. In general it is helpful to warm the camera ahead of time or use an anti-condensation medium to counteract condensation.

13.2.4 Hygiene

The various designs of camera determine the different means of maintaining hygiene. Mouth-mirror video cameras, as described above, are the least problematical in this regard.

Many endoscope cameras have a removable "cap" which covers the lens and possibly the chip; these can be easily sterilized (e.g. Sirocam 2, Sirona). Other systems are supplied with plastic sheets which can be slipped over the camera (Fig. 13.15). This naturally does not improve image quality, but is generally a satisfactory solution as

long as there are no air vents between the lens surface and the plastic cover.
Other endoscope systems are so well encapsulated that the camera unit can be completely immersed in liquid cold sterilization solutions.

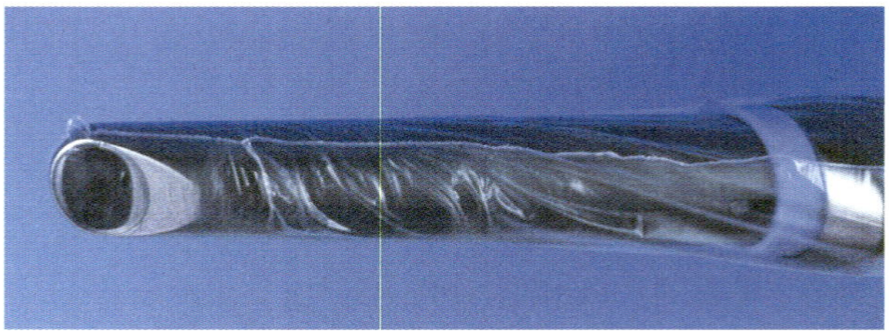

Fig. 13.15 If the camera cap can not or should not be sterilized, plastic covers should be used. It should be ensured that there are no folds in front of the lens.

13.2.5 Correct orientation of image on the monitor/splitscreen function

Particularly initially, the orientation of the image on the monitor can pose a problem. Generally speaking, the lens and the image sensor are coupled. Turning the camera turns the image on the monitor. This not only is confusing to the patient but also to a dentist looking for a particular intraoral detail.
In the case of many systems the objects are reversed on the monitor; these can be "flipped" using an electronic means.
In other systems the image is correctly displayed due to their specially designed optical system.
The DentalScout mouth-mirror video camera has a marking on the camera for correct positioning of the CCD chip which is doing the recording. Depending on the situation the mirror can be turned, keeping the camera position and thus the position of the CCD chip the same.

It is useful to be able to display several images at a time on the monitor. Most systems allow four images to be shown simultaneously, allowing "before and after" images to be compared or several results for a patient to be displayed (Fig. 13.16).

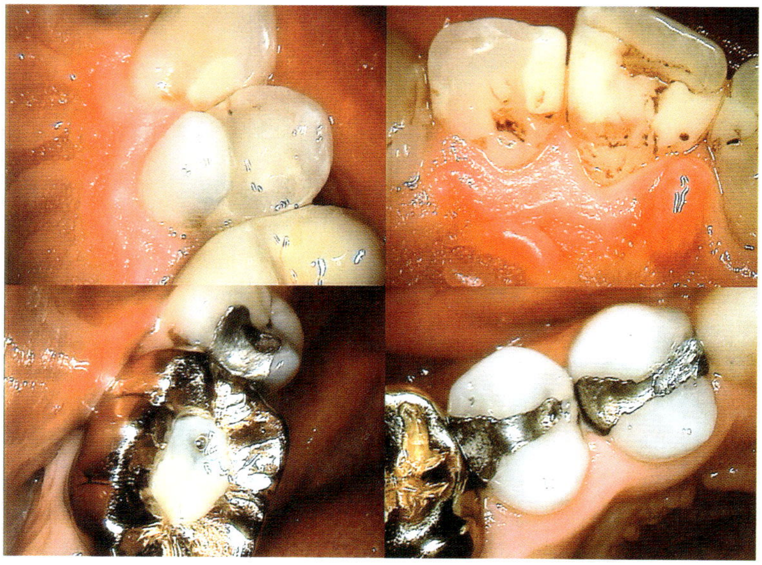

Fig. 13.16 The ability to show several images at one time on a monitor is not merely a gadget, but a useful aid in patient consultations (Photo: NewTech).

13.2.6 Expansion

The various systems differ in their ability to be expanded. Simple systems only allow observation of a "frozen" monitor image (with video resolution) using their integrated electronics or image storage from a video printer.

The next expansion stage entails connection of the system to a PC or a PC network . This allows image archiving and, if necessary, simulation of treatment results (dental imaging). The current trend is toward use of the computer. Intraoral video cameras can be connected to today's powerful computer systems without any problems.

While the expansion capability of cameras with universal lenses has reached its limits, many accessories are now being offered for endoscope cameras which are geared toward special applications (Fig. 13.17). Thus it is possible to use fiber optic technology to visually examine the periodontal sulcus or to examine a plaque scraping under the light microscope on the monitor (Fig. 13.18). While some systems offer small interchangeable lenses (e.g. Reveal) (Fig. 13.19), others (e.g. Lercher, NewTech) have different endoscopic features and accessories.

The degree of expansion should be seriously considered before purchase of any system. Here too, the system which appears at first glance to be the most economical is not always so in the long run when the required expansion capability hits a dead end.

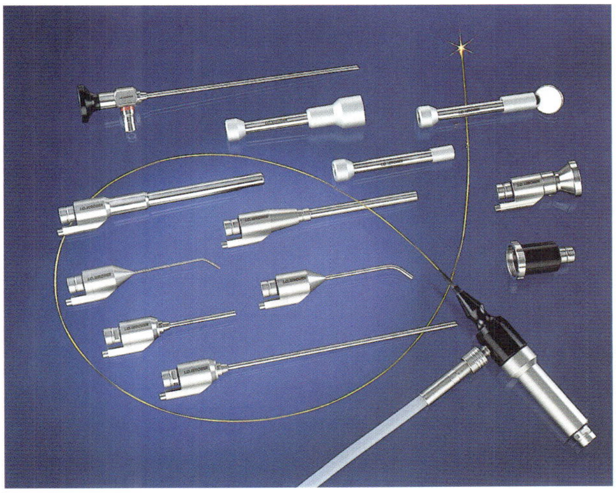

Fig. 13.17 Many manufacturers offer a large variety of endoscope fittings. (Photo: Lercher)

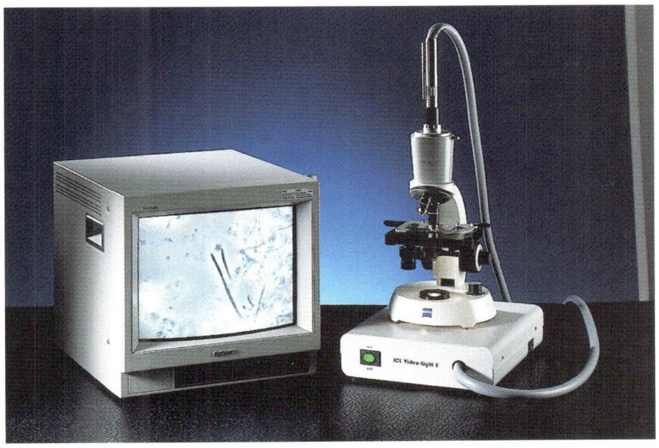

Fig. 13.18 The patient is always impressed by plaque scrapings shown under a microscope. This has less to do with diagnosis than with motivation. (Photo: Lercher)

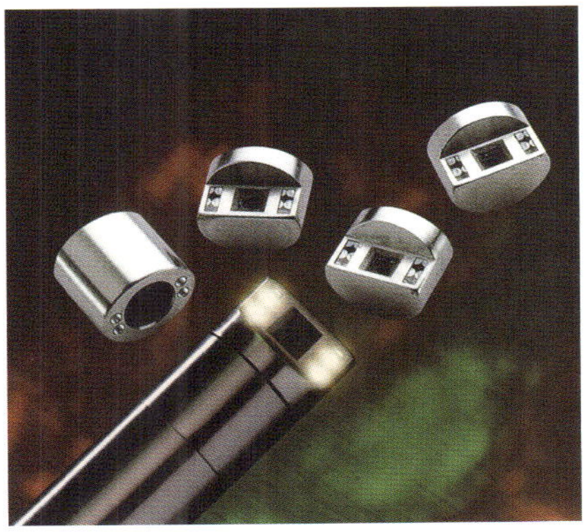

Fig. 13.19 Interchangeable lenses are used to meet the requirements for different images. (Photo: Reveal)

13.2.7 Integration into the dental practice

Integration into the dental practice is currently one of the thorniest problems. Ideally, every dental chair should have a video system. It is easy to imagine, in addition to the handpieces, air turbine and three ways syringe, to have another tube for the intraoral camera, which, when removed, activates the system and switches on a well-designed flatscreen monitor in front of the patient.

Some equipment manufacturers (e.g. KaVo, Planmeca) already offer video systems which are integrated into the dental chair unit(Fig. 13.20).

The system should be integrated into the dental practice's computer network, where also patients' data and possibly also digital X-ray records are stored.

At the moment most dental practices are far removed from this, and therefore the usual video systems appear still somewhat provisional. They are frequently placed on trolleys which are generally in the way.

A fundamental technical problem is that the development cycles for electronic imaging is relatively short, while a dental unit can be used over many years in a dental practice. Module combinations which allow even fixed components to be changed or upgraded are therefore to be recommended.

Many manufacturers offer cameras which can be removed from their base unit and moved into another treatment room, to be docked into another base unit (e.g. Reveal, Lercher, NewTech, Planmeca, CaddyCam from Dentron) (Fig. 13.21 and 13.22). This eliminates the need to purchase several expensive cameras. Thus, for example, the docking station of the Reveal System can accept an intraoral camera, an intraoral X-ray system or an extraoral lighting system which can be attached to the head or the telescopic spectacle.

Another problem which is still to be addressed is the "spaghetti junction" of cables on the floor, since this already has to accommodate the foot controller of the dental unit and that of the camera. The wireless foot switch from CAPAZ, which has a multi-channel infrared transmitter, is a development aimed at solving this problem. The receiver is connected to a PC via a serial port. Using the

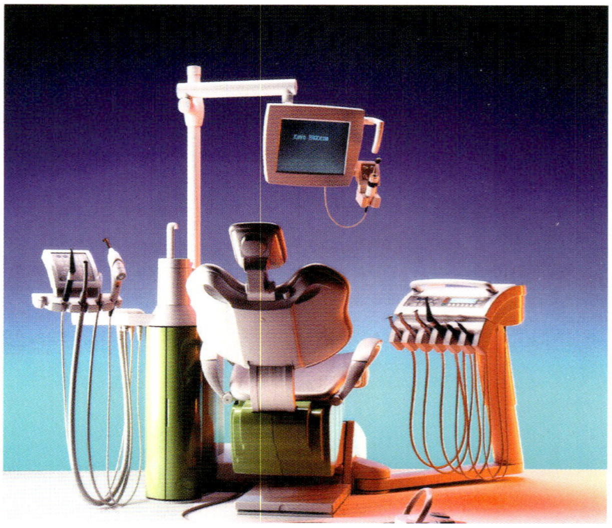

Fig. 13.20 An example of good integration of a monitor into a dental workplace. (Photo: KaVo)

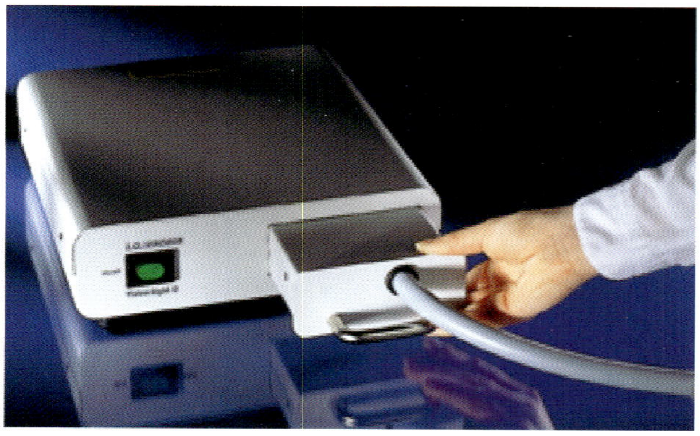

Fig. 13.21 Camera modules which can be docked mean that the camera is available in every treatment room. (Photo: Lercher)

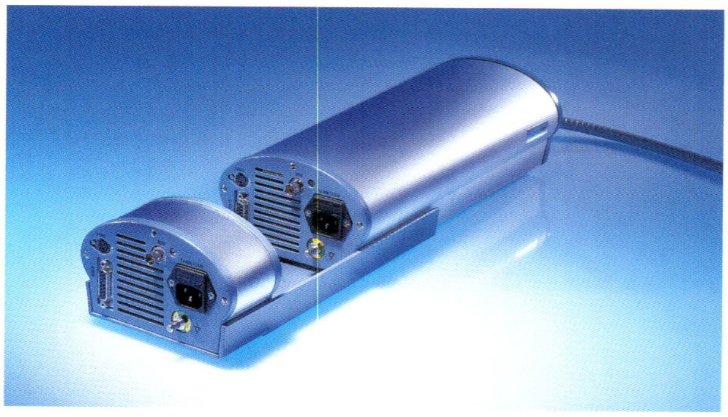

Fig. 13.22 A docking station allows the camera to be quickly connected to the base station. (Photo: Dürr)

software provided, each pedal (variants have two or three pedals) can be assigned to a key or mouse entry. This not only allows a video camera to be addressed, but any software package which does not permit foot control.
Such a wireless connection to a PC also has advantages in regard to certain legal aspects, at least in Germany. If a foot pedal near the patient leads to a PC, it must meet the requirements of the "Medizinproduktegesetz" (MPG). This is not necessary if data transmission is done without a cable. According to the regulations in Germany, only equipment marked CE may be employed within a radius of 1.5 m around the patient. If equipment is used outside this radius which does not conform to the MPG, and which is connected to equipment which is in the immediate vicinity of the patient (for example, a printer), the certificate for use of the entire system is invalidated. To circumvent this, wireless connections can be used or special base stations which securely separate the connections to the non-medical electrical accessories (e.g. Flexi Scope System Safe, from NewTech).
Retrofitting a camera system to a dental unit also presents problems with the interface; the camera's electronics and the monitor have to be connected by cable. Other systems use radio transmission between the monitor and the camera's base station (Dürr, NewTech).
Recent developments are cameras without cables which transmit radio or infrared signals to the base station. The Japanese company RF System lab offers two camera models which allow wireless image transmission to a base station which powers the monitor. Power comes from a battery pack in the camera's grip. According to the manufacturer's technical specifications, the professional model of the two variants has an unusually high resolution of 760,000 pixels (the author has had no personal experience of the cameras to date).

13.3 Requirement Checklist

The market for intraoral video systems has become complex and is rapidly changing. For this reason, a list is given of important points for consideration before purchase of such a system before these are detailed. Their sequence does not denote their importance.

- ✓ High resolution image with good color rendition
- ✓ Easy to use, preferably with one hand
- ✓ Good freeze frame images
- ✓ Possibility of split-screen images
- ✓ Network capable
- ✓ Large zoom range from individual tooth to groups of teeth
- ✓ Autofocus, large depth of field
- ✓ 0 degree lens and 90 degree lens
- ✓ Minimal distortion
- ✓ Hygienic treatment? Sterilizable? Plastic caps?
- ✓ Images reversed?
- ✓ Images upright?
- ✓ System transportable?
- ✓ Noise
- ✓ Reduction of condensation on front of lens
- ✓ Camera size
- ✓ Price
- ✓ Manufacturer's back-up (guarantee, maintenance, etc.)

13.4 Practical Tips

As with any other imaging system, when using intraoral video systems (and other image recording devices), the user should be aware that, from the patient's point of view, the camera is being employed in an intimate zone. Even though most patients are fairly relaxed about this some react dif-

ferently than we expect. This can be prevented through a proper approach.
Before the camera is used for the first time the patient should be informed about its application and use. The patient should be aware of the fact that the camera is a tool which can help him or her improve conditions in the mouth and which also significantly improves diagnosis due to its great magnification. This creates acceptance and thus a quiet and relaxed atmosphere. Avoid starting with negative findings, e.g. with coatings on the lingual surfaces of the lower molars. Start with areas which are perfectly maintained or naturally healthy! Praise the patient for this! Only then can the user carefully begin on negative aspects. These should not be criticized, but suggestions should be made about improvements.
As in the case of any new technology which is being introduced in the practice, this takes experience and also psychological sensitivity (Fig. 13.23)

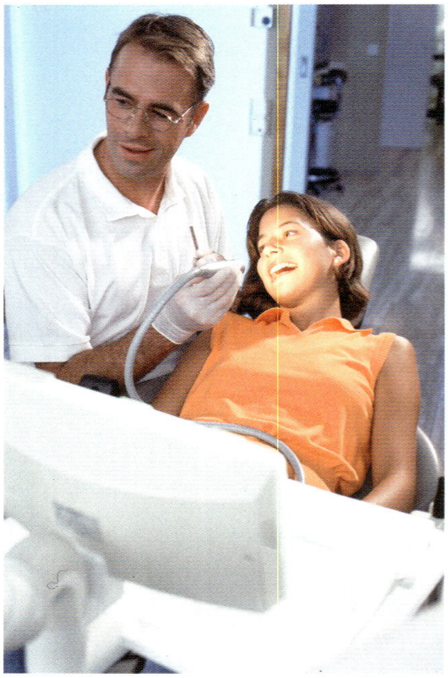

Fig. 13. 23 A relaxed atmosphere is an important prerequisite for work with an intraoral video system. (Photo: Dürr)

13.5 Future Developments

Improvements are to be expected in image resolution and integration into the dental unit. Wireless systems with rechargeable battery packs and radio signals to the base station will replace the "hose cameras". At present, an intraoral video system is used above all to inform and motivate the patient. There are developments in train, however, which are aimed at replacing a direct view with control via a monitor for some procedures, just as is done with endoscopes in many medical applications. It is conceivable that the camera could be mounted on the head of the contra angle handpiece so that treatment could be undertaken without a mirror under monitor control, which would be an advantage in many situations.

13.6 Examples of Intraoral Video Systems

In citing these examples no claim is made for comprehensiveness or an appraisal. Technical details should be obtained from technical specifications.

13.6.1 Mouth-mirror video cameras

Dental Scout (Dentron)
Compact video camera with mouth mirror (see above). The Dental Scout P 2000 has interchangeable lenses (macro-telelens for intraoral detailed views, macro lens for intraoral overviews as well as profile and enface images). ViewBase software for archiving and image enhancement as well as ISDN image transmission.

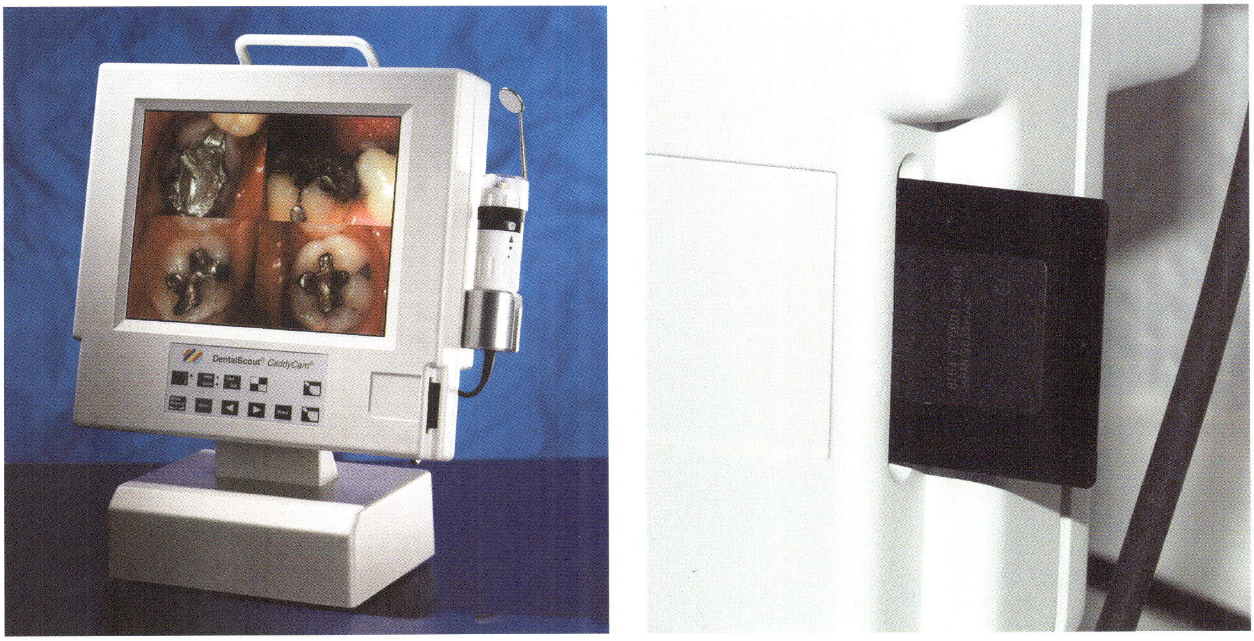

Fig. 13.24 The CaddyCam is an interesting alternative to a camera system which can be wheeled around the practice on a trolley (a). The images are stored on a SmartMedia card and can be read into a computer (b). (Photo a: Dentron)

Dental Scout CaddyCam (Dentron)

Portable, compact system which combines a flat screen monitor and an intraoral video camera in one unit. A docking station is located in the foot which contains a power supply and foot switch connection (Fig. 13.24). If such stations are located in the various treatment rooms, the monitor-camera-unit needs only to be plugged in. This also automatically provides power.

Many images can be stored on the SmartMedia® card and can be transferred without a cable to a PC (BMP file). There they can be stored, enhanced or printed out, thus eliminating the need for an expensive video printer.

The camera is a digital variant of the Dental Scout P 2000. Two lenses are available: one for the mouth mirror and the other as a 0 degree lens for extraoral imaging. A C-mount adapter allows the camera to be easily connected to a microscope (e.g for plaque diagnosis).

Either one or four images can be displayed on the flatscreen monitor. The monitor is also configured for use as either a video or computer monitor.

13.6.2 Cameras with universal lenses

True Vision 2

Easily portable system available in a wall-mount or counter-top configuration. Suitable für multiple-operatory installations.

$^1/_4$" Interline Transfer CCD with 480 TV lines of resolution and automatic white balance. Optically clear sleeve for asepsis. Small and light camera handpiece.Integral sliding focus for macro, intraoral and extraoral viewing.

Vipercam (Integra Medical)

The Vipercam intraoral camera is a state of the art intraoral camera designed specifically for integration with a computer. Vipercam uses a low cost docking station for multi-op installations. Using this approach allows the dentist to carry only the portable hand-piece from operatory to operatory. The NEW Vipercam DV Exam Station allows the capture of four full screen images with the ability to display them one at a time, or as a quad. 470

TV lines of resolution. 768 x 494 pixels- NTSC visible. 752 x 582 pixels- PAL visible. Stainless steel, lens tube with 10.5mm diameter. Well balanced, rear drive focus with 3 detented positions: Macro, Intraoral, Extraoral.

CygnaScope™ (Cygnus Technologies)
The CygnaScope is the world's first intraoral camera with an ultra-high speed CyLink (IEEE-1394/FireWire) digital computer connection, eliminating the need for a video capture card. The camera is plugged into a FireWire-equipped computer. All models also include video outputs for easy connection to any television set, video network, or video printer.
With an on-board computer, images can be captured and frozen in single, dual, or quad mode. Easy integration with most major practice management and dental imaging software allows for effortless storage and capture using a computer.
CygnaScope uses the $^1/_4$" SONY CCD that produces more than 437,664 pixels with full-frame digital output.
The model CygnaScope MICRO, weighing only just 27 oz., offers the ultimate in portability and image quality.

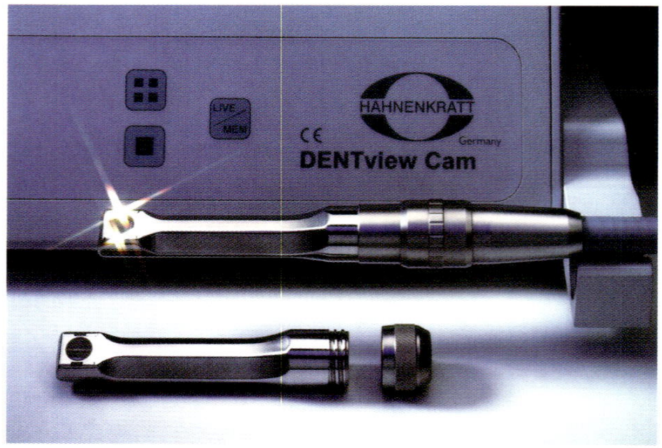

Fig. 13.25 Dentview camera with focusable universal lens. (Photo: Hahnenkratt)

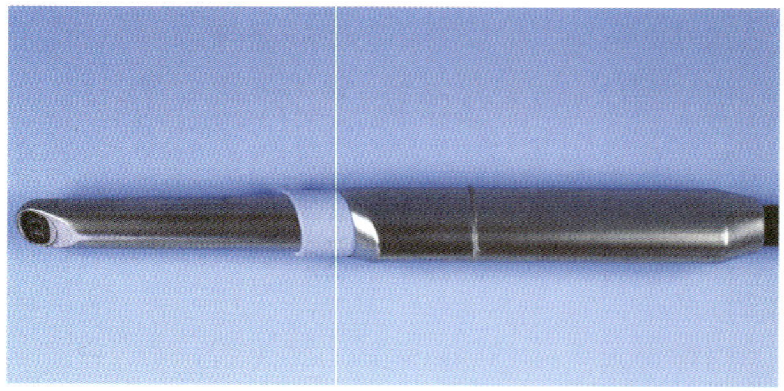
Fig. 13.26 The Sirocam 2 allows images to be framed using a slider.

AcuCam Concept IV (Gendex)
Small and light intraoral video system using a $^1/_4$" CCD. The One Press Function Touch Pad makes the camera easy to use. Can be integrated into VixWin 2000 software. Stainless steel handpiece with intraoral, estraoral and macro settings. A non-inverting roof prism presents images in their true clinical orientation. Resolving power is 80 line pairs per mm. A 72° wide angle lens provides increased depth of field.

DENTview (Hahnenkratt)
Infinitely focusable universal lens with fix-focus function in macro, intraoral and extraoral settings (Fig. 13.25). Aperture angle of the lens is 72 degrees. The program DENTpic is used for archiving and display of images. DENTinfo program is a freely configurable patient information system which can incorporate the user's own images, scanned in images, text and videos.

Intracam (Planmeca)
Camera integrated well in the treatment unit; one-hand operation, correct orientation of images, 90 degree lens, hygienic caps. Intracam S is a portable variant.

Sirocam 2 (Sirona)
Slender video camera with universal lens, 90 degree lens; removable titanium cap can be sterilized (Fig. 13.26). Image is framed using a slider on the handpiece. Three standard views with preset stops: individual tooth, quadrant, full face view.

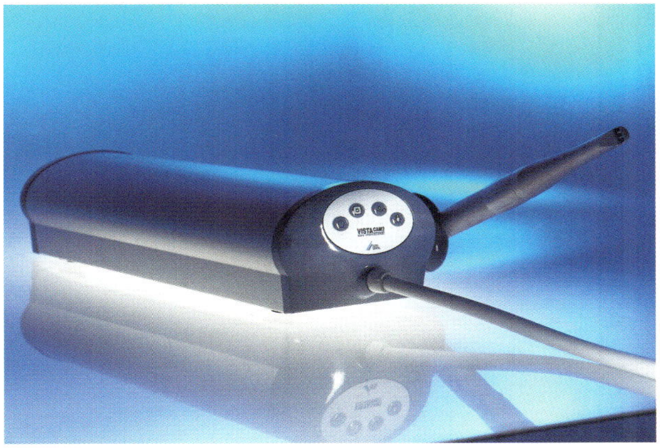

Fig. 13.27 Also well designed: the VistaCam 2. (Photo: Dürr)

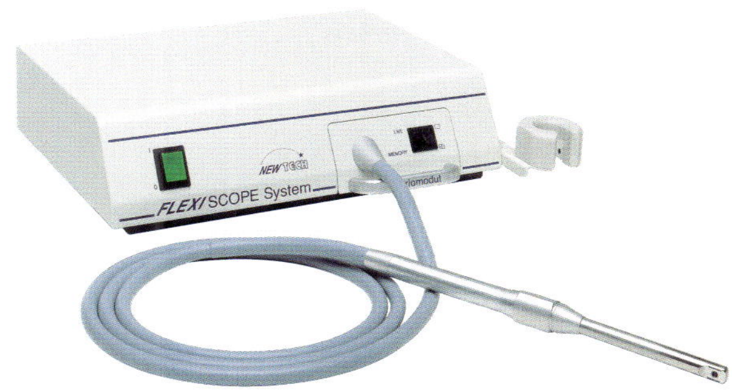

Fig. 13.28 Flexiscope System from NewTech. (Photo: NewTech)

13.6.3 System with interchangeable lens

Reveal Imaging System (Distributor: DMT)
Modular camera system with interchangeable lenses (Fig. 13.19). As an alternative to the intraoral camera, an intraoral X-ray sensor or extraoral lighting system can be connected to the base station. Lighting provided by arc light. Camera head housing can be fully immersed in disinfectant. "Aloisius" software for image display and processing.

13.6.4 Endoscope cameras

VistaCam 2 (Dürr)
New design of intraoral video camera with magnification up to 100 times (object size in relation to monitor display). One-hand operation via rotating ring for macro to portrait setting (Fig. 13.27). VistaCam 2 High Professional model with ability for white balance and selection between spot and integrated metering. The VistaCam 2 available with video freeze solution, PC-supported system, stand alone or networked. Software: DBSWIN.

Flexiscope Cameras (NewTech, Freiburg)
Modular camera system with many accessories. Flexiscope Eco as complete camera system with non-removable endoscopic lens. Flexiscope Classic as entry-level model with interchangeable lenses. Flexiscope Optomodul with interchangeable camera module and lenses. Flexiscope multivision as expandable modular system with special applications (microscope adapter, microdiagnostic probe, etc.)

Video-Light Cameras (I.C. Lercher)
Cameras with many accessories including various lenses and filters. Video-Light E as entry-level model, Video-Light D allows individual settings. Video-Light C with removable camera module for use in several treatment rooms (see Fig. 13.21). Can be connected to a microscope and laboratory conference system.
Software: Dentbase image database for archiving and image processing. Ability to measure object. Imaging software.

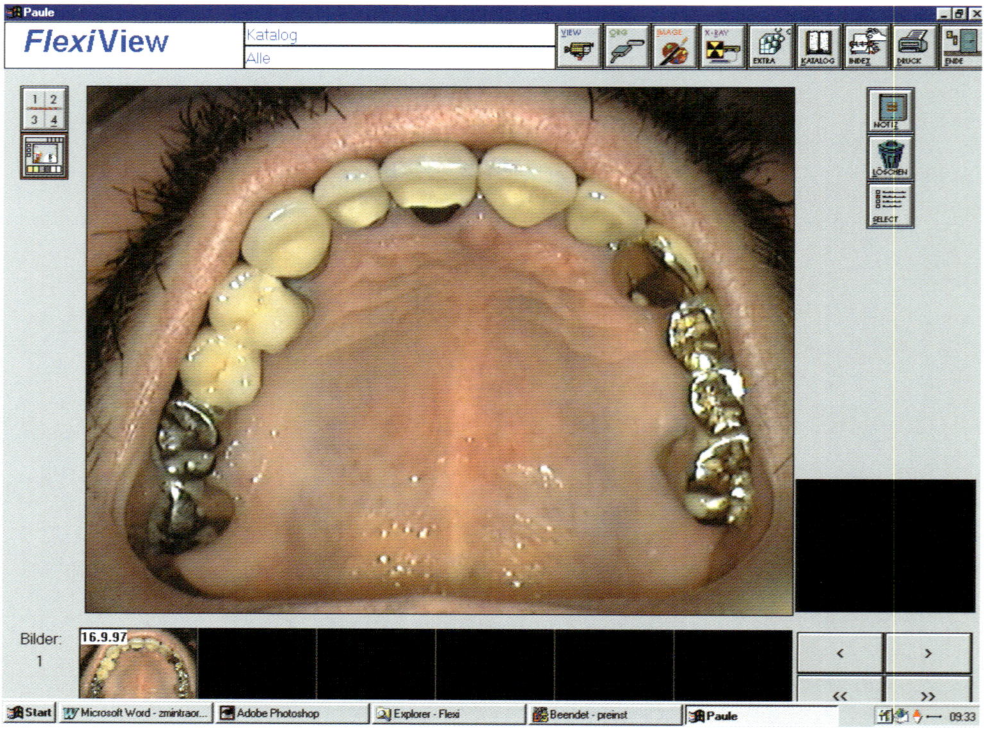

Fig. 13.29
Screen shot of the FlexiView monitor.

13.7 Hardware and Software

Where once "computer system requirements" were always listed for the operation of intraoral cameras this is no longer the case, since the standard computers of today are very high performance.
Most manufacturers also offer software as part of the package. Software is required for image display. If treatment simulations are required then an imaging program is necessary. If images are to be archived, an image database needs to be procured (Fig. 13.29). In all cases with program modules, the user will find that special programs for dentistry are significantly more expensive than commercially available image archive and processing ones (Fig. 13.30). Nevertheless, they sometimes have advantages in terms of operation. Some examples of programs are listed with the individual video cameras. Image archive programs which file images according to patient can be very effectively used for patient consultation if "classic patients" are entered under particular topics (cone crowns, ceramic inlays etc.)

13.8 Dental Imaging

In North America and the United Kingdom the term "imaging" is used to describe all procedures which result in an image regardless of whether the systems used to produce these are conventional or digital. In dental practice, "imaging" refers more specifically to the simulation of the results of treatment on a monitor.
The technical requirements for this are a PC with a high performance graphics card and an imaging program. The latter is a special image processing program which allows image details to be

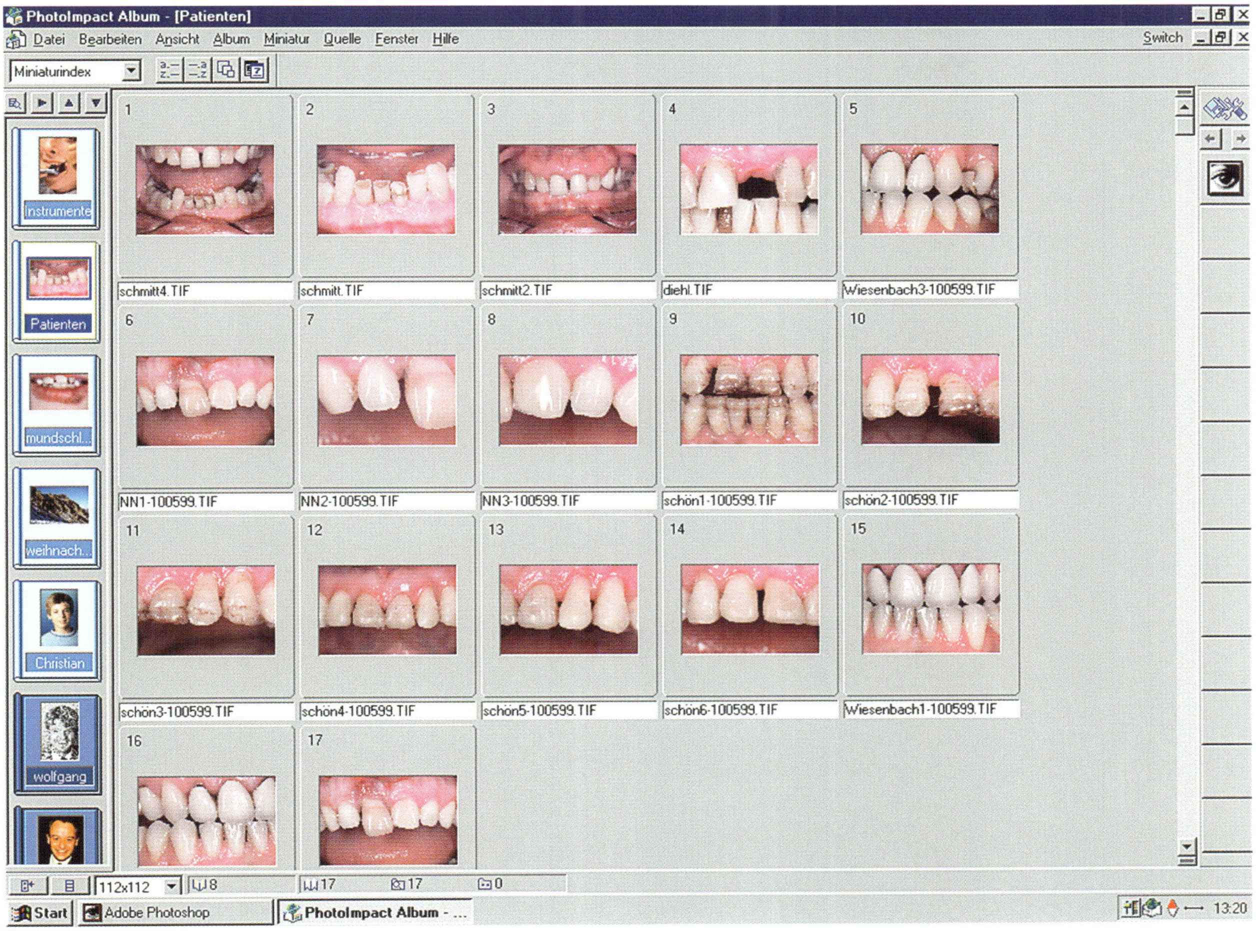

Fig. 13.30 Screen shot from an economical, but powerful image editing software package – PhotoImpact, which also has a basic image archiving facility.

changed quite easily (ViewBase®, Dentron; FLEXI VISION, NewTech; WIN EBV, Lercher, etc.)
Whoever does not need dental imaging on a permanent basis can use commercial image processing programs, which do not offer as many special features but are far less expensive (e. g. PhotoImpact, Corel PhotoPaint, Picture Publisher, Photoshop). If the user does not need the latest version of the software, these programs can be purchased for under $ 100. The latest versions cost between $ 100 and $ 400. The more complex professional programs such as Photoshop (Adobe) are more expensive and are suited to the more ambitious user because of their many features.

The requirements for a treatment simulation is the availability of the initial image on the monitor. Sources of images include:

- ✓ Intraoral video camera with PC connection
- ✓ Digital photographic camera
- ✓ Conventional photograph which must be available on a PC in digitized form

It is not the purpose of this overview to discuss all aspects and possibilities of imaging. This can be found in special literature (e.g. Goldstein). Changes which are frequently simulated are:

Dental Practice of Drs. Beatrix and Wolfgang Bengel
Darmstädter Str. 190a
64625 Bensheim
Tel. 06251-76095 * Fax 06251-76096

TREATMENT SIMULATION

Patient: N.N.
Date: X.X.00

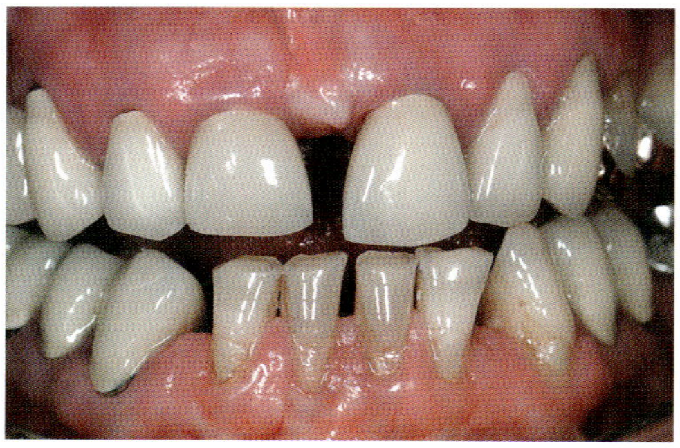

initial situation

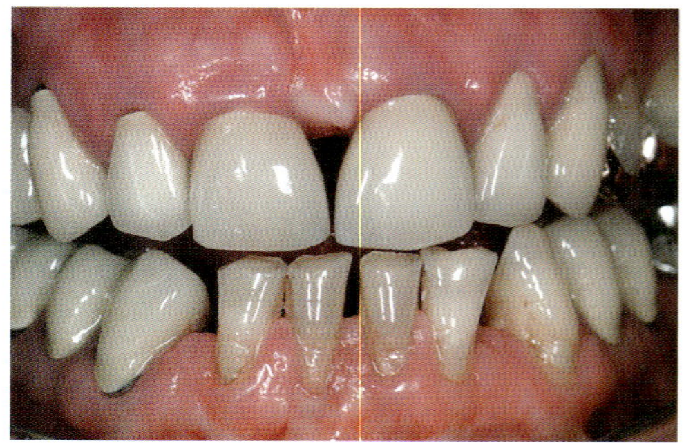

treatment proposal

Dear Mrs. N.N.,

The result of treatment shown here is a computer simulation. This can only be an approximation of later treatment and only serves as point of reference. Anatomical and technical issues may dictate changes from this.

Fig. 13.31 If the results of dental imaging are printed out for the patient it should be emphasized as a matter of course that these results are not binding.

- ✓ Closing gaps between teeth
- ✓ Changing color of teeth
- ✓ Changing tooth shape and gumline
- ✓ Changing existing fillings
- ✓ Changing angle of teeth

This can be achieved by changing the available components of the image, for example through compression, distortion, rotation, moving, etc.
In principle, the mouse, or, even better, a graphic pen, is used to mark and select the area to be changed. This area is then duplicated and changed or moved to a different location. With a little bit of practice good results can be achieved quickly even with commercial image manipulation programs.
Another possibility is to build up a database from

which details can be removed and inserted into the image which is to be altered.
Imaging is time-consuming. It is a responsible activity which demands knowledge of the subject, aesthetic skills and a feeling for psychology. It can not be trusted to an external dental technician but should be done by the dentist him or herself or specially trained personnel under direct supervision. Otherwise there is the risk that unrealistic proposals for treatment are suggested which subsequently prove untenable. This would lead to much disappointment and trouble after treatment. In any case, the patient must be made aware – if possible, in writing – that the results of dental imaging are no guarantee of treatment, and only approach a possible result (Fig. 13.31).

Conclusion

Today the intraoral video system is a tool which significantly improves communication between dentist and patient, simplifies documentation and puts diagnosis on a higher plane in terms of quality.
Even though further improvements in the systems are to be expected, the technology available today can be regarded as being sufficiently mature.
It is not possible to make a general recommendation for "the best" video camera system per se, due to the many types available and the various requirements of users. However, it is highly recommended that the potential user try out the system in the practice before making a decision to purchase. Systems which can be expanded are to be preferred over less expensive complete systems, unless the user is absolutely certain that such a complete system will also meet his or her requirements in future.

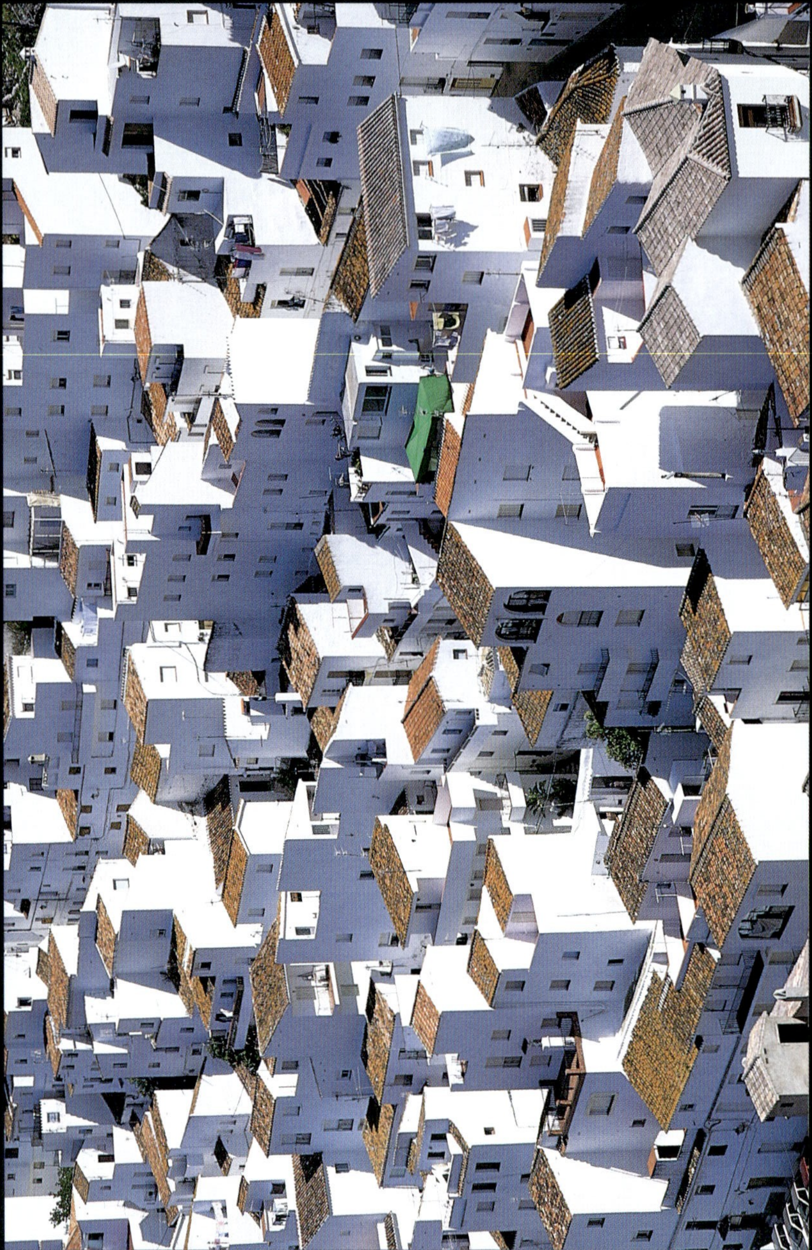

14 Legal Considerations

Anyone who employs photographic documentation in a company or dental practice should be aware that legal issues can arise from his or her photography and be well advised of their significance. The following refers to the legal situation in Germany, but will be similar in other countries.

There are three key issues:

✓ Copyright
✓ Rights to own images
✓ Medical confidentiality

◄ Many effects of light are due to its scattering and reflection. The "white villages" in Andalusia are white to keep out the sun's heat. The color reflects a large portion of the light and the heat is reduced by about 70%. This photograph also illustrates another important aspect of light, which has to do with the psychology of perception. Light falling directly on an object, particularly low angled light, produces clear shadows. The distribution of light and shadow is an important indication to us of three dimensions. Our perception of three dimensions depends less on stereoscopic vision than on other factors which include overlapping, aerial perspective (already covered in Chapter 8) and above all, the distribution of light and shadow. Although this image is only two dimensional it appears to us not as a rendering of different color surfaces, but as a three dimensional impression. The houses appear to be cubic shapes stacked one upon the other.

14.1 Copyright

The person producing the work (image) is entitled to determine the use and manner of its publication, distribution and sales. Misuse can give rise to legal action (copyright law).
Generally, the originator of the image is the person who took it. If, however, the person is only the person implementing this, that is, if he or she is only carrying out the task by operating the camera, that is, he or she is operating only under the instruction of a third party without influencing the content of the image, he is not the holder of the copyright under our law. In practical terms, this means that a dental assistant who takes a photograph under the instruction of the head of the dental practice has no right to claim copyright of the image. The holder of the copyright is the person who has had overall control of the production of the image, in this case, the head of the dental practice.
However, if someone else is tasked with making the image, for example, a photographer, who is free to determine the composition and the techni-

cal means needed to produce it, this person is entitled to hold copyright. In the case of doubt – which is however an exception in a dental practice – a clear agreement should be reached about who holds copyright, or whether the copyright holder assigns the usage rights to the images to another person.

14.2 Right to One's Own Likeness

As part of the general personal rights granted under the constitution, every person has the "right to one's own likeness". This means that "likenesses" can be distributed or publicly displayed only with the consent of the person whose likeness it is. A "likeness" is created when an image of a person is designed to identify him or her.
This means that partial images which do not allow a person to be identified do not apply to the right to one's own likeness. Intraoral images, for example, can thus be published without concern. The same is true for photographs in which the patient's features are obscured. Individual cases have to determine whether it is sufficient just to cover over the eyes.

14.3 Medical Confidentiality

While the "right to one's own likeness" is subject to certain limitations (police matters, historical images), distribution of dental images is further restricted under medical confidentiality. This confidentiality relates to identifiable patient images. Partial images or those which have been rendered unidentifiable so that the patient could not be traced through them, are not subject to medical confidentiality.

14.4 Consent of the Patient

To avoid problems arising under medical confidentiality and the publication of "likenesses," the consent of the patient should be obtained as a matter of course. This presupposes that the patient has been informed about the ramifications of his or her decision and has the mental maturity to give consent. In the case of minors the consent should be obtained from the parent or guardian.

In order to avoid problems from the outset the consent should be in written form, although consent expressed verbally or tacitly are also legally binding. A consent form can be drawn up tailored to the requirements of the individual practice. A suggestion for such a form is shown in Fig. 14.1.

Consent Form

I consent to Dr. X., in Y. taking photographic images of myself (my son, my daughter) for the purpose of better dental diagnosis and treatment, as well as publishing the images for purposes of instruction, teaching or other scientific uses.

I have been informed about the type of the possible publication and have no further questions.

____

Place, Date

____

Signature of patient/parent or guardian

Fig. 14.1

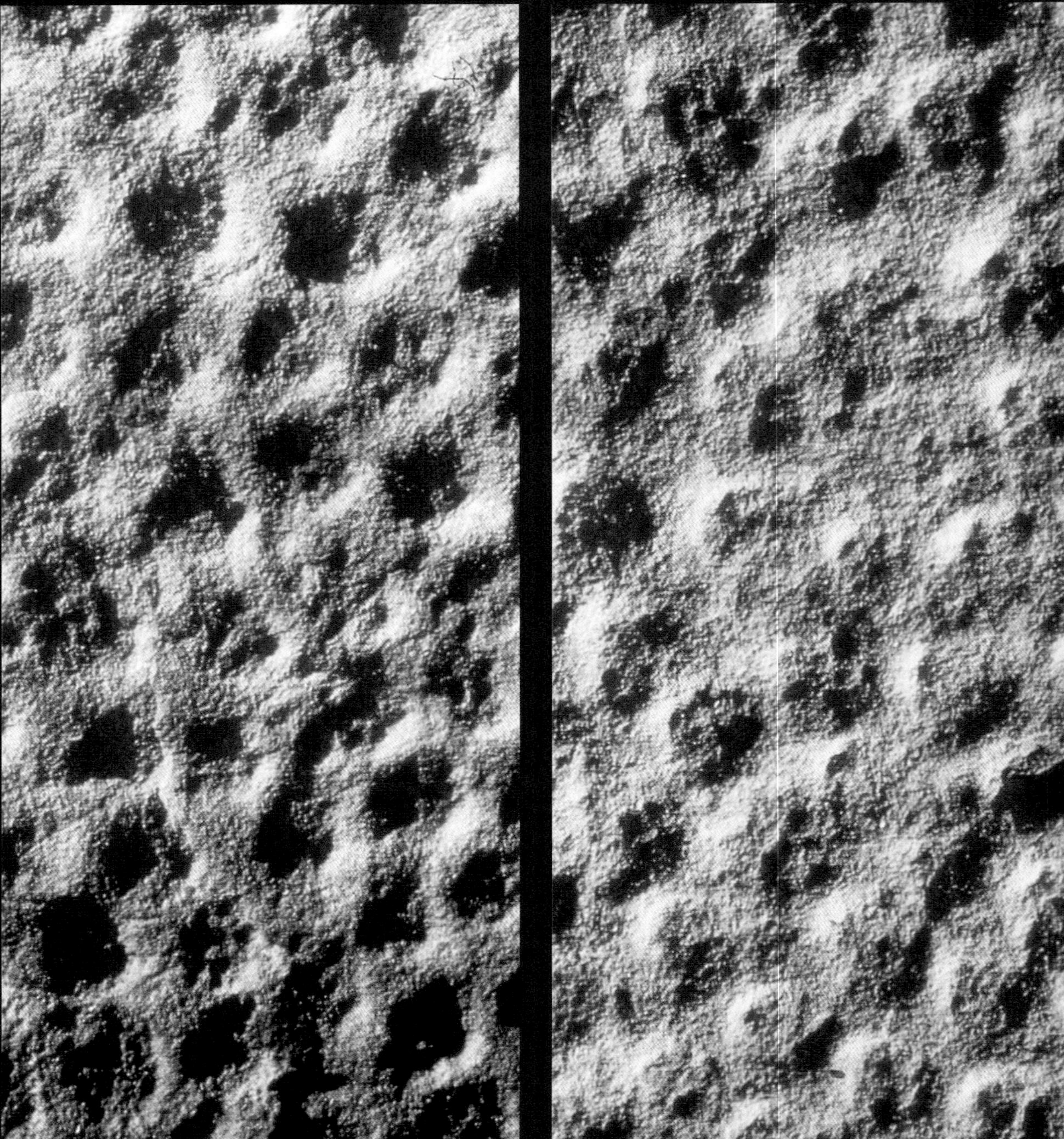

15 Glossary

This glossary is not an exhaustive photographic lexicon. The information herein is merely designed to supplement the text and add material in such a way as not to interrupt the flow of text and facts. Concepts explained in the text are not repeated here.

The direction of light determines whether we perceive a surface to be concave or convex. This photo shows the indentations on a stone at the entrance of a Maltese temple. The edge of light at the lower part of each depression as well as the shadow edge at the upper part makes this very clear. The upside down image appears to have raised areas instead of depressions.
This effect is caused by the fact that during our evolution we became used to a light source from overhead, the sun. Even room lighting today usually comes from above. Thus a certain light-shadow distribution leads us to make conclusions automatically about spatial relationships. The "incorrect" direction of light easily confuses our perception (optical illusion).

Aberrations
Deviation of the original image caused by characteristics of the light and materials used in construction of the lens (Fig. 15.1). Significant imaging errors are spherical (Fig. 15.1) and chromatic aberration (Fig. 10.4a), coma, pincushion distortion, distortion and astigmatism. Aberrations are generally insignificant in dental photography, since lenses are usually stopped way down, which alleviates the problems.

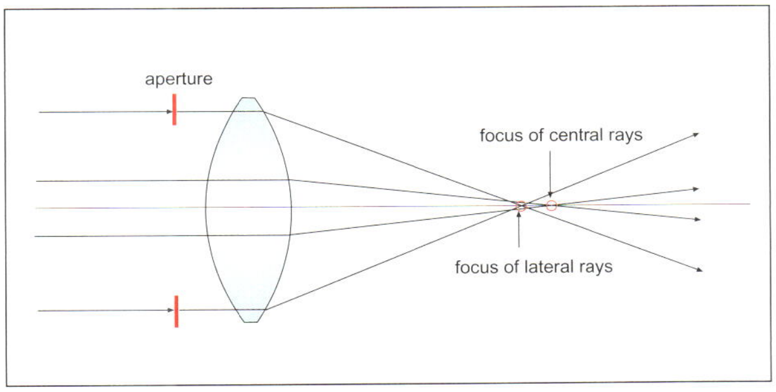

Fig. 15.1 Spherical aberration is a frequent fault in a lens: light rays through the lens axis and those through the edges of a lens are not focused at the same point. This fault is reduced when the lens is stopped down.

Angle of view
The angle that the lens "sees". Normal lenses have an angle of view which roughly corresponds to that of the human eye (ca. 45 – 55 degrees). Wide

angle lenses have a larger angle of view and telephoto lenses a smaller one.

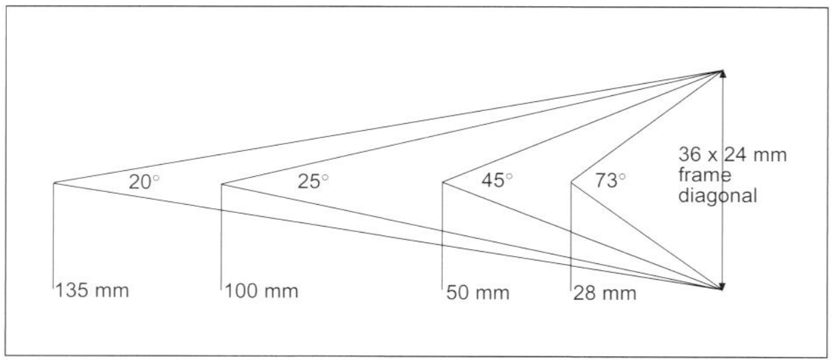

Fig. 15.2 The angle of view of a lens is what it "sees". The diagram shows the angles of view of common lenses.

Aperture
Opening in the lens which regulates the amount of light. Mostly an iris aperture consisting of overlapping metal blades. Stopping down (closing) the aperture reduces the image brightness and increases the depth of field. The next higher aperture reduces the amount of light by half and the next lower one doubles it. The area of a circle increases with the square of the radius. To double the amount of light (= area of circle) the radius has to be increased by the factor of the root of 2 (about 1.4). This produces the aperture numbers.

CCD
Charge coupled device. Semiconductors with light sensitive elements. Linear CCDs are generally found in scanners and those with area sensors in cameras.

CD-ROM
Compact disk – read only memory. Data storage medium comparable to audio CD used for permanent data storage, which can not be changed or erased.

CMOS
Pronounced "C moss". (Complementary Metal Oxide Silicon). Integrated circuit which is increasingly being used as an image sensor in place of CCD chips. It draws less current than a CCD chip, but requires more light. Less expensive to produce than a CCD chip.

Color depth
Color depth describes the ability of a device to render color. A color depth of 1 bit means that only black and white can be reproduced. A color depth of 8 bits allows 256 colors to be reproduced (2^8). A color depth of 24 bits means that more than 16 million colors can be reproduced. A 32 bit color system allows 8 additional databits for transparent options or masks.

Color temperature
The term "color temperature" describes the spectral energy distribution of a light source.
A color slide film registers light as it is, generally coloured. Our brain, however, fools us into seeing white light regardless of the light source (color adaptation of the brain). The color of a radiating object, that is, the spectral composition of the light it emits, is dependent on this temperature. The so-called distribution temperature of an object can be measured in Kelvins (0 degrees C = 273 degrees K). It is compared to the so-called ideal "black body," which is a theoretical temperature radiator, whose color of light changes according to the increasing heat. The distribution temperature is thus the temperature in Kelvins to which a "black body" must be heated to emit light of the same color temperature as the light source to be determined. These values are important in photography to avoid variations in color due to the film's emulsion not being balanced to the color temperature of the light. Daylight and tungsten light film are roughly balanced for color termperature. Daylight balanced film is for a color temperature of 5600 degrees K and tungsten light film for 3200–3400

degrees K. If daylight balanced film is used under tungsten lighting, the light has to be "corrected" by using a blue filter. If a film for tungsten light is used in daylight, an orange filter has to be used. Fine color corrections can be undertaken by using a color temperature meter and the required conversion filters.
The mired scale was introduced to simplify calculations with the Kelvin scale; the mired scale is indirectly proportional (mired = micro reciprocal degree). Mired values are calculated by dividing the number 1 000 000 by the distribution temperature in degrees K (mired = 1 000 000: Kelvin).

Depth of field

Zone of acceptable sharpness, the area in front of and behind the focusing plane selected which appears sufficiently sharp to us.
A point in a subject is reproduced sharply as a point only in the exact focal plane. In front of this and behind this it is reproduced in small circles. The diameter of the circles of confusion and the resolving capabilities of the human eye determine whether a point is perceived as sharp or unsharp. The diameter of the circle of confusion is determined by the diameter of the aperture. The smaller the aperture diameter, the larger the zone of apparent sharpness (depth of field). Furthermore, the diameter of the circle of confusion is also determined by distance of the subject and the focal length of the lens (Fig. 1.25 and 1.26). Both of these define the reproduction ratio. Thus, the depth of field at a given aperture is dependent only on the reproduction ratio. At greater reproduction ratios the depth of field is reduced.
The distribution of the depth of field is important to know for focusing. Normally, about 1/3 of the depth of field is in front of the focusing plane and 2/3 behind it. At a reproduction ratio of 1:1 about one half of the depth of field is in front and one half is behind the point being focused on. Thus in close-up photography the closest part of the subject should not be focused on to avoid "throwing away" large portions of the depth of field.

Digitizer

Also called a frame grabber, is able to convert analog video signals into digital graphic data.

Electronic flash

Standard light source for medical photography which provides short duration, high power lighting.
Powered by rechargeable power packs or commercial batteries. Can be mains powered for stationary applications.
The flash capacitor is charged with a relatively weak current to several hundred volts via a transformer. The flash tubes are connected to the capacitor. The tubes are filled with xenon. The flash is fired instantaneously via the capacitor. This places a charge of about 10,000 volts on the ignition electrode. The gas in the flash tubes is thus ionized and electrically conductive. In about 1/1000th of a second the energy of the capacitor is discharged via the flash tubes. The current briefly illuminates the ionized gas. Discharge time depends on the capacitance of the condenser (capacitor).
Simple electronic flashguns always fully discharge the capacitor. Film exposure must therefore be regulated via the aperture setting. The guide number of the flashgun gives an indication of this. Modern computer flash and TTL-controlled flashguns limit energy output by shutting off the flash. This is done using a thyristor, which shuts off the power to the flash tubes via a sensor in the flashgun - or, in the case of TTL control in the camera – when there is sufficient light from the flash for correct film exposure. This prevents the capacitor from being fully discharged and reduces the time needed to fully recharge the capacitor (recycling time).
TTL-controlled flash is to be preferred over computer flash, since the former measure the light reflected off the film surface.
When using electronic flash it should be ensured that the correct synch speed is set on the camera, otherwise flash duration will be too short and produce a curtain effect on the film. Since the light from an electronic flash is relatively concentrated

and results in a "hard" light, special accessories are used to increase the illuminating surface. These include reflectors, soft boxes, etc., which are particularly useful for portrait and technical photography.
Modern electronic flash units allow several units to be connected which are not only triggered by the camera, but which permit their output to be controlled. Additional flashguns can be fired via slave units which are triggered by the on-camera flash.

Exposure
Alteration of a light sensitive medium by exposure to light. Exposure is the product of light intensity and time. In other words: exposure is the product of aperture and shutter speed at a given film speed. Opening the aperture by one stop or increasing the shutter speed by a step doubles the amount of light falling on the film. In terms of image brightness the result is the same whether the aperture is opened up one stop and the shutter speed halved, or whether the shutter speed is doubled and the aperture stopped down a stop (Bunsen-Roscoe reciprocity law). (Fig. 1.3). The purpose of the image is decisive. If a large depth of field is required, the aperture is stopped down and the shutter speed increased. If camera or subject movement is to be eliminated, the shutter speed must be very short, meaning that the aperture has to be opened up. If the aperture is to be stopped down and the shutter speed reduced at the same time this can only be done with increased light (additional lighting) or by using a faster speed film.

Exposure control
Modern SLRs have various methods of exposure control:

- Shutter priority
- Aperture priority
- Program mode
- Manual exposure

With ***shutter priority*** ("S" symbol) the shutter speed is selected and the camera sets the appropriate aperture.

Aperture priority is the setting of choice for dental photography, since this sets the aperture which controls depth of field (Fig. 1.4). The appropriate shutter speed is set by the camera. When using flash the synchro speed is automatically set and the amount of light controlled by the duration of the flash (with TTL flash).

In *program mode* ("P" symbol) the camera sets both values. Modern cameras have a number of special programs (close-up, backlighting, portrait, etc).

When the camera is set to ***manual*** the exposure values determined by the light meter are set manually on the camera. This is the method of choice for instance in copy work.

Subjects which do not have "normal" brightness require exposure compensation. A small bright object in front of a dark background generally leads to overexposure of the subject. This requires a "minus correction" on the exposure control to obtain the correct exposure. In difficult cases exposure bracketing is recommended. Conversely, a bright subject which fills the frame, such as a ceramic crown at a large reproduction ratio, will require a "plus correction" (Fig. 1.29b).

Exposure measurement
Determination of light intensity using light meters, either as separate hand-held meters or ones integrated into the camera.
There are two methods of measuring light: incident reading and reflected light reading.
To take an **incident reading** the hand held meter is pointed in the direction of the camera. The measuring angle is increased through the use of a spherical diffusor over the light receiving element. One variant of this way of measurement is flash metering using a flash meter.

In taking a **reflected light reading**, the light reflected by the subject is measured. Camera light meters have three different types of measurement depending on the ratio of the measuring surface to the size of the field being measured:

✓ Averaged metering (Fig. 15.3a)
✓ Selective metering
✓ Spot metering (Fig. 15.3b).

With averaged metering the overall brightness of the subject is measured. With selective metering the most important part of the image is measured. Most SLRs have center-weighted averaged metering. This means that although the overall light intensity is measured, the center is given greater prominence (e.g. to 80%). Modern light meters use a matrix; certain parts of the image are given greater prominence in determining the exposure. Spot metering covers an extremely small angle (e. g. 1 degree).
In many instances it makes sense to take a substitute reading, for example, when the subject can not be directly measured because it can not be reached or when a subject varies substantially from an average reading (bright crowns filling the image frame, portrait of a dark-skinned person), or the subject is high-contrast.
The photographer's own hand can be used for a substitute reading. In many instances, for example in technical photography and copy work, the use of a gray card makes sense. This is a piece of cardboard or sheet of plastic which reflects about 18% of a "normal" object. This means that 18% of the light is reflected back from the surface. All meters are set to this medium gray value. The gray card is held as close to possible to the object in a front view, in the direction of the camera, and with side lighting, positioned between the axis of the light and the optical axis (Fig. 15.4). If metering is done with the camera's own light meter, the camera is set to "manual" (manual light reading) and an aperture/shutter speed combination is selected which achieves the correct exposure. Thereafter the gray card is removed and the image is taken using the values set.

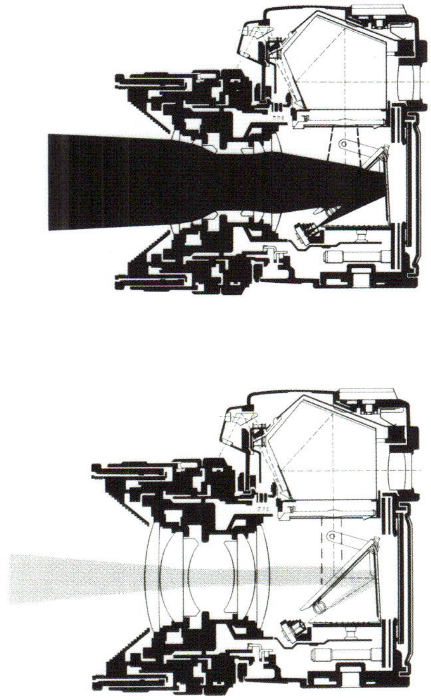

Fig. 15.3 In averaged metering the illumination from the entire image is measured (a); in spot metering (b) only one point in the center of the image (1 degree or 2 degrees) is measured.

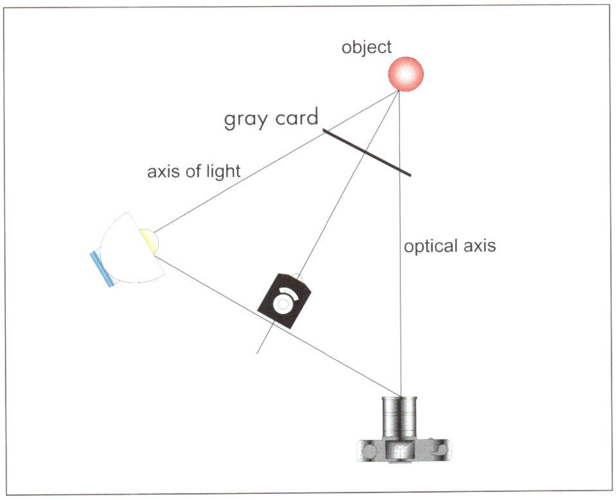

Fig. 15.4 Using a gray card to determine exposure leads to better exposures in many instances. With side lighting, the gray card is placed between the optical axis of the camera and the axis of the light.

Film

The lens on a camera produces a projected image which the film permanently records.
A film consists of a base layer of plastic which ensures its mechanical stability. The next layer of emulsion is the functional one. This light sensitive layer is a suspension of silver halides in gelatine. When light strikes this silver halide layer a latent image is produced which is intensified millions of times through the development process. A reverse image is produced in the silver halide, with light areas appearing dark and vice versa. Fixing converts these unexposed silver halides into colorless salts.
In general, films are divided into:

- ✓ Black and white film
- ✓ Color film
- ✓ Instant print film
- ✓ Instant slide film

Black and white film is used if color rendition is not required or desired. Available as negative and slide film.
"Normal" black and white film has dyes which ensure that all visible colors can be reproduced in gray scales (panchromatic film). Orthochromatic films are "blind" to red. Such films are used as "document films" for reproduction.
Black and white slides (e.g. Agfa Scala) can be used for specific purposes or effects.

Color film has several layers of emulsion, the silver halides of which are sensitive to one third of the color spectrum. Color negative film is less applicable for dental photography.
Color slide film is the standard material for medical documentation. Slide film produces images for projection which are brilliant, crisp and have good color rendition. Daylight balanced slides are normally used which is balanced for a color temperature of 5000–5600 degrees K. Films for artificial light are balanced for a color temperature of 3200–3400 degrees K. If daylight balanced film is used with tungsten lighting a reddish-yellow cast is produced. A film balanced for tungsten light exposed in daylight demonstrates a bluish cast. Both of these can be compensated by using the appropriate correction filters.

Instant color print films produce a self-developed color photo within minutes. These come in two sheet and one sheet versions. Instant slide films are available in the 35mm autoprocess slide film series from Polaroid. They are of lesser significance for practical dental photography.
The films are distinguished by their light sensitivities among other features. The table shows the film speeds. Generally these are designated in ISO (International Standards Organization) numbers which encompass the arithmetic ASA numbers and the DIN numbers (ISO = ASA/DIN).

ASA arithmetical	DIN logarithmic
25	15
32	16
40	17
50	18
64	19
80	20
100	21
125	22
160	23
200	24
250	25
320	26
400	27

Firewire

(IEEE 1394) High speed interface developed by Apple and Texas Instruments which is currently the fastest means of data transfer. Up to 63 devices can be connected. Professional SLR digital cameras (e.g. Kodak DCS cameras, Nikon D1X) can be connected to a PC via a Firewire interface.

Focal plane shutter

Usual type of shutter in 35mm cameras, consisting of two fabric or slatted metal blinds placed immediately in front of the film plane. The amount of light is controlled by the width between them. The slit between both curtains can travel vertically or horizontally in front of the film and successively expose the image (Fig. 15.5).

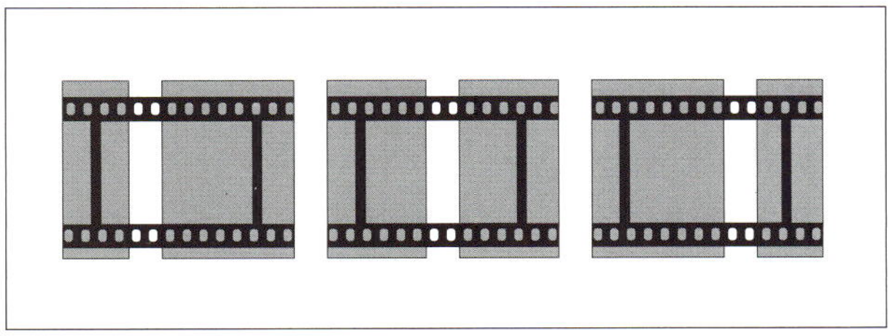

Fig. 15.5 In a focal plane shutter the exposure is determined by the width between the curtains, which travel either vertically or horizontally in front of the film plane.

Focal point/focal length

Distance between the focal point to the lens plane (Fig. 15.6). The back focal length, which differs from the front focal length in asymmetrical lenses, is engraved on the front of lenses. In normal lenses the focal length is approximately equal to the diagonal of the picture frame. In 35mm cameras with 24 x 36mm film format this is about 43.5mm. Lenses with a shorter focal length are termed wide-angle and those with a longer length, telephoto lenses.

Focusing

In order to achieve a sharp image on a film it is necessary for the focusing plane of the lens and film plane to be the same. The focusing plane is defined as a plane which is vertical to the optical axis and running through the focusing point.
For very distant objects the lens is focused on "infinity" so that the film plane and the focal plane coincide. Thus the distance between the lens and the film plane is the same as the focal length of the lens. If the camera is moved closer to the object, the distance between the lens and the film plane must be increased in order to achieve a sharp image. This is done by moving the lens away from the film plane using the focusing ring or by accessories which increase the distance to the film plane.

Focusing screen

Part of the viewfinder system of the camera on which the image is displayed correctly after being reversed by the mirror. Generally viewfinders have a split image rangefinder which is surrounded by a microprism. Neither of these are particularly useful for close-up photography. It is strongly recommended that the standard focusing screen be replaced with a grid focusing screen which aids in correct positioning of the camera (Fig. 1.5a)

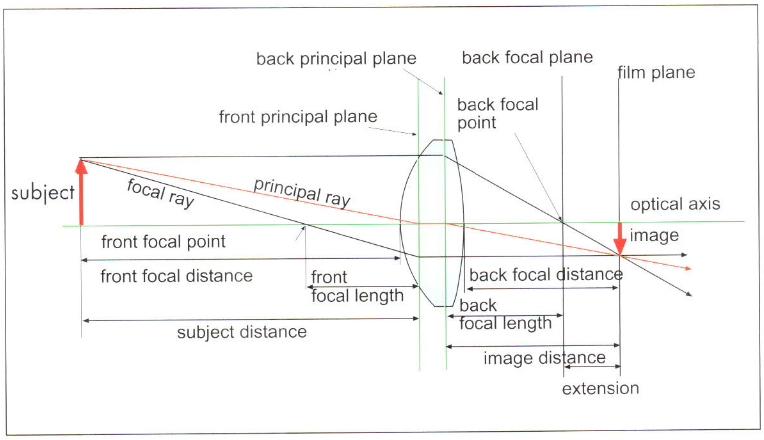

Fig. 15.6 Diagram of key optical terms.

Guide number

Value which indicates the light output of a flashgun. It is based on a film speed of ISO 100 and equals the product of the flashgun-subject distance (in m) and the aperture:

Guide number = distance (m) x aperture

Example: For a flashgun with a guide number of 32 and a subject distance of 4m an aperture of f/8 must be set (Fig. 15.7).

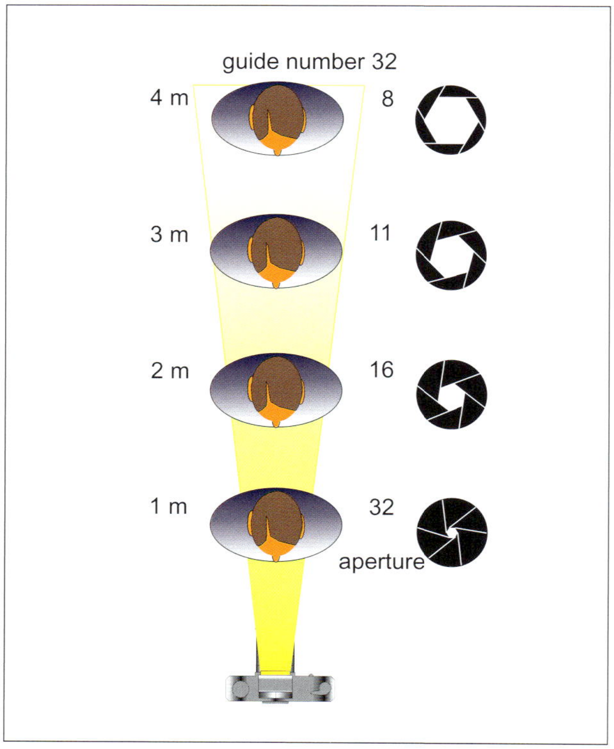

Fig. 15.7 The guide number indicates the performance of a flashgun. The required lens aperture is calculated by dividing the guide number into the subject distance (in m).

At close ranges calculations with guide numbers are inexact. In order to achieve the correct values, exposure bracketing series are recommended. It is simpler to use TTL controlled flashguns.
If two flashguns with the same output are fired in the same direction (e.g. a twin flash system), the overall guide number is calculated by multiplying the guide number of one flashgun times 1.4.

Instant camera

An instant camera exposes instant film, which is subsequently developed and available within minutes. The disadvantages of an instant camera are the higher cost per image, limited settings and picture format and lack of a negative.

Lens speed/relative aperture

The maximum aperture ratio of a lens is called lens speed or relative aperture. This is cited in the ratio of 1:X. A 50mm lens with an aperture diameter of 27mm thus has a lens speed of 27:50 = 1:1.8. Lenses with extremely wide apertures are not recommended for dental photography as they are not only very expensive, but have a very shallow depth of field. The advantage is their very bright image in the viewfinder. When the shutter release is pressed this depth of field becomes of course greater, as focusing is always done with the aperture wide open. When the shutter is pressed, the lens is stopped down to the selected aperture. Nevertheless, a very shallow depth of field in the viewfinder often causes the operator to overlook some details of the subject.

Lens stop

Reciprocal of the aperture ratio. The lens stop is the ratio of the diameter of the opening (aperture diameter) and the lens focal length lens. F/4 for instance means that the aperture diameter fits four times in the focal length of the lens (Fig. 15.8). The aperture settings form the "international aperture sequence" of 1, 1.4, 2, 2.8, 4, 5.6, 8, 11, 16, 22, 32, 45.

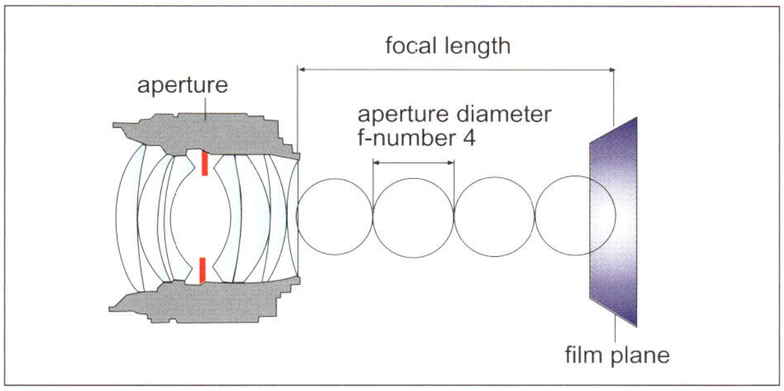

Fig. 15.8 The aperture number indicates the number of how many times the aperture diameter fits in the focal length of the lens. In this case the aperture is f/4.

Macro lens

Lenses between 50mm and 200mm which are specially designed for close up photography (clear color rendition, good resolution, lack of distortion, good field flattening). Today most macro lenses have floating elements which are coupled to the distance setting and allow large reproduction ratios, mostly 1:1, without the use of additional accessories, achieving good image quality. Since these lenses can also be set to "infinity" they can also be used in normal photography.

Magnification ratio

Size ratio between the image on the film and the object (Fig. 1.9). A reproduction ratio of 1:2 means that in reality the object is twice as large as it is on the film (0.5x magnification). Reproduction ratios in dental photography are usually between 1:10 (portrait photography) and 2:1 (image of two teeth which fill the frame). Macro lenses commonly used today without accessories have reproduction ratios of 1:1. With accessories (extension tubes, auto-macro tubes, bellows units) or optical means (teleconverters, close-up lenses) the maximum reproduction ratio can be further increased.

The reproduction ratio can be determined fairly accurately by measuring the image in the viewfinder in millimeters. It should be noted, however, that there are small deviations between the image in the viewfinder and that on the film. This can be determined from the camera's technical specifications.

The table allows the reproduction ratio to be determined by measuring the image in the viewfinder (horizontal format).

Measurement in horizontal format	magnification ratio
9	4:1
10	3.6:1
11	3.3:1
12	3:1
13	2.8:1
14	2.6:1
15	2.4:1
16	2.3:1
17	2.1:1
18	2:1
19	1.9:1
20	1.8:1
21	1.7:1
22	1.6:1
23	1.5:1
24	1.5:1
25	1.4:1
26	1.4:1
27	1.3:1
28	1.3:1
29	1.2:1
30	1.2:1
31	1.2:1
32-34	1.1:1
35-38	1:1
66-80	1:2

Medical lenses

Macro lenses with integrated ringflash or sector flash. They can either be purchased individually for use with system cameras (example: Nikon Medical Lens) or in a fixed camera-lens combination (example: Yashica Dental Eye). They are most frequently used in medical photography for photography in body cavities because they provide lighting without any problems.

PCMCIA card
Personal Computer Memory Card International Association. A card about the size of a check card which can be inserted in the PCM-CIA slots of notebook computers or special readers. Depending on design, these cards can have various functions (modem, network connection, data storage). Storage cards are of interest in digital photography; these are found in professional digital cameras and allow rapid image transfer to the notebook or a PC (via a reader). Three standards available: Type I with 3mm, Type II with 5.5mm and Type III with 10mm density.

Polarizing filter
Neutrally colored filter which only lets light through which is vibrating parallel to the polarizing plane of the filter (Fig. 5.16b). This increases contrast and achieves images with greater color saturation and separation. Its significance in dental object photography is the fact that polarizing filters can eliminate reflections from shiny, non-metallic surfaces which consist of polarized light. The reduction of reflections depends on the angle of the polarizing filter to the reflecting surface. An angle of about 35 degrees is the optimum, depending on the type of material. It is possible to completely eliminate reflections, even from metallic surfaces, by also polarizing the light used to make the image. Cross polarizing filters are available for opthalmology, but these create unnatural and strange looking images in dental photography.
Cameras with TTL measurement which has polarizing elements in the camera meter's light path which therefore absorb this light being measured (semi permeable mirrors, beam splitters, etc) need circular polarizing filters. In contrast to the normal linear polarizing filter, a circular polarizing filter splits the light into two phase shifted components which vibrate at 90 degrees to each other which permit exposure measurement independently of the polarization direction.
Aside from eliminating reflections, special applications for polarizing filters include photoelastic study of stresses and the representation of double refractive phenomena.

RAM
Random access memory of a computer.

Resolution
In electronic imaging and editing, resolution is the measure of pixel density. Resolution is expressed as pixels per inch (ppi) for images and as dots per inch (dpi) for input or output devices. When using scanners, a distinction is made between optical, physical and interpolated resolution.

Resolution ability
Ability of an optical system to distinctly render two points of an object or lines in close proximity (Fig. 12.6).

SCSI
Small Computer System Interface is a standardized, high speed data transfer interface which allows connection of up to eight additional devices (scanner, CD- ROM drives etc.).

Shutter
Device in the camera which controls the duration and instant of exposure. Together with the aperture, the shutter speed controls the image brightness. There are two designs of shutter: central shutters (of no significance in small format photography) and focal plane shutters.

Single lens reflex camera
Most versatile type of camera in which the light passing through the lens is directed by a mirror angled at 45 degrees to the optical axis onto a matte screen (Fig. 15.9). By looking at this matte screen the photographer is able to frame the picture, check its sharpness and depth of field. At present

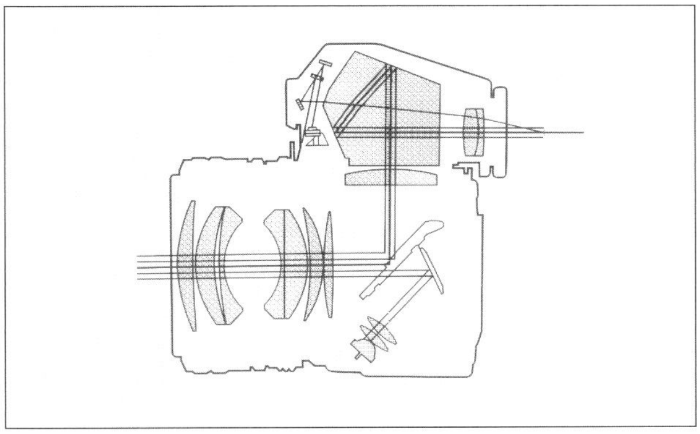

Fig. 15.9 Diagram of a single lens reflex camera.

only single lens reflex cameras are of significance, in which the subject is viewed through the taking lens. In medical documentation with only few exceptions only small format (24 x 36mm) SLR cameras are used.

Subject distance/image distance

Distance between the subject and the external main plane of the lens, or the distance between the film plane and the internal main plane (see Fig. 15.6). When the lens is set on "infinity" the image distance is equal to the focal length of the lens. Up to a reproduction ratio of 1:1 the subject distance is longer than the image distance; with greater magnification on the film, however, it is shorter. At a reproduction ratio of 1:1 the image distance is equal to twice the focal length of the lens.

Thumbnail

Small, low resolution version of an image used for indexing and visualization in photo archive programs.

USB

Universal Serial Bus. High speed connection which allows 127 devices to be connected to the computer. Used by most modern digital cameras.

Viewfinder camera

Camera with direct vision viewfinder, in contrast to an SLR. The viewfinder and lens are not optically connected in non-reflex cameras (Fig. 1.2). Viewfinder cameras have only limited application in close-up work due to the discrepancy between the image in the viewfinder and the actual image (parallax). Moreover, the depth of field can not be visually checked in close-up work. For these reasons viewfinder cameras are not suitable for serious work in medical photography.

Appendix

Important Addresses

This listing is not exhaustive. The presence or absence of a company does not indicate any judgement.

Adobe Systems GmbH
Ohmstraße 1
D-85716 Unterschleissheim
Tel: +49 - 89 - 317 05 - 0
Fax: +49 - 89 - 317 05 - 05

Agfa-Gevaert AG
D-51301 Leverkusen
Tel.: +49 - 214 - 30 - 1
Fax: +49 - 214 - 30 4880

Archivtechnik Kunze
Walkmühlenweg 45-47
D-75365 Calw
Tel.: +49 - 7051 - 127 62
Fax: +49 - 7051 - 400 36

Bonacker GmbH
Postfach 71 01 30
D-28761 Bremen
Tel.: +49 - 421 - 65 85 70
Fax: +49 - 421 - 65 85 723

Canon Euro-Photo GmbH
Siemensring 90-92
D-47877 Willich
Tel.: +49 - 21 54 - 495 - 0
Fax: +49 - 21 54 - 495 - 499

Cullmann GmbH
Kapell-Leite 2
D-90579 Langenzenn
Tel.: +49 - 91 01 - 700 - 0
Fax: +49 - 91 01 - 700 35

Dental-Foto-Technik Arthur Binz
Gemeindestraße 2
CH-8967 Widen
Tel.: +41 - 56 - 631 64 14
Fax: +41 - 56 - 631 64 15

Dent-o-care Dentalvertriebs GmbH
Ahornstraße 2
D-85635 Höhenkirchen
Tel.: +49 - 81 02 - 4112
Fax: +49 - 81 02 - 6523

Deutsche Gesellschaft für Photographie e.V.
Rheingasse 8 – 12
D-50676 Köln

Epson Deutschland GmbH
Zülpicher Str. 6
D-40549 Düsseldorf
Tel.: +49 - 211 - 5603 - 0
Fax: +49 - 211 - 504 77 87

Filtrop AG
Schlossweg 24
FL-9496 Balzers
Liechtenstein

Fuji Photo Film (Europe) GmbH
Heesenstraße 31
D-40549 Düsseldorf
Tel.: +49 - 211 - 5089 - 0
Fax: +49 - 211 - 5089 - 344

Hama GmbH & Co.
Dresdner Str. 9
D-86651 Monheim
Tel.: +49 - 9091/502-0
Fax: +49 - 9091/502 - 274

JVC Professional Products
Grüner Weg 10
D-61169 Friedberg
Tel.: +49 - 60 31 - 6050
Fax: +49 - 60 31 - 605-280

Kaiser Fototechnik GmbH & Co. KG
Im Krötenteich 2
D-74722 Buchen
Tel.: +49 - 62 81 - 407 - 0
Fax: +49 - 62 81 - 407 55

Kodak AG
Hedelfinger Str. 60
D-70327 Stuttgart
Tel.: +49 - 711 - 406 0
Fax: +49 - 711 - 406 5397

Leica Kamera AG
Oskar-Barnack-Str. 11
D-35606 Solms
Tel.: +49 - 64 42 - 208 0
Fax: +49 - 64 42 - 208 333

Lester A. Dine Inc.
351 Hiatt Drive - Palm Beach Gardens -
Florida 33418
Tel.: +1-561 624-9100
Fax: +1-561 624-9103

Minolta GmbH
Kurt- Fischer-Str. 50
D-22923 Ahgrensburg
Tel.: +49 - 41 02 - 701
Fax: +49 - 41 02 - 401 78

Nikon GmbH
Tiefenbroichger Weg 25
D-40472 Düsseldorf
Tel.: +49 - 211 - 94 14 - 0
Fax: +49 - 211 - 94 14 - 330

Novoflex Präzisionstechnik GmbH
Brahmsstraße 7
D-87700 Memmingen
Tel.: +49 - 83 31 - 88888
Fax: +49 - 83 31 471 74

Olympus Optical Co. (Europa) GmbH
Wendenstraße 14-16
D-20097 Hamburg
Tel.: +49 - 40 - 237 73 - 0
Fax: +49 - 40 - 233 7 65

Pentax GmbH
Julius- Vosseler-Str. 104
D-22527 Hamburg
Tel.: +49 - 40 - 561 92 - 0
Fax: +49 - 40 - 561 92 - 23

Photomed International
15500 Erwin Street, Suite 1021
Van Nuys, CA 91411
Tel.: +1-800-998 7765

Polaroid GmbH
Sprendlinger Landstraße 109
D-63069 Offenbach
Tel.: +49 - 69 - 8404 - 1
Fax: +49 - 69 - 8404 204

Ulead Systems Inc.
Wolfenbütteler Str. 33
D-38102 Braunschweig
Tel.: +49 - 531 - 220 79 - 0
Fax: +49 - 531 - 220 79 - 99

Yashica Kyocera GmbH
Eiffestraße 76
D-20537 Hamburg
Tel.: +49 - 40 - 251 50 70
Fax: +49 - 40 - 250 32 11

Internet Addresses

This listing is not exhaustive. The presence or absence of a company does not indicate any judgement.

Industry
www.agfa.com
www.canon. com
www.casio. com
www.epson. com
www.fujifilm. com
www.fotowand. com
www.jvc. com
www.kaiser-fototechnik.de/en/index.htm
www.kodak.com
www.leica-camera.com
www.minolta. com
www.nikonusa.com
www.olympus.com
www.polaroid.com
www.ricoh-europe.com
www.siliconfilm.com
www.sony.com
www.toshiba.com
www.yashica.com

Scanners
www.avision.com
www.epson.com
www.microtek.com
www.mustek.com
www.plustek.com
www.umax.com

Storage media
www.crucial.com
www.ibm.com
www.iomega.com
www.lexarmedia.com
www.sandisk.com
www.simpletech.com

Software
www.adobe.com
www.corel.com
www.download.com
www.gimp.org
www.grafik-software.de
www.lemkesoft.com
www.micrografx.com
www.microsoft.com
www.photoshopuser.com/
www.ulead.com

Companies
ptv.polaroid.com/realweb/dentalimaging/pol001b/video100_rm/main.htm
www.bitsinstyle.de
www.chriscamera.com/dental.htm
www.digident.com/camerachoices.htm
www.digitale-fototechnik.de
www.dinecorp.com
www.discdirekt.com
www.d-store.com/d-store/Digi-Slave/rf50.html
www.foto24.de
www.kodak.com/US/en/health/dental/products/digPho/digiPhoKit.jhtml
www.ny-camera.net
www.photomed.net
www.tiffen.com

Magazines/Communities/Information
www.digit.de
www.dpreview.com
www.fotoline.ch
www.megapixel.net/
www.pcphotoreview.com/
www.peimag.com
www.photolink.de
www.photoweb.de
www.robgalbraith.com/
www.shortcourses.com/
www.tambcd.edu/res/photo.html

Organizations
www.photosuisse.ch
www.psa-photo.org

Bibliography

Adams, C.P.: Dental Photography, John Wright&Sons Ltd., Bristol, 1968

Baker CM: Introducing dentistry to the 21st century via the intraoral camera. Dent Today15, 94-5 (1996)

Baumann, H.D.: Digitale Mal- und Grafiktechniken. DuMont, Köln, 1993

Bengel, W.: Die Photographie in Zahnmedizin und Zahntechnik. Quintessenz, Berlin, 1984

Bengel, W.: Sailwind MacroMate: Für Objektbeleuchtung im Nahbereich. Photomed' 5: 90-93 (1992)

Bengel, W.: Einfache Fotografie kleiner Objekte unter Verwendung einer neuen Faserlichtquelle. Quintessenz 43, 2,293-309 (1992)

Bengel, W.: Zahnärztliche Sach- und Reprofotografie. Zahnärztliche Mitteilungen 87, 2044-2050 (1997) Heft Nr. 17, 01.09.1997

Bengel W.: Möglichkeiten der digitalen Fotografie in der Zahnheilkunde. Quintessenz 48, 4,517-536 und 5,671-683 (1997)

Bengel, W.: Bildschirmfotografie. Quintessenz 48,10,1381-1387 (1997)

Blaker, A.A.: Handbook for Scientific Photography. 2nd Ed. Focal Press, Boston, 1989

Brown, E.M.: Medical Photography of Patients. Lewis & Co., London, 1968

Claman L.J., Rashid, R.: Techniques for Dental Photography. In: Vetter, J.P. (Hrsg.): Biomedical Photography. Butterworth-.Heinemann, Boston, 1992

Deininger, H.K.: Die Reproduktion von Röntgenaufnahmen. Photomed' 6, 19-24, 1993

DiSaia J.P.: Digital photography for the plastic surgeon. Plast Reconstr Surg. 102, 569-573 (1998)

Enk, D. und T. Filler: Optimierte Bildschirmfotografie. Photomed' 5: 42-49, 1992

Fan, P.P.: Choosing the Right Clinical Camera. Part I-III. Oral Health, 4-6/1998,

Farr C.: Video Imaging. Dentistry Today November/December 1993

Fleischer, G.: Dia-Vorträge. Thieme, Stuttgart, 1986

Freehe, C.L.: Symposion on Dental Photography. Dent. Clin. North Am. Part II. Philadelphia, 1968

Freeman, M.: The Photographer's Studio Manual. Collins, London, 1984

Freund, U.: Picture Publisher 4.0 - das offizielle Handbuch. te-wi-Verlag, München, 1994

Frey, S.: Die Macht des Bildes. Huber, Bern, 1999

Gehrman, R.E.: Dental Photography. PennWell, Tulsa, 1982

Goldstein, CE, Goldstein, RE, Garber DA: Imaging in Esthetic Dentistry. Quintessence, Chicago, 1998

Gradias, M.: Computergrafik in der Praxis. Reihe: Medien in der Wissenschaft (Band 3). Gesellschaft für Medien in der Wissenschaft e.V. (Hrsg.) Göttingen, 1994

Händel, K.: Rechtsfragen der medizinischen Photographie. Photomed' 3, 281-286, 1990

Hansell, P. (Hrsg.): A Guide to Medical Photography. MTP Press, Lancaster, 1979

Kraus, H.: Das große Buch zu Photoshop 2.51. Data Becker, Düsseldorf, 1994

LeBeau, L.J.: Photography of Small Laboratory Objects. In: Vetter, J.P. (Hrsg.): Biomedical Photography. Butterworth-.Heinemann, Boston, 1992

LeBeau, L.: Fotografie kleiner biomedizinischer Objekte. Photomed' 6, 159-167, 1993

Maro, F.: Sicher Präsentieren. Econ, Düsseldorf, 1994

Meyer, T.: Die Inszenierung des Scheins. Suhrkamp, Frankfurt, 1992

Nathanson O: Dental imaging by a computer: a look at the future. JADA 1991 122: 45-46

Rashid, R., Claman, L.J.: Equipment for Dental Photography. In: Vetter, J.P. (Hrsg.): Biomedical Photography. Butterworth-.Heinemann, Boston, 1992

Riedel, H.: Fotorecht für die Praxis. Verlag Photo Technik International, München 1988

Schirra, Chr., Haak, R.: Bitte lächeln! Die zahnärztliche Fotografie als Hilfsmittel bei der Patientendokumentation und -kommunikation. Quintessenz 50, 4, 377-384 (1999)

Schlicht, H.-J.: Digitale Bildverarbeitung mit dem PC. Addison-Wesley, 1993, 1993

Schlicht, H.-J.: Anwendung und professionelle Nutzung der Kodak Photo CD. Addison-Wesley, Bonn, 1995

Schröder, G.: Technische Fotografie. Vogel, Würzburg, 1981

Seino, H. et al.: Dental Imagination - A Record of Techniques and Feelings. Quintessence, Tokyo 1988

Spanik, C.: Elektronische Bildverarbeitung mit dem PC. Würzburg, Vogel, 1994

Thomas JR et al.: Analysis of patient response to preoperative computerized video imaging. Arch Otolaryngol Head Neck Surg 115, 793-796 (1989)

Van der Veen, G.: Die Archivierung von Dias und Videobändern: Ein Minimalansatz. Photomed' 1, 285-288, 1988

Vetter, J.P. (Hrsg.): Biomedical Photography. Butterworth-Heinemann, Boston, 1992

Vonow, P.: Zahnärztliche Fotografie: Das Contax-Dental-System. Schweiz. Mschr. Zahnheilk. 93, 252-7 (1983) 4

Walz, P.: Photo-CD mit dem PC. Würzburg, Vogel, 1994

Wander, P., Gordon, P.: Dental Photography. BDJ, London, 1987

Wesche, H.: Photoaufnahmen abseits der Routine – ein Praxisbericht. Photomed' 2, 191-194, 1989

Wesche, H.: Diakopie mit dem Farbmischkopf. Photomed' 3, 49-54, 1990

Wesche H.: Das Illumitran 3 S von Bowens im klinischen Alltag: Ein Praxisbericht. Photomed' 6, 201-207, 1993

Williams, A.R.: Medical Photography Study Guide. MTP Press, Lancaster, 1984

Williams, A.R.: Positionierung und Beleuchtung für die Patientenphotographie. Photomed' 4, 21-34, 1991

Williams A.R., Nieuwenhuis, G.: Clinical and Operating Room Photography. In: Vetter, J.P. (Hrsg.): Biomedical Photography. Butterworth-.Heinemann, Boston, 1992

Woerrlein, H., Neumann, G.: Perfekt präsentieren. Markt & Technik, München, 1993

Wolf, H.: Zwei Makroblitzgeräte im Test: Nikon Macro Speedlight SB-21 und Minolta Macro-Flash 1200 AF. Photomed' 1, 111-124, 1988

Index

G

N

O

P

R

S